Hepatic Encephalopathy in Chronic Liver Failure

Hepatic Encephalopathy in Chronic Liver Failure

Edited by

Livio Capocaccia

University of Rome
Rome, Italy

Joseph E. Fischer

University of Cincinnati Medical Center
Cincinnati, Ohio

and

Filippo Rossi-Fanelli

University of Rome
Rome, Italy

Plenum Press • New York and London

Library of Congress Cataloging in Publication Data

Italian Association for the Study of the Liver. Congress (1982: Rome, Italy)
    Hepatic encephalopathy in chronic liver failure.

    "Proceedings of the 1982 Congress of the Italian Association for the Study of the
Liver, held November 19–20, 1982, in Rome, Italy" – T.p. verso.
    Includes bibliographical references and index.
    1. Hepatic coma – Congresses. I. Capocaccia, Livio. II. Fischer, Joseph E. III.
Rossi-Fanelli, Filippo. IV. Title. [DNLM: 1. Hepatic encephalopathy – Congresses. 2.
Hepatic encephalopathy – Etiology – Congresses. WI 700 A849h 1982]
RC848.H4I86   1982   616.3′62   84-4893
ISBN-13: 978-1-4684-4789-7   e-ISBN-13: 978-1-4684-4787-3
DOI: 10.1007/978-1-4684-4787-3

Proceedings of the 1982 Congress of the Italian Association for the Study
of the Liver, held November 19–20, 1982, in Rome, Italy

© 1984 Plenum Press, New York
Softcover reprint of the hardcover 1st edition 1984

A Division of Plenum Publishing Corporation
233 Spring Street, New York, N.Y. 10013

PREFACE

The meeting which took place in Rome on November 19th and 20th of 1982 is easily the best meeting on hepatic coma that I have ever attended, and I have attended many. It was an exceedingly well-planned meeting with prolonged opportunity for discussion, and there was genuine interplay and exchange of ideas (not the usual picture of a rushed meeting with investigators presenting their own point of view and talking past each other without a meaningful exchange) which took place in Rome.

My co-editors and I hope that the published transcript, which of course can only reflect what transpired in Rome on those two days, does justice to a very intellectually exciting and gratifying exchange of ideas.

L. Capocaccia,
J. E. Fischer and
F. Rossi-Fanelli

CONTENTS

INTRODUCTION

J. E. Fischer

Department of Surgery, University of Cincinnati Medical

Center, Cincinnati, Ohio

Hepatic encephalopathy remains a distressing complication of hepatic failure. It is a syndrome of malfunction of the central nervous system occurring in the presence of liver disease. In the acute situation it can make patient care extremely difficult, as well as being extremely upsetting to both the patient and his family. In the chronic situation, such as seen following portalsystemic shunt or in progressive liver disease, the loss of judgment, disturbance in day/night rhythm and inability of patient to function in society may be distressing, indeed.

The consideration of hepatic encephalopathy and its etiology has undergone a radical turn within the past decade. No longer is hepatic encephalopathy considered a toxic hypothesis brought about by the presence of some "poison" such as ammonia; at present, hepatic encephalopathy is seen in the context of severe metabolic derangements, which failure of the liver, the central biochemical powerhouse of the organ, must bring with it. There is increased awareness of a variety of influences, hormonal, circulatory and metabolic, as well as the realization that several mechanisms may be involved.

Although it is clear that no conclusion was reached in the conference that follows, it is gratifying to me to hear terms such as neurotransmitters, amino acids, hormones (of which insulin and glucagon are examples), receptors and the words "synaptic cleft" come up as often in the discussion of the etiology of hepatic encephalopathy as they have in this conference. While the etiology remains controversial, it is clear that if we better understand how the brain functions we may be able to provide more comprehensive and more successful therapy for hepatic encephalopathy.

As we increase our understanding of this disease, or as we test specific hypotheses, it is clear that therapeutic innovations will result. One of these, the administration of branched chain enriched amino acid solutions in the correction of amino acid imbalance, which are thought by some to have etiologic significance in the genesis of hepatic encephalopathy is the subject of intensive discussion at this meeting. This is, of course, particularly gratifying to me as one of the originators of the concept. Yet the meeting has additional value for both myself and the other participants by giving us the opportunity for discussion of a wide range of topics and for a genuine exchange of ideas concerning one of the most complicated diseases in existence today.

SECTION 1

PATHOGENETIC PROBLEMS IN HEPATIC ENCEPHALOPATHY

AMMONIA: THE OLD AND THE NEW

L. Zieve

Hennepin County Medical Center, University of Minnesota
Minneapolis, MN, USA

INTRODUCTION

Experimental evidence relating increased blood ammonia to cerebral dysfunction dates back to 1877 when Eck first created a portocaval shunt. In the 1930's Van Caulert and Kirk described mental disturbances in cirrhotics receiving ammonium salts.[1] However, it wasn't until 1952 that Gabuzda, Phillips, Schwartz, and Davidson[2,3] recognized that symptoms and EEG changes indistinguishable from hepatic encephalopathy could be produced in cirrhotics given ammonium-containing cation-exchange resins, ammonium salts, urea, or protein orally. Two years later a patient with a normal liver who had a portocaval shunt following a Whipple procedure for carcinoma of the pancreas was reported by McDermoff and Adams[4] to have recurrent episodes of irrationality, confusion, disorientation, incontinence, drowsiness, apathy, stupor, and sometimes coma Blood ammonia and EEG abnormalities were correlated with the manifestations, which were reproducible by feeding the patient meat, urea, ammonium-containing cation-exchange resin, or ammonium chloride. Such observations in cirrhotics and in patients with portacaval shunts have been confirmed many times since these early reports, so a relationship between ammonia and the clinical syndrome of hepatic coma is well established.

SOURCES

In hepatic encephalopathy ammonia and glutamine are increased in blood, muscle, brain, spinal fluid and urine (Figure 1). Glutamine is derived from ammonia and glutamate in the tissues. Most of the ammonia in blood and tissues is of dietary origin. The major sources of blood ammonia are 1. ammonia in the food eaten, 2. small intestinal digestion of dietary protein and metabolic utilization of the absorb-

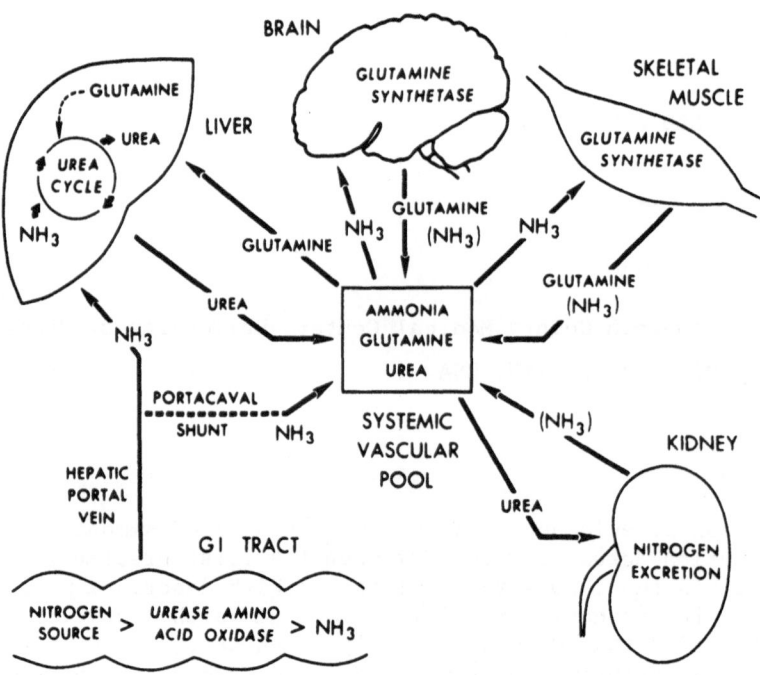

Fig. 1. Diagram of ammonia generation and disposition. (From
Lockwood et al. J. Clin. Invest. 63: 449, 1979).

ed glutamine, 3. metabolic utilization of endogenous glutamine by
the small intestine, 4. colonic bacterial metabolism of dietary
protein or its products and of urea secreted into the intestine
(about 25-30% of all the urea formed). 5. Amino acid metabolism in
tissues. It appears from studies of germ-free animals and studies
with isolated bowel segments that about one-half (or less) of the
ammonia coming from the gut is a result of bacterial action, the
remainder coming from the small intestine.This applies to both
fasting and non-fasting conditions.[5] In the presence of azotemia
increased amounts of ammonia are generated from the breakdown of
increased urea in the intestine.

Nitrogenous food substances have varying effects on blood ammonia or encephalopathy depending upon the protein source and amino
acid content.[6,7] Milk and cheese protein is better tolerated than
meat protein by patients susceptible to encephalopathy. Dogs with

portacaval shunts also tolerate milk protein better than meat protein. In cirrhotics, blood in the gut causes a greater rise in blood ammonia than equivalent amounts of casein and milk. Amino acids have varying ammoniagenic potency in cirrhotics susceptible to hepatic encephalopathy. Those that raise the blood ammonia the most are threonine, serine, glycine, glutamine, histidine, lysine, and asparagine. Alanine, phenylalanine, tyrosine, proline, leucine, isoleucine, and valine have about 1/8 the effect of the highest group. Arginine, aspartic acid, glutamic acid tryptophan and urea have only a slight effect comparatively.

Under fasting conditions ammonia coming from kidney, muscle and brain, which are ordinarily relatively minor sources, has more significance. Ammonia release from kidney is greater than normal in patients with encephalopathy and is further increased in the presence of hypokalemia. Ammonia is released from muscle with exercise. The amount released for a given amount of exertion is greater than normal in encephalopathic patients.[5,8]

METABOLISM, DISPOSITION, TOXICITY

When blood ammonia levels are increased, brain and muscle uptake of ammonia is increased. The amount taken up is proportional to the arterial blood level. The brain ammonia utilization rate is also closely correlated ($r = 0.93$) with the arterial blood level (Figure 2).[9] The ammonia utilization reactions apparently take place in a compartment that includes less than 1/5 of all brain ammonia. In encephalopathic patients the brain ammonia utilization rate is increased by two-thirds. The primary disposition of ammonia is by the formation of glutamine. Studies in noraml cats receiving labeled ammonia by carotid artery infusion indicate that the newly formed glutamine is derived from a small but metabolically active compartment of glutamic acid.[10] The observation of a small active compartment of ammonia utilization in man and of glutamine formation from a small active compartment of glutamic acid in the cat is probably more than coincidence.

In patients with liver disease there is a fairly good correlation between blood (arterial or venous) and spinal fluid ammonia, but those with hepatic coma cannot be differentiated from those not in coma. In general the correlation between blood ammonia and the degree of hepatic encephalopathy is poor, and a single blood ammonia determination is of little clinical value (Figure 3). This poor correlation probably stems from the fact that skeletal muscle is a much larger metabolic site than brain for circulating ammonia.[9] Thus under constant conditions of formation of ammonia, muscle removal largely determines blood levels. This is particularly true in the presence of portal-systemic shunts. However, in an individual patient, fluctuations in blood ammonia often correlate fairly well with changing neuropsychiatric status so serial blood ammonia

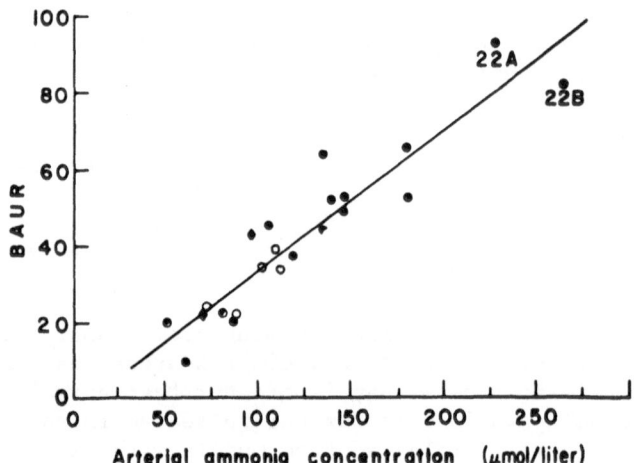

Fig. 2. Relationship of brain ammonia utilization rate (BAUR) to
        arterial ammonia concentration. (From Lockwood et al. J.
        Clin. Invest. 63: 449, 1979 .)

determinations may be of value.

    Acute ammonia intoxication in animals stimulates oxidative metab-
olism of the brain, but brain energy balance is maintained.[7] Studies
of isolated cerebral or spinal cord neurons in the cat indicate that
ammonium ions abolish the hyperpolarizing action of post-synaptic
inhibition by blocking the active outward extrusion of chloride ions.
The effect is a loss of post-synpatic inhibition, depending to some
extent on previous depolarizations of the neuron.[11] After chronic
ammonia intoxication much smaller amounts of NH_4 are needed to produce this effect.

    Pure ammonia intoxication is thus a hyperkinetic state with a
convulsive phase. The severity of the encephalopathy due to NH_3 is
related exponentially to the brain concentration of NH_3. In pure
ammonia coma in rats the brain NH_3 is about 5 times normal, whereas
in experimental hepatic coma it is only 3 times normal. Also in pure
ammonia coma the correlation between blood and brain NH_3 is good
(Figure 4), whereas in experimental hepatic coma it is poor (Figure
5). By reducing the amount of NH_4 injected, and giving simultaneously
small amounts of a mercaptan and a fatty acid, coma can be induced
in normal rats with brain NH_3 levels that are similar to those of
experimental hepatic coma. Since these three substances accumulate
during hepatic failure, it seems likely that synergistic interaction
among them may have a significant pathogenetic role in experimental
hepatic coma.

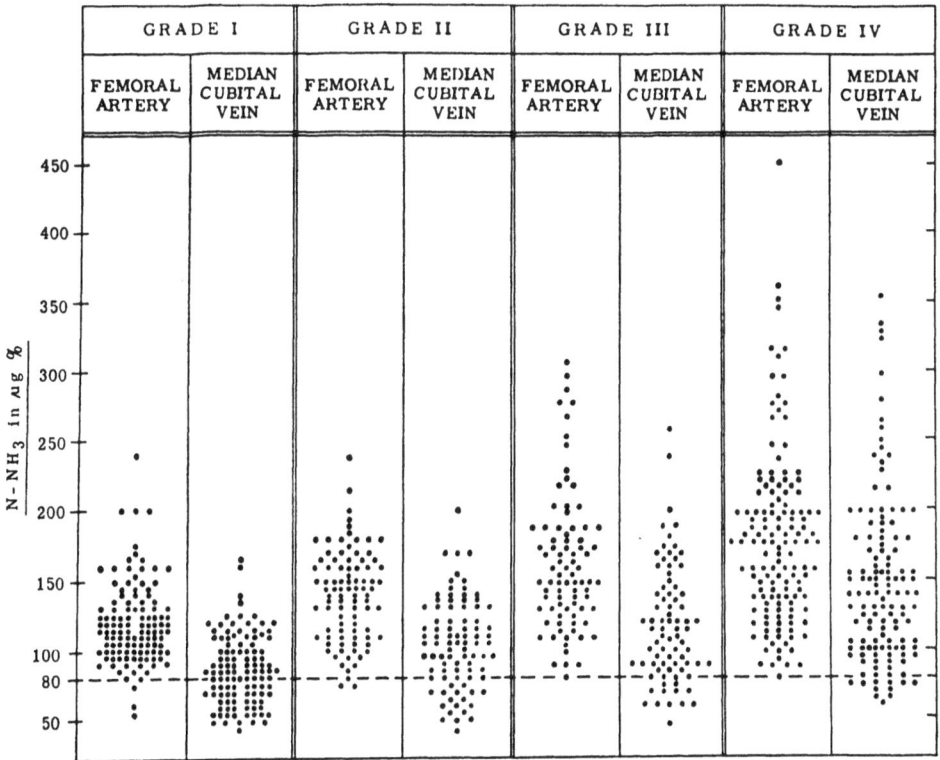

Fig. 3. Relationship of blood ammonia concentration to clinical
severity of hepatic encephalopathy. Grade IV patients were
deeply comatose. (From Stahl. Ann. Int. Med. 58: 1, 1963.)

Chronic hyperammonemia associated with prolonged infusion of
ammonium salts or with a portacaval shunt results in Alzheimer Type
II astrocytosis in the brain and diffuse slowing on the EEG similar
to that seen in hepatic coma.[6] Brain α-ketoglutarate is reduced.[12]
Animals that are chronically hyperammonemic following a portacaval
shunt are more susceptible than non-shunted animals to the toxic
effects of additional acute ammonia loads. A smaller dose of ammonia
causes coma, and cerebral depression lasts longer. Cerebral dysfunction occurs before any evidence of primary energy failure as
reflected by changes in the brain adenine nucleotides.[13] Cerebral
blood flow and oxygen consumption are reduced, and the concentrations of glutamate and aspartate in the brain are decreased.[14] The
EEG develops high-voltage slow waves.

The formation of glutamine and of urea are the two ways of

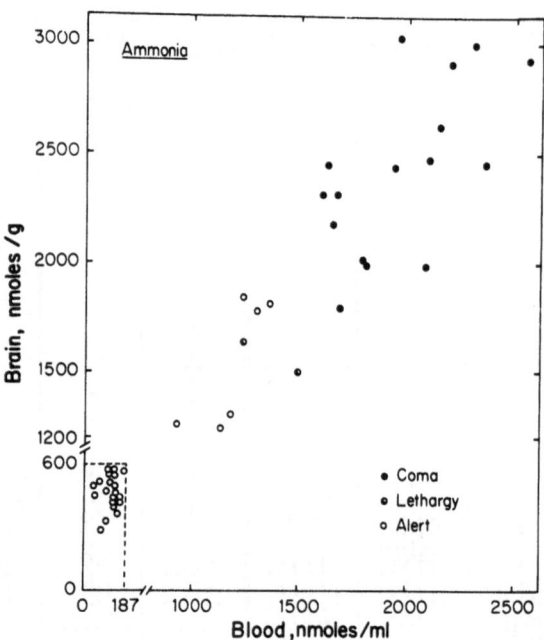

Fig. 4. Correlation between brain and arterial blood ammonia concentrations in rats injected with varying doses of NH_4Cl.

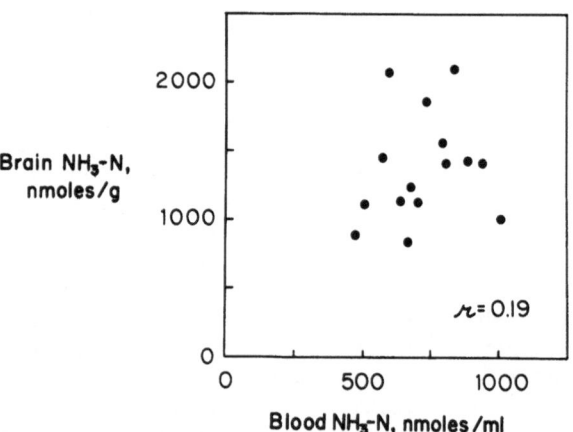

Fig. 5. Correlation between brain and arterial blood ammonia concentrations in rats in hepatic coma following massive
ischemic hepatic necrosis.

disposing of ammonia (Figure 6). From studies in normal rats it
appears that glutamine synthesis is the major mechanism for disposal
of ammonia (about 80%) at low concentrations of ammonia, but that the
capacities of the urea - and glutamine - synthesizing systems are
approximately equivalent in the presence of a large excess of ammonia.[15] Recent dynamic studies in man using isotopically labeled ammonia indicate the importance of the glutamine pathway, since about 50%
of the arterial ammonia was metabolized by muscle, and the fraction
going to brain was approximately equivalent to that going to liver.[9]
If the urea pathway is lost as in the totally hepatectomized dog,
glutamine synthesis expands to largely, but not entirely, handle the
increased ammonia load (Figure 7).[16] Presumably in patients with
moderate or severe liver disease, in whom the maximum rate of urea
synthesis is depressed,[17] glutamine synthesis expands similarly.

In patients with hepatic encephalopathy the correlation between
spinal fluid glutamine and severity of the encephalopathy is good,
though far from perfect (Figure 8).[18] Cerebrospinal fluid glutamine
is presumably the spill-over from brain glutamine which accumulates
as the brain ammonia increases. α-Ketoglutaramate in derived from
glutamine by removal of an amino-group from the α-carbon. Like glutamine it is increased in the spinal fluid in hepatic encephalopathy,[19,20]
and has about as good a correlation as glutamine with severity.
The spinal fluid concentration of glutamine in these patients is
about 30-50 times that of α-ketoglutaramate, which probably has the
same significance as glutamine. There is no good evidence that either
has a role in pathogenesis. However, no parameter has correlated
better with severity of encephalopathy than these two substances,
and any hypothesis of pathogenesis must account for this correlation.

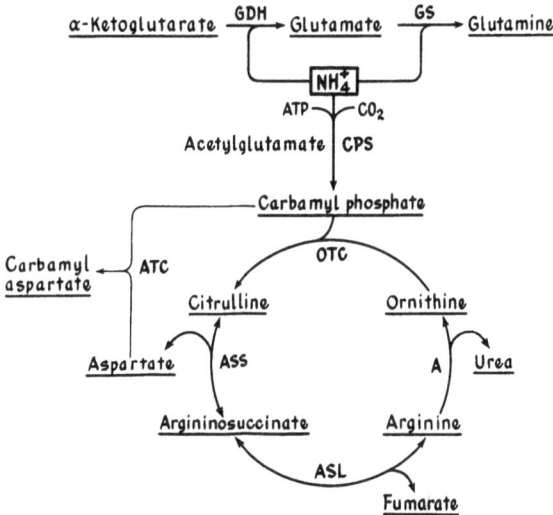

Fig. 6. Pathways for disposition of ammonia.

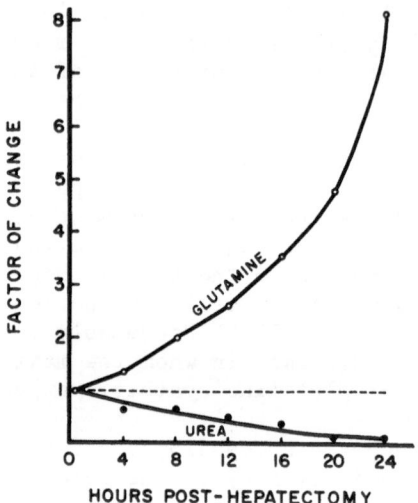

Fig. 7. Geometric rise in blood glutamine following total hepatectomy
        in the dog. (From Drapanas et al. Ann. Surg. 162: 621,1965.)

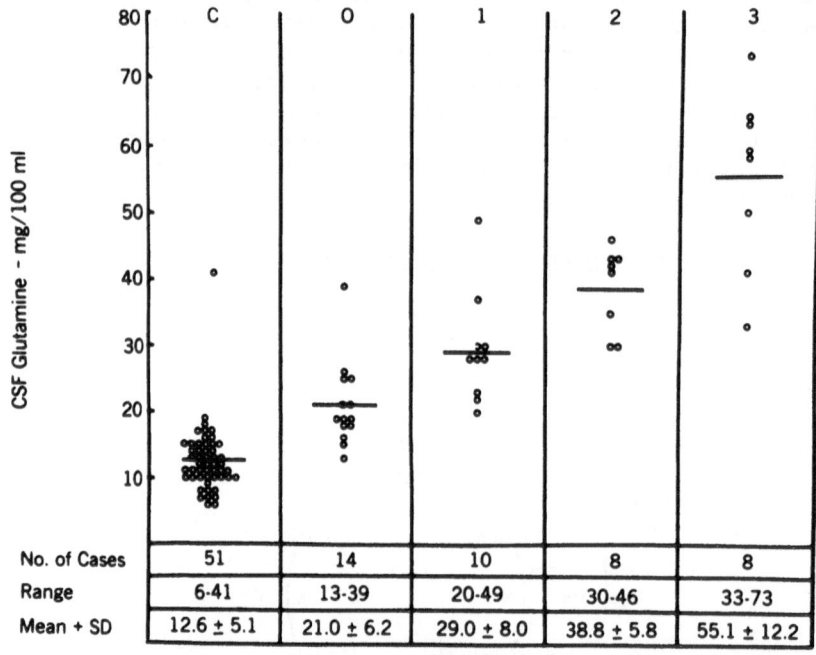

	C	O	1	2	3
No. of Cases	51	14	10	8	8
Range	6-41	13-39	20-49	30-46	33-73
Mean + SD	12.6 ± 5.1	21.0 ± 6.2	29.0 ± 8.0	38.8 ± 5.8	55.1 ± 12.2

Fig. 8. Relationship of cerebrospinal fluid glutamine concentration
        to clinical severity of hepatic encephalopathy. Grade 3 pa-
        tients were unconscious. (From Hourani, Hamlin, and Reynolds.
        Arch. Int. Med. 127: 1033, 1971.)

CONCLUSION

By way of summary I will recapitulate the evidence for a pathogenetic role of ammonia in hepatic encephalopathy. Of the various candidate toxins, ammonia is probably most important, and has most cumulative evidence supporting its role as an etiologic factor, in patients with cirrhosis ammonium salts and substances that generate or release ammonia cause encephalopathy or coma. Removal of the ammonia producers or releasers results in improvement in the encephalopathy. Patients without liver disease who have portacaval shunts have been observed to develop encephalopathy that worsened or improved in relation to the rise or fall in the blood ammonia. A good correlation is observed in unselected patients between severity of encephalopathy and the cerebrospinal fluid concentration of glutamine or α-ketoglutaramate, substances that reflect brain ammonia. In diseases characterized by urea cycle abnormalities, e.g. Reyes syndrome and congenital hyperammonemic states, encephalopathy occurs in association with high blood ammonia levels. The conclusion that disturbed ammonia metabolism is a basic casual factor in hepatic encephalopathy is unavoidable. However, from clinical inconsistencies that are observed, and from experimental observations, it is clear that ammonia excess alone cannot entirely account for the encephalopathy in the typical case.

REFERENCES

1. G. J. Gabuzda, Hepatic coma: Clinical consideration, pathogenesis, and management, in "Advances in Internal Medicine", Dock, W. and Snapper I. eds., Vol. II, Chicago Year Book, pp. 11-73 (1962).
2. G. J. Gabuzda, G. B. Phillips, and C. S. Davidson, Reversible toxic manifestations in patients with cirrhosis of the liver given cation-exchange resins, New Eng. J. Med. 246: 124(1952).
3. G. B. Phillips, The syndrome of impending hepatic coma in patients with cirrhosis of the liver given certain nitrogenous substances, New Eng. J. Med. 247: 239 (1952).
4. W. V. McDermott and R. D. Adams, Episodic stupor associated with an Eck fistula in the human with particular reference to the metabolism of ammonia, J. Clin. Invest. 33: 1 (1954).
5. G. R. Onstad and L. Zieve, What determines blood ammonia? Gastroenterology 77: 803 (1979).
6. H. O. Conn and M. M. Lieberthal, The hepatic coma syndromes and lactulose. William and Wilkins, Baltimore (1979).
7. L. Zieve and D. M. Nicoloff, Pathogenesis of hepatic coma, Ann. Rev. Med. 26: 143 (1975).
8. A. M. Dawson, Regulation of blood ammonia, Gut 19: 504 (1978).
9. A. H. Lockwood, The dynamics of ammonia metabolism in man. Effects of liver disease and hyperammonemia, J. Clin. Invest. 63: 449 (1979).

10. S. Berl, G. Takagaki, D. D. Clarke, and H. Waelsch, Metabolic compartments in vivo. Ammonia and glutamic acid metabolism in brain and liver, J. Biol. Chem. 237: 2562 (1962).

11. W. Raabe and R. J. Gumnit, Disinhibition in cat motor cortex by ammonia, J. Neurophysiol. 38: 347 (1975).

12. G. M. Clark and B. Eiseman, Studies in ammonia metabolism. IV. Biochemical changes in brain tissues of dogs during ammonia-induced coma, New Eng. J. Med. 259: 178 (1958).

13. B. Hindfelt, F. Plum, and T. E. Duffy, Effect of acute ammonia intoxication on cerebral metabolism in rats with portacaval shunts, J. Clin. Invest. 59: 386 (1977).

14. A. Gjedde, A. H. Lockwood, T. E. Duffy, and F. Plum, Cerebral blood flow and metabolism in chronically hyperammonemic rats: Effect of an acute ammonia challenge, Annals of Neurology 3: 325 (1978).

15. G. D. Duda and P. Handler, Kinetics of ammonia metabolism in vivo, J. Biol. Chem. 232: 303 (1958).

16. T. Drapanas, R. H. McMenamy, W. J. Adler, and J. O. Vang, Intermediary metabolism following hepatectomy in dogs, Ann. Surg. 162: 621 (1965).

17. J. D. Ansley, J. W. Isaacs, L. F. Rikkers, M. H. Kutner, B. M. Nordlinger, and D. Rudman, Quantitative tests of nitrogen metabolism in cirrhosis: Relations to other manifestations of liver disease, Gastroenterology 75: 570 (1978).

18. R. T. Hourani, E. M. Hamlin, and T. B. Reynolds, Cerebrospinal fluid glutamine as a measure of hepatic encephalopathy, Arch. Int. Med. 127: 1033 (1971).

19. T. E. Duffy, F. Vergara, and F. Plum, α-ketoglutaramate in hepatic encephalopathy, in: "Brain Dysfunction in Metabolic Disorders," F. Plum ed., Res. Publ. Assoc. Nerv. Ment. Dis. 53: 39 (1974).

20. F. Plum and B. Hindfelt, The neurological complications of liver disease, in: "Handbook of Clinical Neurology," P. H. Vinken and G. W. Bruyn, Vol. 27, Metabolic and Deficiency Diseases of the Nervous System, Part I. American Elsevier, New York Publishing Co. Inc., pp. 349-377 (1976).

ROLE OF SYNERGISM IN THE PATHOGENESIS OF HEPATIC ENCEPHALOPATHY

L. Zieve

Hennepin County Medical Center, University of Minnesota
Minneapolis, MN, U.S.A.

PATHOGENETIC FACTORS

My thesis is that the accumulation of certain toxins having synergistic interactions with each other lead to the development of hepatic encephalopathy, and that other endogenous abnormalities augment the toxicity of these substances (Figure 1). Four of the substances that accumulate during hepatic failure have been shown unequivocally to cause coma in experimental animals. These are ammonia, mercaptans, fatty acids, and phenols. The role of ammonia in human HE is well recognized, and has been discussed (see chapter by Schenker). However, ammonia excess alone cannot entirely account for the encephalopathy seen in a typical case, though it is an important factor.[1]

Like ammonia, mercaptans that accumulate during hepatic failure come largely from the gut. Mercaptans are thio-alcohols. The prototype is methane-thiol(CH_3SH). Two important derivatives are dimethyl sulfide (CH_3SCH_3) and dimethyldisulfide (CH_3S-SCH_3). Challenger & Walshe in 1955 isolated methane-thiol from the urine of a patient in coma due to fulminant hepatic failure.[2] They were looking for the cause of fetor hepaticus, and suspected a mixture of the 3 substances previously mentioned. No better suggestion has been made, but there is no direct proof of this hypothesis. In 1970, we measured mercaptans in the breath for the first time and found a 4-fold increase of methanethiol.[3] We also found an increase in breath dimethylsulfide in cirrhotics following the feeding of methionine. The intensity of the odor was closely related to the concentration of dimethylsulfide in the breath. However this odor was not the typical fetor hepaticus of hepatic coma.

Synergistic Variables

Primary Toxins	Augmenting Abnormalities
Ammonia	Hypoxia
Mercaptans	Hypovolemia
Fatty Acids	Hypotension
Phenols	Hypoglycemia
Possibly AA abn.	Decreased albumin, Na, K, or Mg

Fig. 1. Pathogenetic variables that probably interact synergistically
with each other in various forms of hepatic encephalopathy.

Mercaptans are quite toxic. The occurrence of coma is one of
the toxic manifestation of methanethiol.[4] The blood level of methanethiol at which coma occurred in normal rats was 3000 picomoles/ml.
Blood methanethiol values observed in fulminant hepatic failure in
rats, and in patients with hepatic encephalopathy following chronic
cirrhosis with failure, who were run at the same time, averaged
approximately 1000 pmoles/ml.[5] Blood methanethiol in 94 consecutive
decompensated cirrhotics with and without hepatic encephalopathy
(PSE) showed a pattern of change on the average that was similar to
that with the blood ammonia.[6] As with the blood ammonia measurement,
serial determinations of blood methanethiol are more valuable than
an isolated single measurement. As the grade of encephalopathy
worsens, the methanethiol concentration generally rises. Thus in
13 consecutive patients who died in hepatic coma II or 85% had blood
MT changes that correlated significantly with the clinical deterioration (Figure 2). The best and the worst grade of encephalopathy
are recorded for each patient in this graph. Only one half of these
patients had changes in blood ammonia consistent with the clinical
changes.

The significance of fatty acids in hepatic failure is at
present an enigma. No consistent relationship could be established
between the clinical course and the elevated plasma level of short
and medium chain fatty acids. Experimentally, such fatty acids in
sufficient dosage cause coma that is reversible. At very low concentrations in vitro they depress the activity of a variety of
enzymes. At pathologic concentrations in vivo, they interfere with
the disposition of ammonia and they augment the coma potential of
both ammonia and mercaptans.[7,8] Excess of fatty acids also predispo-
ses the animal to hypoglycemia, an opposite effect to that of NH_4
alone (Figure 3).[9] In Reyes syndrome fatty-acidemia is of major
direct significance. In hepatic failure its role is probably indirect,
perhaps operating through fatty acid synergism with ammonia and
mercaptans.

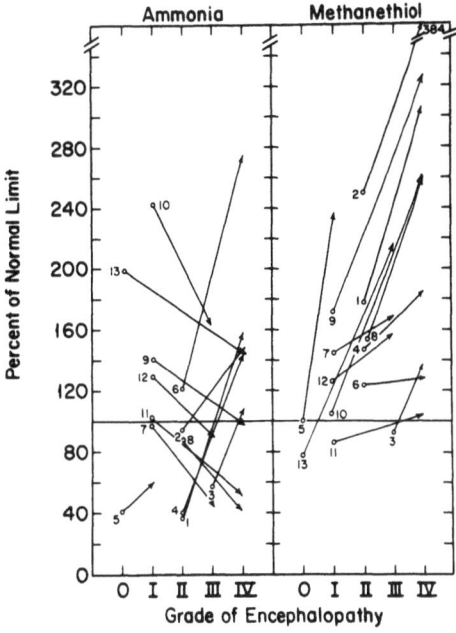

Fig. 2.   Changes in blood ammonia and methanethiol in relation to
          changes in grade of hepatic encephalopathy in patients who
          died after progression of their encephalopathy. In grade
          IV encephalopathy the patients were unconscious. Arrows
          indicate the direction of change and the values when the
          encephalopathy was at its worst. Circles indicate values
          when the encephalopathy was the least. Numbers identify
          individual patients. The values of ammonia and methane-
          thiol on the ordinate are expressed as a percentage of
          their upper limits of normal (90 mmole/ml and 550 pmole/
          ml, respectively).
          (From Gut 21: 318, 1980.)

     The significance of phenols is also uncertain at present. A
modest relationship between blood phenols and severity of encephalopathy has been demonstrated,[10] but the diffuse rapid and persistent
tremor seen with relatively small doses of phenol in the experimental animal is not a characteristic of human hepatic coma. Like fatty
acids, its role in hepatic failure is probably indirect.

SYNERGISM

     I would like now to review the experimental data that demon-
strate synergisms among the coma-producing effects of these substances as well as their interaction with other endogenous abnormal-

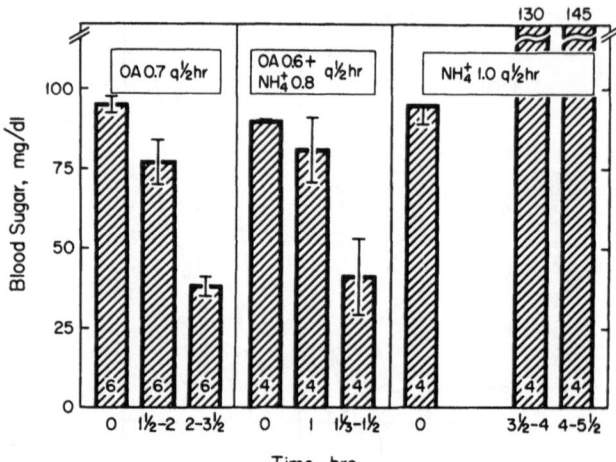

Fig. 3. Effect of multiple subcoma intraperitoneal (IP) doses of
         octanoic acid (OA 0.7 mmole/½ hr), NH$_4$Cl (NH$_4^+$ 1.0 mmole/
         ½ hr), or a combination (OA 0.6 + NH$_4^+$ 0.8 mmole/½ hr) on
         the blood sugar. Bars give means ± SEMs.
         (From J. Lab. Clin. Med. 101: in press.)

ities.   These studies have been performed on rats primarily. Since
I will refer repeatedly to the occurrence of coma in rats, I want
first to define coma as a state of unconsciousness in which the rat
is unresponsive to pain and its righting reflex is lost; i.e. when
placed on its back the rat remains there. Dose-response curves have
been constructed giving the incidence of coma in response to various
doses of a given toxin or of a combination of toxins.

Methanethiol and ammonia come largely from the same source, the
bowel, and influence each other's coma-producing potential as well
as that of fatty acids such as octanoic acid. Figure 4 shows the
effect of subcoma doses of methanethiol and of dimethylsulfide on
the dose-response curve for NH$_4^+$ in normal rats.[4] The CD50 of NH$_4^+$
(dose causing coma in 50% of animals) was reduced by 68% in the
presence of a subcoma dose of methanethiol. Dimethylsulfide had a
similar though not as prominent an effect. When the dose of NH$_4^+$ was
reduced to 1.0 mmole, the coma incidence went from 0 to 100% as long
as a small amount of methanethiol was also given. The effect of a
subcoma dose of methanethiol on the dose-response curve for the
fatty acid, octanoate, was similar. The CD$_{50}$ was again reduced by
2/3.

The same sort of synergism was demonstrated between fatty acids
or phenol and NH$_4^+$. A subcoma dose of octanoate reduced the NH$_4^+$ coma
dose by 30-50%, and conversely.[4] Blood and brain levels of ammonia
at which coma occurred in some of the rats were also significantly

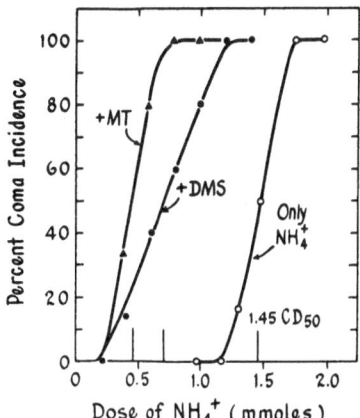

Fig. 4.   Coma-induction dose-response curves in rats for NH_4^+ in the
presence or absence of an inhaled dose of methanethiol
(0.12% by volume) or dimethylsulfide (6.36% by volume).
CD_{50} = dose causing coma in 50% of rats.
(From J. Lab. Clin. Med. 83: 16, 1974.)

reduced when a subcoma dose of octanoate was injected simultaneously
with the NH_4^+ (Figure 5). However the levels at which coma occurred
in all of the rats remained the same, though the dose of NH_4^+ was
reduced.[11] Plasma levels of octanoate at which coma occurred in
some of the rats were also reduced. A subcoma dose of phenol reduced
the NH_4^+ coma dose by 25%, and conversely.[12] Blood and brain levels
of ammonia at which encephalopathy occurred in some of the rats were
reduced slightly when the subcoma dose of phenol was injected simultaneously with the NH_4^+. However the close curvilinear relationship
between brain ammonia and severity of encephalopathy was unaffected
(Figure 6).

Since the brain's energy source is primarily glucose, one might
expect a lack of glucose to affect the neurotoxicity of substances
like ammonia. One can in fact demonstrate a synergism between ammonium ion-induced coma and hypoglycemia. Rats with blood sugars
between 25 and 45 mg% following injections of insulin were more
sensitive to the effects of NH_4^+. The CD_{50} for NH_4^+ was reduced by
approximately 30%. A subcoma dose of 1.2 mmoles NH_4^+ caused coma in
100% of animals who had hypoglycemia insufficient in itself to cause
coma.[9] The synergism between hypoglycemia and octanoate was similar.
Warren and Schenker have likewise shown in mice that hypoxia has a
similar augmenting effect on the toxicity of NH_4^+.[13]

Subcoma doses of fatty acids and of mercaptans influence the
occurrence of coma by influencing the blood level of ammonia as
well as by their cellular effects. Figure 7 shows that very small

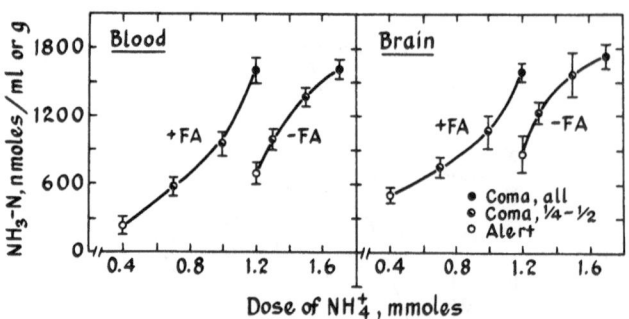

Fig. 5. Relationships of blood and brain ammonia concentrations
         to the IP dose of NH_4^+, the presence or absence of a
         simultaneous IP dose of octanoate (FA), and the presence
         or absence of coma in 300 $\pm$ 30 g mole rats. Means $\pm$ SEMs
         are plotted.
         (From Cerebral Energy Metabolism and Metabolic Encephalo-
         pathy, D. W. McCandless, ed. 1983, Plenum Publishing Corp.,
         New York.)

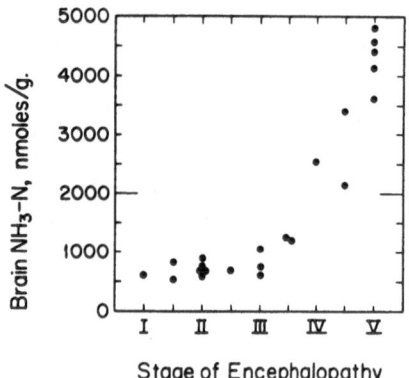

Fig. 6. Relationship of brain ammonia concentration to stage of
         encephalopathy in rats receiving a subcoma IP dose of
         phenol (450 μmoles) plus IP doses of NH_4^+ varying between
         0.5 and 2.0 mmoles. Stage I: incipient stage of overt
         encephalopathy; II: precoma; III: borderline coma; IV:
         unconsciousness with some response to stimuli; V: deep
         coma unresponsive to anything.

subcoma doses of the fatty acid, octanoate, and of methanethiol,
when given with the highest subcoma dose of NH_4^+ increased the blood
ammonia two-fold and in the process put the rats in coma. Other

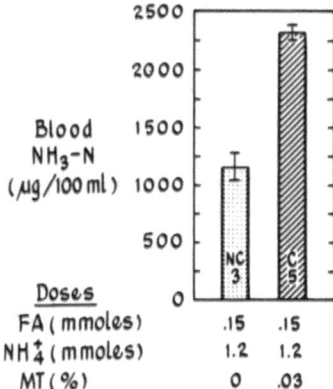

Fig. 7. Blood ammonia concentrations in 300 g rats after IP injections of the highest subcoma dose of NH_4Cl simultaneously
with very small subcoma doses of IP octanoate (FA) and
inhaled methanethiol (MT). Number of rats indicated at base
of each bar. NC = no coma. C = coma induction.
(From J. Lab. Clin. Med. 83: 16, 1974.)

fatty acids such as hexanoic, decanoic, and oleic acids had similar
effects. We found an explanation for these in vivo effects by demonstrating in vitro in a liver homogenate system that fatty acids in
appropriately low concentrations depressed carbamylphosphate synthetase and glutamate dehydrogenase activities, the key enzymes involved
in the disposition of ammonia.[8] In similar fashion, we found that
subcoma doses of methanethiol or dimethylsulfide influenced the
occurrence of coma by influencing the blood level of ammonia. An
explanation for this rise in blood ammonia was sought and found in
a study of the urea cycle. In an isolated perfused rat liver system,
as little as 0.5 μM MT reduced urea formation from ammonia by 62%
over a period of 2 hours.[14] In this perfused liver system, 10 mM
octanoate reduced urea formation by 50% over a period of 2 hours.

The average brain and blood levels of ammonia and methanethiol
in rats in hepatic coma following acute massive liver necrosis are
much lower than the levels required to produce coma in normal rats
with each of these substances individually.[15] In experimental hepatic
coma the increase in brain ammonia is 3-fold and brain methanethiol
5-fold. The corresponding figure in pure ammonia coma is 4 to 5-fold
and in pure methanethiol coma 23-fold.

Normal rats become comatose when they are given a suitable
combination of doses of NH_4^+, methanethiol and octanoic acid, which
result in brain levels of both ammonia and methanethiol that are
similar to those observed in the rat with experimental hepatic coma.
We reasoned that if this combination of brain levels is sufficient

to cause coma in normal rats, it should be sufficient to do so in rats with badly damaged livers. Therefore, the encephalopathy that occurs following experimental acute ischemic fulminant hepatic failure may be explained by the synergistic interaction of these three toxic substances without invoking other factors. These experimental observations on synergism have implications for human hepatic encephalopathy, because ammonia, mercaptans and fatty acids accumulate simultaneously in patients with hepatic failure. The only other substances that both accumulate in hepatic failure and have been either shown or claimed to cause reversible coma in experimental animals are phenol derivatives, the combination of Phe and Tryp, and GABA.

CONCLUSION

Coma following liver failure in patients is a complex phenomenon with many facets, and a whole spectrum of variations depending on the circumstances and rate of its development. In addition to the accumulation of potential coma-producing toxins such as ammonia, mercaptans, fatty acids, and phenols, endogenous metabolic abnormalities such as hypoxia, hypovolemia, hypotension, in some circumstances hypoglycemia, and depletion of albumin, sodium, potassium, magnesium and zinc are commonly present. The closest thing to our animal model of acute ischemic hepatic necrosis is fulminant hepatic failure with massive necrosis. One would anticipate that synergistic interactions among toxins and endogenous abnormalities play an important role in such cases. In Reye's syndrome, where abnormalities of fatty acids and ammonia are particularly prominent, and where hypoglycemia and hypoxia may augment their toxicity, synergistic interactions seem of particular importance in pathogenesis. However, in the usual case of chronic liver disease with gradual deterioration leading ultimately to hepatic coma, endogenous factors affecting the mental state of the patient are more subtly involved. A direct relationship between the presence of toxins and the development of encephalopathy is much more difficult to establish, and synergistic interactions may be obscured. I believe however, that in that circumstance also, encephalopathy results from synergistic effects of toxins and various endogenous metabolic abnormalities of a subacute or chronic nature.

REFERENCES

1. L. Zieve, Hepatic encephalopathy, in "Diseases of the Liver", L. Schiff and E. R. Schiff, eds., J. B. Lippincott Co., Philadelphia, pp. 433-459 (1982).
2. F. Challenger and J. M. Walshe, Methyl mercaptan in relation to factor hepaticus, Biochem. J. 59: 372 (1955).
3. S. Chen, L. Zieve, and V. Mahadevan, Mercaptans and dimethyl sulfide in the breath of patients with cirrhosis of the liver, J. Lab. Clin. Med. 75: 628 (1970).

4. L. Zieve, W.M. Doizaki, and F.J. Zieve, Synergism between mercap-
    tans and ammonia or fatty acids in the production of coma:
    A possible role for mercaptans in the pathogenesis of hepatic
    coma, J. Lab. Clin. Med. 83: 16 (1974).
5. W. M. Doizaki and L. Zieve, An improved method for measuring
    blood mercaptans, J. Lab. Clin. Med. 90: 849 (1977).
6. C. J. McClain, L. Zieve, W. M. Doizaki, S. Gillerstadt, and G.R.
    Onstad, Blood methanethiol in alcoholic liver disease with
    and without hepatic encephalopathy, Gut 21: 318 (1980).
7. F. J. Zieve, L. Zieve, and W. M. Doizaki, , Synergism between
    ammonia and fatty acids in the production of coma: implica-
    tions for hepatic coma, J. Pharmacol. Exp. Therap. 191: 10
    (1974).
8. R. F. Derr and L. Zieve, Effect of fatty acids on the disposi-
    tion of ammonia J. Pharmacol. Exp. Therap. 197: 675 (1976).
9. L. Zieve, C. Lyftogt, and K. Draves, Toxicity of a fatty acid
    and ammonia: interactions with hypoglycemia and Krebs cycle
    inhibition, J. Lab. Clin. Med. 101: in press (1983).
10. D. Muting and H. Reikowski, Protein metabolism in liver disease,
    in: "Progress in Liver Diseases", Vol II, H. Popper and F.
    Schaffner eds., Grune and Stratton, New York, pp. 84-94
    (1965).
11. L. Zieve, Encephalopathy due to short and medium chain fatty
    acids, in: "Cerebral Energy Metabolism and Metabolic Ence-
    phalopathy", D. W. Mc Candless, ed., Plenum Publishing Corp.
    New York, in press (1983).
12. G. Windus-Podehl, C. Lyftogt, L. Zieve, and G. Brunner, Ence-
    phalopathic effect of phenol in rats, J. Lab. Clin. Med.
    101: 586 (1983).
13. K. S. Warren and S. Schenker, Hypoxia and ammonia toxicity, Am.
    J. Physiol. 199: 1105 (1960).
14. R. F. Derr and L. Zieve, Methanethiol and fatty acids depress
    urea synthesis by the isolated perfused rat liver, J. Lab.
    Clin. Med. 100: 585 (1982).
15. L. Zieve and W. M. Doizaki, Brain and blood methanethiol and
    ammonia concentrations in experimental hepatic coma and
    coma due to injections of various combinations of these
    substances, Gastroenterology 79: 1070 (1980).

γ-AMINOBUTYRIC ACID RECEPTORS IN EXPERIMENTAL HEPATIC ENCEPHALOPATHY

M. L. Zeneroli, M. Baraldi° and E. Ventura

Istituti di Clinica Medica III e di Farmacologia

Università di Modena - 41100 Modena - Italy

INTRODUCTION

Studies on the pathogenesis of hepatic encephalopathy (HE) following fulminant hepatic failure (FHF) have focused on biochemical changes occurring in blood, in cerebrospinal fluid or in brain with the aim of recognizing the primary factors leading to the central nervous system (CNS) dysfunction of coma. Because of the numerous metabolic abnormalities found in this pathology a congeries of theories has been generated, but none of these is so fully proved as to be accepted.

Our philosophy in studies on pathogenesis of experimental HE was guided by the following rationale: 1) to choose an animal model that closely approximates the huamn pathology 2) to electrophysiologically characterize the model 3) to reconcile the electrophysiological findings with altered activity of neurotransmitter systems at the synaptic level in the CNS and, in turn, receptor alterations 4) to study whether the alterations of receptors (if any) are related to changes in the environment of the synaptic membranes 5) to demonstrate that peripheral factors, that are increased in FHF, are really able to fully reproduce, when injected in normal animals, behavioral, electrophysiological and biochemical changes in the CNS similar to those of HE.

ANIMAL MODEL OF FULMINANT HEPATIC FAILURE

D-Galactosamine has been proved to produce experimental FHF similar to the human pathology.[1-4] Male Sprague Dawley rats (weighing 100-125 g) were intraperitoneally injected with 3 g/kg of D-Galactosamine-HCl. Following a single injection about 70-80% of rats develop

FHF leading to a gradual appearance of encephalopathy. The encephalopathy is characterized by mild confusion, agitation, drowsiness and stupor in the stage that we term "mild" followed by a "severe" stage characterized by flaccidity, lethargy, areflexicity to pain stimuli and full coma. A small percentage of rats can recover from the mild stage owing to liver regeneration.

In this animal model we documented a plasma amino acid imbalance,[5] indicating the possibility that an increased quantity of aromatic amino acids enter through the blood brain barrier.[6] In fact, the assay of tyrosine in striatal tissue of these rats showed a 5 fold increase in the severe stage parallel with a decrease of Dopamine and Norepinephrine in the presence of increased levels of octopamine.[5] Moreover, we have documented a progressive increase in brain ammonia levels rising by 7 times in the severe stage.[7]

ELECTROPHYSIOLOGICAL STUDIES

A crucial point in studies performed in animal models of HE is the evaluation of the coma state. In fact, objective assessment of unconsciousness is not possible using arbitrary judgement by the observers. On the other hand the use of EEG in animals does not discriminate the degree and the kind of unconsciousness,[2] whereas waves of abnormal form, such as triphasic waves, that appear during the development of coma prove to be unspecific to HE.[8]

With the above mentioned considerations in mind, we used Visual Evoked Potentials (VEP) to evaluate neuronal changes that progressively take place during the development of HE since VEPs were proved to reflect demyelinization processes and changes in neurotransmitters.[4,7,9-12]

As shown in Figure 1, VEPs recorded in control rats were characterised by four waves positive and negative labelled P_1, N_1, P_2 and N_2. Rats in mild stage of HE galactosamine-induced showed a reduction of N_1 and P_2 amplitudes without changes in the latencies, whereas rats in severe HE showed a decrease in the amplitudes of N_1, P_2 and N_2 waves, a significant increase of the latency of N_1 (P < 0.05 vs controls) with a shortening of the latency of N_2 (P < 0.05). The reliability of VEP to discriminate different stages of HE was an useful tool to select animals at the same degree of encephalopathy for biochemical and binding studies.

To demonstrate the specificity of VEP pattern and its capacity in discriminating different states of unconsciousness, we performed experiments using different agents. A tolbutamide-induced hypoglycemic coma in rat proved different from VEP recorded in HE.[12] Moreover injection of drugs such as barbiturates, benzodiazepines and aminooxyacetic acid in normal animals (Figure 1) induced VEP patterns similar to each other, but different from the VEP recorded in rats

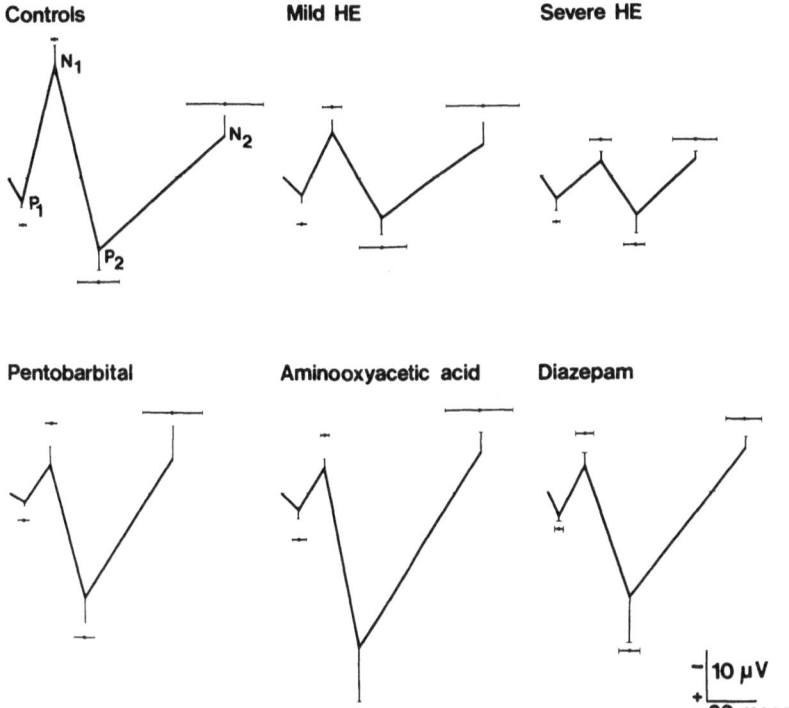

Fig. 1.   Composite mean flash evoked responses recorded in control
          rats, in rats with galactosamine-induced FHF in mild and
          in severe stage of HE and in normal rats i.p. injected
          with pentobarbital sodium (32 mg/kg), aminooxyacetic acid
          (50 mg/kg), diazepam (5 mg/kg). Vertical bars represent 1
          SD of the amplitudes, horizontal bars represent the mean ±
          1 SD of the latency of the near peak.

during HE. These results contradict the report of D. F. Schafer and
E. A. Jones.[13,14] The similarity of VEP pattern induced by the
injection of barbiturates, aminooxyacetic acid or diazepam seems to
prove the reliability of VEP recording since all of them are known
to potentiate the inhibitory action of γ-aminobutyric acid (GABA)
at the synaptic level.[15-17]

     Incidentally, this last observation allows us to state that a
simple increase of inhibitory GABAergic activity in animals with
intact synaptic structures does not lead to a comatose state similar
to that of HE.

     On the basis of these observations we tested in normal animals
substances claimed to be primary factors in causing HE, such as
tryptophan plus phenylalanine,[18] tryptophan plus octopamine,[19]

separate injections of ammonia, of dimethyldisulfide and of octanoic
acid and subacute treatment with ammonia + dimethyldisulfide + octanoic acid.[20] None of these substances reproduced behavioral and VEP
pattern of HE[4,7,12] except the last mentioned subacute administration
of ammonia, mercaptans and short chain fatty acids,[7] suggesting a
pathogenetic role of these toxins acting in a synergistic fashion
in the induction of HE.

STUDIES ON GABA RECEPTOR COMPLEX

Since HE is mainly characterized by a generalized depression
of CNS, few authors have hitherto considered the hypothesis that
GABA might be implicated in this pathology (for review see[20-22]).
The assay of GABA levels in blood and in spinal fluid both in animals
and in men gave conflicting results without convincing evidence in
support of a direct role of GABA in the development of coma.[23,24]
Recently it has been suggested that an increased production of GABA
deriving from gut in a rabbit model of galactosamine-induced FHF
could be the primary agent in the pathogenesis of HE.[13,14] This
hypothesis assumes that the increased peripheral GABA passing through
a permeable blood-brain barrier leads to an increased level of GABA
in brain. However it has not been convincingly shown that authentic
GABA can penetrate through the blood brain barrier in this pathological condition and no assay of GABA has been done in brain tissue.

It is well known that GABA poorly penetrates the blood brain
barrier in normal conditions.[25] Utilizing ^{3}H-GABA, we have recently
demonstrated[26] that after an intravenous injection of this neurotransmitter in normal rats and in rats with severe HE, GABA is
rapidly metabolized in blood. In fact, 30 minutes after i.v. injection the levels of ^{3}H-GABA were markedly decreased whereas ^{3}H-me-
tabolites concentrations were enhanced. In blood of comatose rats
the rate of disappearance of ^{3}H-GABA was slightly delayed and paralleled by a reduction in ^{3}H-metabolites, probably related to a
reduction of mitocondrial GABA-transaminase activity caused by the
massive necrosis of the liver.

When the level of ^{3}H-GABA was determined in brain, as shown
in Figure 2, the content of authentic GABA was constantly lower in
comatose rats than in controls (maximum recovery: 0.033% in controls,
0.029 in rats with severe HE) indicating that there is no increased
permeability of the blood brain barrier for GABA during HE. In fact,
an altered blood brain barrier has been described in HE only for
substances that are not metabolized at this level and that freely
diffuse through the barrier such as insuline and glucose.[27] By
contrast GABA is metabolized at the level of the barrier by GABA-
transaminase strategically located in the endothelial cells of the
barrier to prevent its entering the brain.[25] This metabolization
invalidates the use of a non-metabolizable isomer of GABA to support
its hypothetical increased entering in brain.[13,14]

Furthermore the direct assay of GABA in blood and in brain of
normal rats and of rats with HE using a gas chromatographic mass-
spectrometric technique did not show any change of GABA level in HE
either in blood or in brain, indicating that this neurotransmitter
was at steady-state level in rats with HE as in control animals.[26]
On the other hand, it is well known that a simple assay of the level
of GABA in brain does not predict its functional activity at the
synaptic level, since there are at least three different pools of
this neurotransmitter in the brain. A more reliable index is given
by the assay of glutamic acid decarboxylase (GAD), the target enzyme
of the GABA synthesis in nerve terminals. GAD levels in rat with HE
were found to be significantly lower compared with values found in
normal rats, indicating the presence in this pathological state of
a decreased synthesis of GABA.[26]

All the above-mentioned findings, taken together, seem to
indicate that peripheral GABA cannot be regarded as a primary factor
in this pathology.

The reduction of GAD activity found in several brain areas
prompted us to carry out GABA binding studies with the aim of demon-

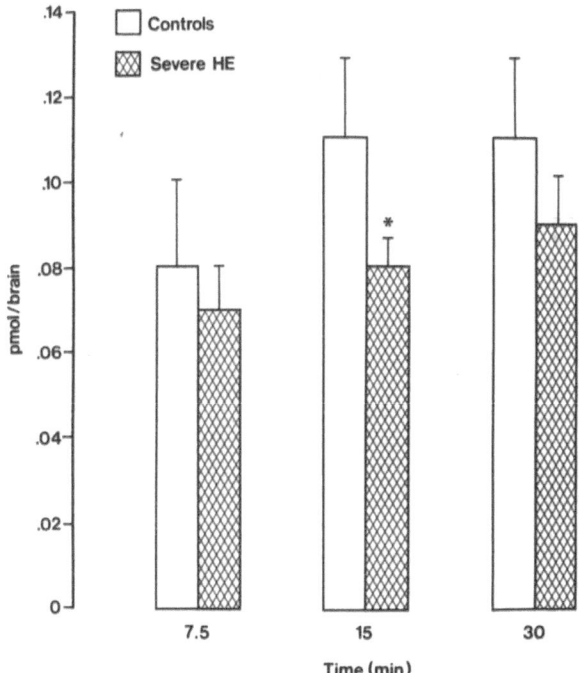

Fig. 2. Levels (mean+1 SD) of ^{3}H-GABA in brain of control rats and
of rats with severe HE after i.v. injection of 2.5 nM/Kg of
^{3}H-GABA (145 µCi/Kg) and 1 µM of unlabeled GABA. Student's
t-test: *P < 0.01 vs controls.

strating whether or not this biochemical change could reflect degenerative processes at the synaptic level. We have recently described
[28-30] that in the mild stage of HE there is an increase in both low
and high affinity GABA binding sites, providing evidence that in
this stage of encephalopathy a denervation supersensitivity phenomenon could be present.[31-33] In the severe degree of HE, when the
animals are in agonal status, a situation in which their cellular
mechanism could be too severely damaged, we detected a selection of
high affinity GABA binding sites. This finding strongly supports
the idea that the disappearance of the low affinity receptors could
be due to a degeneration phenomenon.

This finding and its interpretation are not surprising since
there is a substantial body of morphological studies performed on
animal models and on man indicating both transformation of astrocytes
(Alzheimer type II) and loss of neurons and of oligodendrocytes in
the most severe stage of HE (for review see[34]). As shown in Figure
3, GABA binding saturation curves performed in triton x 100 treated
brain membrane preparations[29] from normal rats or from rats in mild
and in severe degree of HE show a progressive change in the binding
capacity of GABA receptors. Briefly, in the mild stage we found an
increase in both low and high affinity GABA receptors without any
change in the affinity constants, while in the severe stage there
is a loss of low affinity binding sites. This finding was further
confirmed by GABA binding studies in several brain areas of rats.
The results shown in Table 1 indicate that the selection of only
high affinity GABA binding sites is a phenomenon involving all the
major brain areas investigated. Moreover GABA binding studies
carried out on GABA receptor solubilized using the method described
by Massotti et al.[35] from brain synaptic membranes of rats in severe
HE we found only high affinity GABA receptors and approximately a
30% reduction in proteins as a further demonstration of the loss
of low affinity binding sites.

The possibility of a direct toxic effect of galactosamine on
brain GABA receptors was excluded by the finding of normal kinetic
characteristics of ^{3}H-GABA binding performed on membranes of the
brains of rats that received D-galactosamine but did not develop
FHF and consequently did not develop HE.[29]

Using membrane preparations frozen, thawed, incubated for 30
minutes at 37°C and extensively washed, we found in the mild stage
an increase in benzodiazepine (Bz) receptors. In fact, ^{3}H-diazepam
binding studies revealed an increased number of receptors in the
mild stage that parallels the increased in GABA binding sites. The
same study performed on membranes of brain in the severe stage
showed that Bz receptors are still increased, indicating that these
receptors are linked with the high affinity GABA receptors. Moreover,
as shown in Figure 4, we detected the same result in cortical membrane preparation.

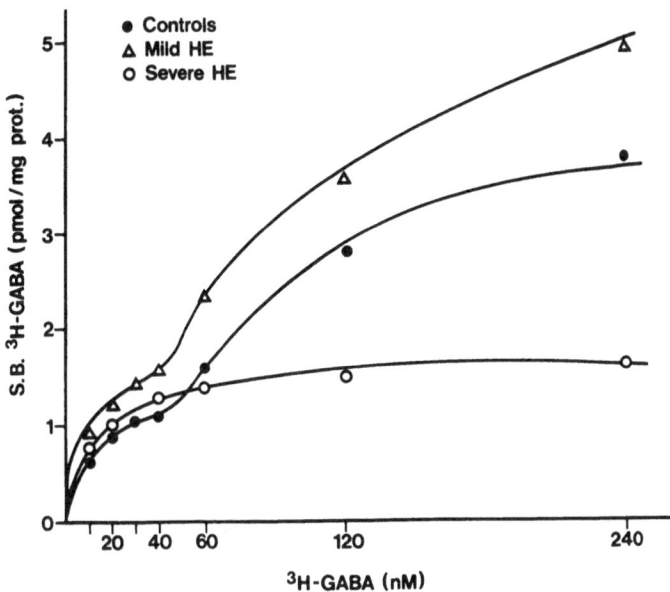

Fig. 3. Saturation curve of ^{3}H-GABA binding to triton x 100 treated synaptic membranes from brain of normal rats and of rats in mild and in severe stage of HE. The values are the mean of 6 separate experiments. Kinetic constants (mean $\pm$ 1 SD) computed from the Scatchard plots of the single experiments in controls were: B_{mx1} 6.0 $\pm$ 0.9 pmol/mg prot., K_{D1} 218+15 nM, B_{mx2} 1.3+0.3 pmol/mg prot., K_{D2} 19.6+6 nM. In rats with mild HE: B_{mx1} 8.1+0.2* pmol/mg prot., K_{D1} 311+6 nM, B_{mx2} 1.9+ 0.2** pmol/mg prot., K_{D2} 24.0 $\pm$ 4 nM. In rats with severe HE: B_{mx1} and K_{D1} undetectable, B_{mx2} 1.9+0.1** pmol/mg prot., K_{D2} 22.9 $\pm$ 4. Student's t-test: * P < 0.05, **P < 0.01 vs controls.

Incidentally, since there are controversial opinions on the linkage of Bz receptors with low or high affinity GABA binding sites [36-38] this is the first direct demonstration that Bz receptors are coupled with high affinity GABA receptors.[37]

D. F. Schafer and E.A. Jones[13-14] have reported an increased number of GABA and Bz receptors in an undefined stage of HE in brain of rabbits with galactosamine-induced FHF and have attributed these findings to an increased entering of gut-derived GABA into brain. These findings apparently seem to be in parallel agreement with our data although a comparison is difficult since no full data have been shown in their reports. Moreover, since an up-regulation of GABA receptor has been described only in the presence of a decrease of GAD and GABA in brains,[31-33] their hypothesis seems to be a

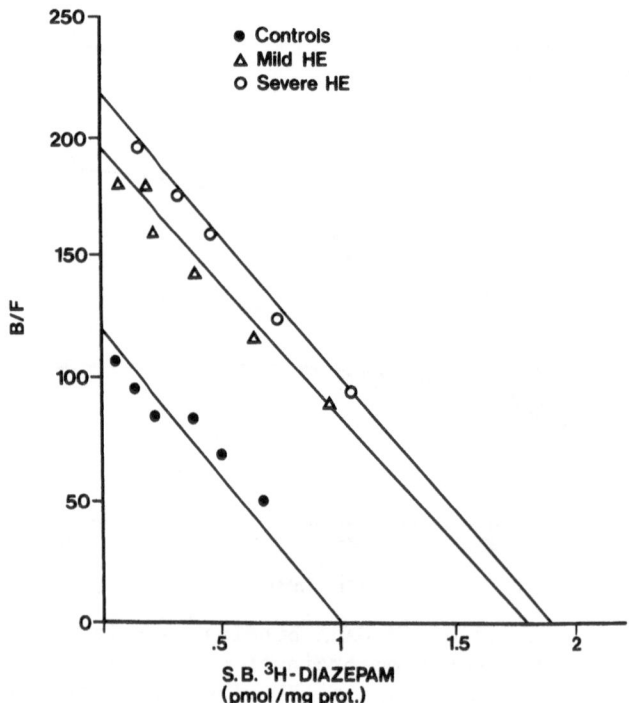

Fig. 4.   Scatchard plot analysis of ^{3}H-diazepam binding to synaptic
          membrane preparation from cortex of control rats and of
          rats in mild and severe HE. Each value represents the mean
          of 3 Scatchard plot of 3 separate experiments done in
          triplicate. Mean $\pm$ 1 SD of the kinetic constants computed
          from the plot of the single experiments were: controls K_D
          9.2 $\pm$ 0.9 nM, B_{mx} 1.0 $\pm$ 0.16 pmol/mg prot.; Mild HE: K_D
          9.0 $\pm$ 0.75 nM, B_{mx} 1.80 $\pm$ 0.15* pmol/mg prot.; Severe HE:
          K_D 8.7 $\pm$ 0.8 nM, B_{mx} 1.85 $\pm$ 0.19* pmol/mg prot. Student's
          t-test: *P < 0.001 vs controls.

contradiction in terms and does not fit our data.

        Following our observation both in vitro and in vivo[39] of the
presence of supersensitive GABA receptor system and bearing in mind
the mutual interaction between GABA and dopaminergic processes in
the nigro-striatal pathway, we performed studies on dopamine (DA)
receptors using striatal membrane preparations of rats in mild and
in severe stage of HE.[5] The results of this investigation demonstrated the presence of a reduction of DA receptor affinity in the
mild stage followed by a down regulation phenomenon in the severe
stage. This last finding seems to give further support to the concept
of the presence in HE of degenerative processes involving different
neuronal receptor systems.

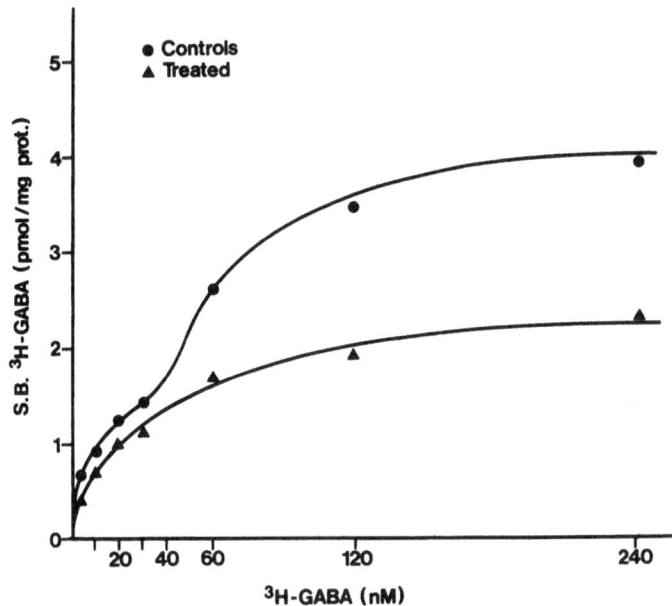

Fig. 5.   Saturation curve of ^{3}H-GABA binding to triton x 100 treated
membranes from brain of control rats and of rats subacutely
i.p. injected with ammonia + mercaptans + octanoic acid
as indicated in Table 2. Mean values ($\pm$ 1 SD) of dissociation
constants computed from the plot of the single experiments
were: Controls B_{mx1} 6.0 $\pm$ 0.9 pmol/mg prot., K_{D1} 218 $\pm$ 15
nM, B_{mx2} 1.3 $\pm$ 0.5 pmol/mg prot., K_{D2} 19.6 $\pm$ 6 nM; Treated
rats B_{mx1} and K_{D1} undetectable, B_{mx2} 2.3 $\pm$ 0.4 pmol/mg prot.
K_{D2} 34 $\pm$ 6 nM.

Our finding of a loss of low affinity GABA receptors with a
selection of high affinity GABA recognition sites concomitant to a
down regulation of DA receptors could be indicative of an imbalance
between inhibitory and excitatory systems of the CNS leading to a
prevalence of the former.

MEMBRANE ENVIRONMENT STUDIES

In search of an explanation of the changes in the protein that
express the low affinity receptor binding capacity, we focused our
attention on the possibility that alterations in the membrane components such as phospholipids and cations could occur during the development of HE.

In this context preliminary results from studies on the
phospholipid composition of homogenates of synaptic preparations
from brain areas of normal rats and of rats in severe HE seem to

Table 1. Kinetic characteristic of ^{3}H-GABA binding in frozen, triton X 100 treated membranes from various brain areas of control rats and of rats with severe degree of hepatic encephalopathy

Brain areas	Low affinity				High affinity					
	K_{D1} (µM)		B_{max1} (pmol/mg prot.)		K_{D2} (µM)		B_{max2} (pmol/mg prot.)		$\dfrac{B_{max\ 2}}{B_{max\ 1}}$	
	Control	Coma	Control	Coma	Control	Coma	Control	Coma	Control	Coma
Cortex	262	(°)	5.2	(°)	14	38.0	0.9	1.9	0.17	0
Hypothalamus	187	(°)	6.0	(°)	19	35.2	1.2	2.7	0.20	0
Striatum	209	(°)	8.5	(°)	28	32.4	2.2	3.7	0.25	0
Cerebellum	162	(°)	9.0	(°)	21	31.3	3.0	4.7	0.33	0

The reported values are the means of separate Scatchard plot analysis obtained from three experiments done in pooled tissue of 18 control rats and of 18 rats with severe degree of HE. The values differed from mean by less than 10%. In the tested areas of comatose rats K_{D1} and B_{max1} were undetectable (°).

Table 2. Zinc levels in brain areas of control rats, of rats with
          galactosamine-induced severe HE and in normal rats with
          an ammonia+mercaptans+octanoic acid-induced[a] coma-like
          state

Brain areas	Controls	Severe HE	Coma-like state
Cerebellum	76 + 27	44 + 25°	57 + 3°
Brainstem	76 + 31	38 + 6°°	29 + 4°°
Hypothalamus	75 + 20	42 + 25°°	60 + 6
Striatum	67 + 11	48 + 6°°	54 + 3°°
Hippocampus	104 + 36	45 + 13°°°	45 + 14°°
Cortex	75 + 28	51 + 6°	11 + 3°°°
Restbrain	67 + 17	42 + 12°°	52 + 6

Values are reported as μg/g dry weight (mean $\pm$ SD); t-test; °P< 0.05,
°°P < 0.01, °°°P < 0.001 vs controls.
(a) Rats were injected every 6 h with NH_4Cl, dymethyldisulfide and
    octanoic acid at the doses of 0.23 mmoles + 23 μmoles + 0.05
    mmoles/rat/x 4 times; 0.70 mmoles + 70 μmoles + 0.15 mmoles/rat
    a 5th time respectively.

indicate that there are neither quantitative nor qualitative changes
of phospholipids.[39]

    There is evidence that free divalent cations are important
factors in the regulation of several enzymatic systems in CNS, and,
in particular, that zinc and, to a lesser extent, copper, inhibit
GAD and GABA transaminase activity, thus regulating the steady state
of GABA.[40,41] Moreover zinc has been regarded as an integral part
of biomembranes and as a stabilizing factor for the tissue integ-
rity.[42] Experiments undertaken to evaluate the levels of zinc,
copper and calcium in tissues of different brain regions in normal
rats and in rats with HE showed a marked decrease of zinc in all
tested areas (Table 2), while no changes were detected in copper
and calcium levels. This phenomenon was paralleled by a decrease of
zinc in liver tissue and by a significant enhancement of zinc in the
blood during mild and severe HE.[43] Thus we have demonstrated that a
decrease of zinc in brain tissue and an increase in blood parallels
a reduction of GAD in nerve terminals and changes in GABA receptors.

    These concomitant phenomena might be regarded as an expression
of lesions induced in nerve terminals by toxins coming from the
failing liver. In fact, since it is well known that zinc is very
tightly bound to intrinsic components of protein membranes, its
decrease in tissue could be a marker of neuron degeneration involving a destabilization of protein complexes that express receptor
binding sites.

ROLE OF PERIPHERAL NEUROTOXINS

Behavioral observation[20,44] and electrophysiological studies performed with VEP[7] demonstrated that ammonia, mercaptans and octanoic acid, when subacutely injected together at low doses, can reproduce a coma-like state similar to HE acting synergistically.

Considering that zinc physiologically stabilizes the biomembranes by reacting with -SH groups of the membrane proteins and since at least one of the components of the toxin mixture, mercaptans, with their -SH groups could act as chelating agents for zinc, we tested the level of this cation in several brain areas of normal rats subacutely injected with the above-mentioned combination of the three toxins. As shown in Table 2, the zinc content of brain tissues fell approximately to the same values as in HE, while its level increased in blood. This finding seems to lend further support to the importance of these substances as primary neurotoxic agents of encephalopathy.

Following this observation, we performed GABA binding studies in synaptic brain membranes of rats in a coma-like state due to the injection of the three toxins. As shown in Figure 5, a marked decrease has been detected in low affinity binding sites resembling the loss of low affinity GABA receptor found in the severe stage of HE.

Although this finding is a further demonstration that, indeed, the injection of ammonia, mercaptans and short-chain fatty acids seems to reproduce the full pattern of HE, we believe that a complete analysis of the effect of each of these toxins on brain GABA receptor must be better characterized and we are presently working on it.

CONCLUSIONS

This review of our studies on experimental hepatic encephalopathy due to FHF provides evidence that the neurological disturbances leading to HE are characterized by degenerative processes demonstrated by a denervation supersensitivity of GABA receptors in the mild stage followed by a selection of distinct high affinity receptors in the severe stage of HE. This concept is further supported by a concomitant down regulation of DA receptors.

All these data taken together seem to indicate that HE results from an imbalance between inhibitory and excitatory receptor systems leading to a functional prevalence of the inhibitory GABA receptor complex.

Moreover we provide some evidence that seems to indicate that zinc is involved in the molecular mechanisms implicated in the changes of receptor binding capacity.

Finally, we lend support to Zieve's theory[20,44] that peripheral toxins such as ammonia, mercaptans and short-chain fatty acids acting synergistically can induce in normal animals behavioral, electrophysiological and biochemical effects that lead to a comatose state strongly resembling HE due to FHF.

To conclude, the direct demonstration of a pathology of brain receptors in experimentally induced HE seems to provide a new insight into the understanding of the CNS disturbance due to primary peripheral metabolic diseases.

REFERENCES

1. D. Keppler, R. Lesch, W. Reutter, and K. Decker, Experimental hepatitis induced by D-galactosamine, Exp. Mol. Path. 9: 279 (1968).
2. B. L. Blitzer, J. G. Waggoner, E. A. Jones, H. R. Gralnick, D. Towne, V. Weise, I. J. Kopin, I. Walters, P. F. Teichenne, D. Goodman, and P. D. Berk, A model of fulminant hepatic failure in rabbit, Gastroenterology 74: 664 (1978).
3. E. Chirito, C. Lister, and T. M. S. Chang, Biochemical, hematological and histological changes in a fulminant hepatic failure rat model for artificial liver assessment, Artif. Organs 3: 42 (1979).
4. M. L. Zeneroli, A. Penne, G. Parrinello, C. Cremonini, and E. Ventura, Comparative evaluation of Visual Evoked potentials in experimental hepatic encephalopathy and in pharmacologically induced coma-like states in rat, Life Sci., 28: 1507 (1981).
5. M. Baraldi, M. L. Zeneroli, P. Ricci, E. Caselgrandi, and E. Ventura, Down regulation of striatal dopamine receptors in experimental hepatic encephalopathy, Life Sci. (in press)
6. J. E. Fischer and R. J. Baldasserini, Pathogenesis and therapy of hepatic coma in: "Progress in Liver Diseases", H. Popper and F. Schaffer eds., Grune and Stratton, New York (1975).
7. M. L. Zeneroli, E. Ventura, M. Baraldi, A. Penne, E. Messori, and L. Zieve, Ammonia, mercaptans and short chain fatty acids as pathogenetic agents of hepatic encephalopathy: evaluation by visual evoked potentials, Hepatology 2:532 (1982).
8. H. Conn and M. M. Lieberthal, The syndrome of portal-systemic encephalopathy, in: "The Hepatic Coma Syndromes and Lactulose". H. Conn and M. M. Lieberthal eds., Williams and Wilkins, Baltimore (1979).
9. W. A. Coob and G. D. Dawson, The latency and form in many of the occipital potentials evoked by bright flashes, J. Physiol. 152: 108 (1960).
10. D. F. Schafer, L. E. Brody, and E. A. Jones, Visual evoked

potentials: an objective measurement of hepatic encephalopathy in the rabbit, Gastroenterology 77, A38 (1979).

11. I. Bodis-Wollner, Evoked potentials, Ann. N.Y. Ac. Sci. 388: 1 (1981).

12. M. L. Zeneroli, C. Cremonini, C. Gollini, G. Pinelli, A. Penne, E. Messori, and M. Baraldi, Effects of hyperammoniemia and of hypoglycemia on visual evoked potentials in rat: comparison with hepatic encephalopathy, Riv. Farmacol. Terap. 13: 35 (1982).

13. D. F. Schafer and E. A. Jones, Hepatic encephalopathy and the γ-aminobutyric acid neurotransmitter system, Lancet 1: 18 (1982).

14. D. F. Schafer and E. A. Jones, Potential neuronal mechanisms in the pathogenesis of hepatic encephalopathy in: "Progress in Liver Diseases", H. Popper and F. J. Schaffner eds.,Grune and Stratton, New York (1982).

15. R. A. Nicoll, J. C. Eccles, T. Oshima, and F. Rusia, Prolongation of hippocampal postsynaptic potentials by barbiturates, Nature 258: 625 (1975).

16. R. H. Evans, Potentiation of the effects of GABA by pentobarbitone, Brain Res. 171: 113 (1979).

17. A. Guidotti, M. Baraldi, and E. Costa, 1-4 benzodiazepines and gamma-aminobutyric acid: pharmacological and biochemical correlates, Pharmacology 19: 267 (1979).

18. F. Rossi-Fanelli, H. Freund, R. Krause, A. R. Smith, J. H. James, S. Castorina-Ziparo, and J. E. Fischer, Induction of coma in normal dogs by the infusion of aromatic amino acids and its prevention by the addition of branched-chain amino acids, Gastroenterology 83: 664 (1982).

19. A. P. Bernardi, W. Chance, and J. E. Fischer, Depression of neurological function by intraventricular octopamine and tryptophan, Gastroenterology 82: 1222 (1982).

20. L. Zieve, The mechanism of hepatic coma, Hepatology 1: 360 (1981).

21. S. Schenker, K. Breen, and A. M. Hoyumpa, Hepatic encephalopathy: current status, Gastroenterology 66: 121 (1974).

22. H. Conn and M. M. Lieberthal, Pathogenesis of portal-systemic encephalopathy, in: "The Hepatic Coma Syndromes and Lactulose", H. Conn and M. M. Lieberthal eds., Williams and Wilkins, Baltimore (1979).

23. E. Polli, Il coma epatico, in "Quaderni di Neurofarmacologia", V. Andreoli, A. De Maio, and M. P. Nielsen eds., Ravizza, Milano (1972).

24. A. M. Mans, S. J. Sanders, R. E. Kirsch, and J. F. Biebuyck, Correlation of plasma and brain amino acid and putative neurotransmitter alterations during acute hepatic coma in the rat, J. Neurochem. 32: 285 (1978).

25. S. S. Oja, P. Kontro, and P. Lahdesmaki in: "Amino Acids as Inhibitory Neurotransmitters" S.S. Oja, P. Kontro, and P. Lahdesmaki eds., Gustav Verlag, Stuttgart, New York (1977).

26. M. L. Zeneroli, E. Iuliano, G. Racagni, and M. Baraldi, Metab-
    olism and brain uptake of γ-aminobutyric acid in galactosa-
    mine-induced hepatic encephalopathy in rats, J. Neurochem.
    38: 1219 (1982).
27. A. S. Livingstone, M. Potwin, C. A. Goresky, M.H. Finlayson,
    and E. J. Hinchey, Changes in the blood-brain barrier in
    hepatic coma after hepatectomy in the rat, Gastroenterology
    73: 697 (1977).
28. M. Baraldi and M.L.Zeneroli, ^{3}H-GABA binding in galactosamine-
    HCl induced hepatic encephalopathy in rat: a denervation
    supersensitivity phenomenon, Soc. Neuroscience 7: 511A (1981).
29. M. Baraldi and M. L. Zeneroli, Experimental hepatic encepha-
    lopathy: changes in γ-aminobutyric acid, Science 216: 427
    (1982).
30. M. Baraldi and M. L. Zeneroli, Experimental hepatic encepha-
    lopathy: a model to study a distinct high affinity GABA
    receptors, in "Dynamics of Neurotransmitter Function" I.
    Hanin ed., Raven Press, New York, in press.
31. J. I. Waddington and A. J. Cross, Denervation supersensitivity
    in the striato-nigral GABA pathway, Nature 276: 618 (1978).
32. A. Guidotti, K. Gale, A. Suria, and G. Toffano, Biochemical
    evidence for two classes of GABA receptors in rat brain,
    Brain Res. 172: 556 (1979).
33. K. Kuriyama, E. Kuriahara, Y. Iti, and Y. Yoneda, Increase in
    striatal ^{3}H-Muscimol binding following intrastriatal injec-
    tion of kainic acid: a denervation supersensitivity pheno-
    menon, J. Neurochem. 35: 343 (1980).
34. N. H. Dierner, Glial and neuronal changes in experimental
    hepatic encephalopathy. A quantitative morphological inve-
    stigation, Acta Neurol. Scand. 71: 58 (1978).
35. M. Massotti, A. Guidotti, and E. Costa, Characterization of
    benzodiazepine and γ-aminobutyric recognition sites and
    their endogenous modulators, J. Neurochem. 1: 409 (1981).
36. A. Guidotti, M. Baraldi, A. Leon, and E. Costa, Benzodiazepines:
    a tool to explore the biochemical and neurophysiological
    basis of anxiety, Fed. Proc. 39: 3039 (1980).
37. M. Brower, J. W. Ferkany, and S. J. Enna, Biochemical identi-
    fication of pharmacologically and functionally distinct GABA
    receptors in rat brain, J. Neuroscience 1: 514 (1981).
38. M. Baraldi, Evidence that benzodiazepine receptors are coupled
    with high affinity GABA binding sites in rat brain,
    Neuroscience Letters 10 (Suppl.): S-58 (1982).
39. M. Baraldi, E. Caselgrandi, P. Borella, C. Cremonini, and M.
    L. Zeneroli, Zinc content in brain tissue and GABA receptor
    function in experimental hepatic encephalopathy, in: "Appli-
    cation of Behavioral Pharmacology in Toxicology" V. Cuomo
    and G. Racagni eds., Raven Press, New York, in press.
40. J. Y. Wu and E. Robert, Properties of brain L-glutamate decarbo-
    xylase: inhibition studies, J. Neurochem. 23: 759 (1974).
41. Th. De Boer, J. Bruinels, and I. L. Bonta, Differential effects

of GABA analogues and zinc on glutamate decarboxylase, 4-aminobutyric-2-oxoglutaric acid transaminase and succinate semildehyde dehydrogenase in rat brain tissue, J. Neurochem. 33: 597 (1979).

42. M. Chvapil, New aspects in the biological role of zinc: a stabilized of macromolecules and biological membranes, Life Sci. 13: 1041 (1973).

43. M. Baraldi, E. Caselgrandi, P. Borella, and M. L. Zeneroli, Decrease of brain zinc in experimental hepatic encephalopathy, Brain Res., in press.

44. L. Zieve, W. M. Doizaki, and F. J. Zieve, Synergism between mercaptans and ammonia or fatty acids in the production of coma: a possible role for mercaptans in the pathogenesis of hepatic coma, J. Lab. Clin. Med. 83: 16 (1974).

A POSSIBLE ROLE FOR EXCITATORY NEUROTOXIC AMINO ACIDS IN THE PATHOGENESIS OF HEPATIC ENCEPHALOPATHY

F. Moroni, G. Lombardi, G. Moneti[x], D. Pellegrini, and
C. Cortesini[xx]

Departments of Pharmacology, [xx]Surgery and [x]The Mass-Spectrometry Centre of the Medical School, Viale G.B. Morgagni, 65 50134 Firenze, Italy

INTRODUCTION

Extensive research in the past few years has been directed towards understanding the role of acidic excitatory amino acids in the pathogenesis of several neurological and psychiatric disorders.[1-3] However, relatively little information is available on the role of glutamic acid (GLU), the prototype of acidic excitatory amino acids, in the pathogenesis of hepatic encephalopathy.[4]

An important finding of this pathological condition is the increased concentration of ammonia in the blood and in the brain.[5-7] Ammonia inhibits the formation of GLU from glutamine (GLN) "in vitro"[8] and it has been suggested that hepatic encephalopathy and hepatic coma are associated with a depletion of the neurotransmitter pool of GLU and a lack of appropriate stimulation of GLU receptors.[9]

However the concentration of ammonia in the blood or in the cerebrospinal fluid (C.S.F.) increases;[9,10] in rats bearing a surgically constructed portocaval anastomosis, a widely used model to study the pathogenesis of hepatic encephalopathy, while the levels of GLU in their brain are either normal or slightly modified.[11-13] In a similar way, patients suffering from hepatic encephalopathy or hepatic coma have increased ammonia concentration in their biological fluids[14-16] and relatively high GLU concentration both in the plasma and in the C.S.F.[17,18]

Moreover, the administration of large doses of ammonium salts (10-20 mmoles/kg i.p.) to several animal species can induce a pattern of tonic and clonic convulsions, which are very similar to those

41

evoked by intracerebroventricular administration of relatively low
doses of GLU, aspartate or quinulinate (an excitatory amino acid originating from the metabolism of tryptophan).

Furthermore, hyperexcitability, agitation, tremor, hyperventi-
lation, hyperreflexia and spasticity are typical signs and symptoms
of hepatic encephalopathy and hepatic coma.[4] It is difficult to as-
sociate these signs and symptoms with decreased functioning of
excitatory neurons. They rather suggest a general increase in nerve-
cell excitability and activity.

With the aim of shedding light on the role of excitatory amino
acid transmitters in the pathogenesis of hepatic encephalopathy, we
studied the synthesis and release of GLU in two experimental models
"in vivo":

1) rats receiving large amount of ammonium acetate intraperitoneally;

2) rats bearing a surgically constructed portocaval anastomosis.

The results of our investigation indicate an increased synthesis
and availability of GLU in several brain areas, in both experimental
models studied, and they suggest that when ammonia levels increase
in the biological fluids and in the brain, GLU receptors are exposed
to increased concentrations of their endogenous ligand.

Measurement of the release synthesis and content of glutamic acid and GABA

The effects of ammonium salt administration on the release of
the neurotransmitter amino acids GABA and GLU from the rat cerebral
cortex were studied using cortical cups and a mass-fragmentographic
method.[19] In the experiments here reported urethane (10 mmol.Kg^{-1})
anaesthetized rats were used. The dura mater was surgically removed
in order to facilitate the output of glutamic acid and a perspex
cylinder was carefully placed on the exposed frontoparietal cortex.
A Ringer solution (0.4 ml) was placed in the cylinder and substituted
every 20 min. In order to identify and measure the output of GLU
and GABA, the following procedures were used: a) purification of the
collected fluid through a Dowex (AG 50x8 100-200 mesh; H^+); b) deri-
vatization of the amino acids with 1,1,1,3,3,3 hexafluoroisopropanol
and pentafluoropropionic anhydride; c) injection of the derivatized
amino acids into a GC-MS 2091 equipped with a multiple ion detector.
The following ions were recorded: m/z 230 and 232 for endogenous GLU
and GABA and m/z 235-238 for the deuterated internal standards
(d_5 GLU and d_6 GABA). In order to measure the content and synthesis
of the amino acids, rats were infused with ^{13}C glucose (uniformly
labelled, isotopic enrichment of 80%) for 10 minutes at a dose of
50 nmol/kg/min.[20,21] At the end of the infusion period the animals

were killed by microwave radiation.[22] Several brain regions were
homogenized in an 80% aqueous ethanol solution. The homogenate was
processed as previously described for the measurement of GLU content
or synthesis.[20,23] The same approach was used to calculate GABA
turnover in the caudate nucleus.[21,24]

The effects of ammonium administration on the release synthesis and content of brain glutamic acid and GABA

Increased arterial ammonia concentration is the "sine qua non"
of hepatic encephalopathy. The administration of a large amount of
ammonium to several animal species has been widely used to study the
modifications of the brain function in the course of the disease. A
dose of 8 mmoles/kg of ammonium acetate in rats decreases the spontaneous motor activity and increases the heart rate and the frequency
of respiration. Higher doses of this salt (12 mmoles/kg i.p.) are
lethal in approximately 90% of the animals. Death occurs few minutes
(10-20) after its administration and it is usually preceded by typical
clonic and tonic convulsions. Most of the experiments here reported
were performed using a dose of 8 mmoles/kg of ammonium acetate. The
intraperitoneal injection of this dose of the salt increased the
output of GLU from the surface of the brain by 125%. This effect
reached its maximum during the first twenty minutes, but it was still
present 40 minutes later. The GABA release was not modified (Fig. 1)
The administration of a lower dose of ammonium acetate (4 mmoles/kg)
increased GLU release by 50% in two out of five rats. On the other

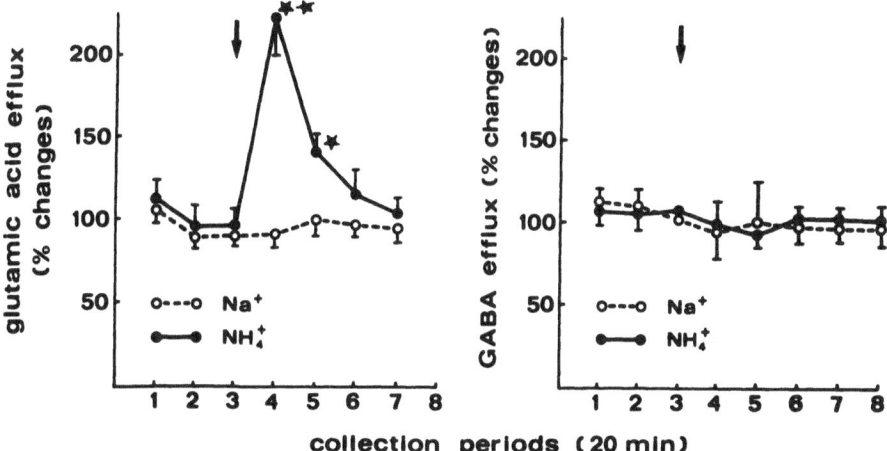

Fig. 1. Time course of the effects of ammonium or sodium acetate
(8 mmoles/kg) on the release of GABA and GLU from the rat
brain surface. The basal release of GABA was 0.07+0.01 and
that of GLU was 9.1+0.8 (nmoles.cm^2.20 min mean +S.E. of at
least six animals). The arrows indicate the time of the injection (i.p.) of the salts * P < 0.05; ** P < 0.01.

hand the basal release of GLU and GABA did not change when sodium
acetate (8 mmoles/kg) was injected. This indicates that the ammonium
ions are responsible for the observed effect (Fig. 1). These ions not
only modified the output of glutamic acid from the brain surface, but
also decreased its content in the parietal cortex by 25% and in the
caudate nucleus by 15% (Table 1). On the other hand, the amount of
$^{13}C_2$ labelled glutamate found in the parietal cortex was 65% greater
when the rats were pretreated with the ammonium salt. A small, but
not statistically significant, increase in the $^{13}C_2$ glutamate content
was also found in the caudate nucleus of the same animals (Table 1).
Sodium acetate did not modify the incorporation of $^{13}C_2$ into the
molecule of GLU.

The effects of portocaval anastomosis (PCA) on the brain synthesis and content of glutamic acid and GABA

Rats bearing a portocaval shunt[25] display anatomical[26,27] behavioral[28] and biochemical[13,29] changes similar to patients affected
by chronic liver disease. For these reasons they have been widely
used as models for studying the metabolic aberrations associated with
liver cirrhosis. The experiments here reported were performed on rats
four weeks after PCA. As previously reported[9,30] the body weight of
these rats was 15-25% lower than that of sham operated animals, and
the percentage of the weight of the liver in comparison to the weight
of the whole animal had also decreased by 20-30%.

Table 1. The effects of intraperitoneal injections of ammonium or
sodium acetate on the content and synthesis of GLU

	GLU content			GLU synthesis		
	Control	Ammonium acetate	Sodium acetate	Control	Ammonium acetate	Sodium acetate
Caudate nucleus	94+5	80+4^x	95+3	2.1+0.2	2.5+0.3	2.0+0.2
Parietal cortex	98+5	76+6^x	100+6	2.3+0.2	3.7+0.3^{xx}	1.9+0.3

The GLU-content values are expressed as nmoles/mg protein and are
the mean of at least six animals for each group.
The GLU-synthesis values are the means ± SE of at least 5 animals
and indicate the percentages of GLU containing two atoms of ^{13}C in
their molecule with respect to the non-labelled amino acid. The labelled compound was synthetized during 10 min of infusion of the
animals with ^{13}C glucose.
^{x}P < 0.05; ^{xx}P < 0.01

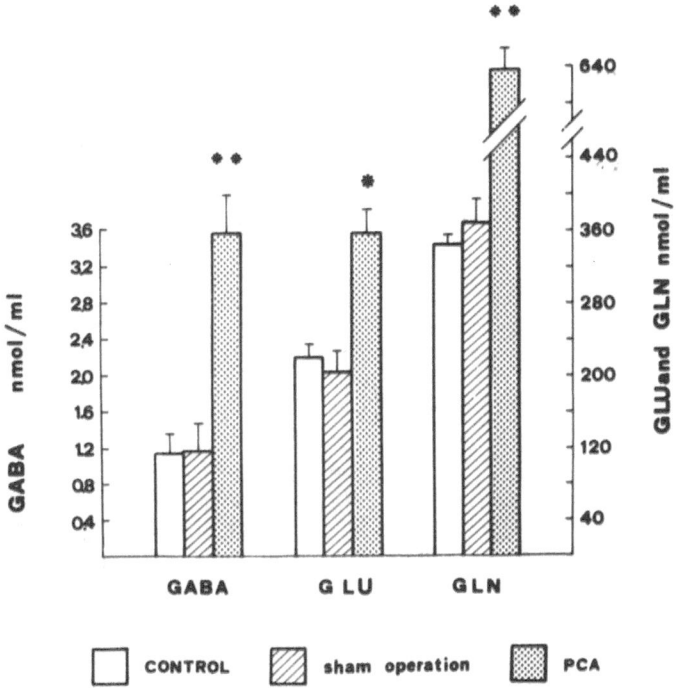

Fig. 2. GABA, GLU and GLN concentration in the blood of PCA rats. Each column is the mean ± SE of at least 6 animals. * P < 0.05; ** P < 0.01.

In these rats, the blood concentration of GABA, GLU and glutamine (GLN) was measured using GC–MS methods and Fig. 2 shows that the blood concentration of GABA increased by 250%, that of GLN by 180% and that of GLU by 50%. The GLN content had also significantly increased in several brain areas (Fig. 3). Moreover, when these animals were fed ad libitum, with a standard laboratory diet, the GLU content in several brain areas had increased by 15-25% (Table 2). After the infusion of ^{13}C glucose, the incorporation of ^{13}C$_2$ into the molecule of GLU had approximately doubled. This suggests a sharp increase in the neosynthesis of this amino acid. The highest increase in the levels of GLU and in its neosynthesis was found in the parietal cortex. On the other hand, neither the portocaval anastomosis, nor the administration of ammonium acetate modified the content of GABA or its turnover rate in the caudate nucleus (Table 3).

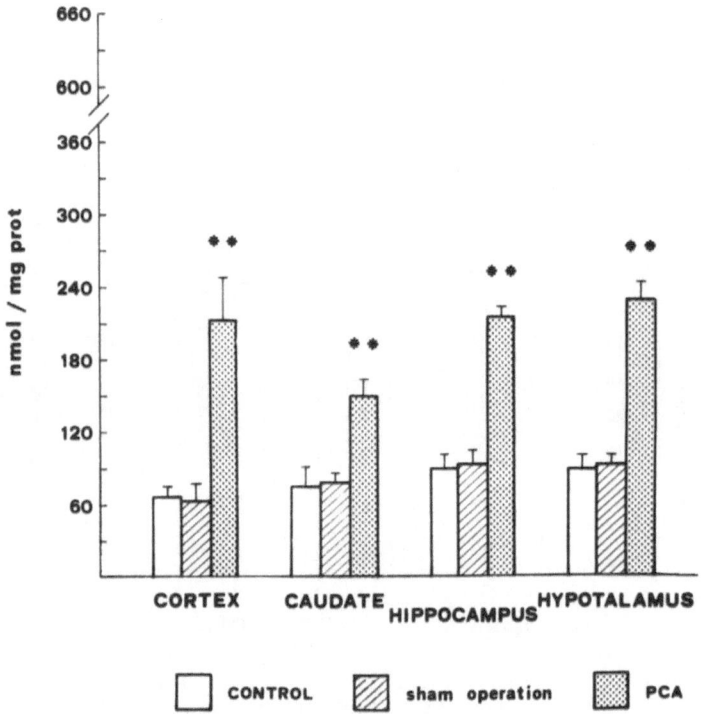

Fig. 3. The content of GLN in several brain areas of rat bearing a PCA. Each column is the mean ± S.E. of at least 6 animals. **P < 0.01.

Table 2. Effect of PCA on the levels and synthesis of glutamic acid in rat brain areas and blood

	GLU content			GLU synthesis	
	Control rats	Sham operated rats	PCA rats	Control rats	PCA rats
Parietal cortex	86+6.8	72+7.8	130+15^{xx}	2.1+.15	5.3+.28^{xx}
Caudate nucleus	77+6.3	71+10	108+10^{xx}	2.4+.19	5.4+.35^{xx}
Hippocampus	105+7.0	99+3.5	135+7.0^{xx}	1.4+.18	2.8+16^{xx}
Hypothalamus	70+6.3	70+8.0	98+8.2^{xx}	1.8+.16	3.5+20^{xx}
Blood (nmol/ml)	.22+.014	.20+.012	.35+.030^{xx}		

Each value is the means ± S.E.M. of at least 6 animals. See legend to table 1. ^{xx} P < 0.01 compared with controls.

Table 3. Lack of effects of P.C.A. or of ammonium administration on
the caudate content and turnover of GABA

	Content	Turnover rate
Saline	25 + 1.2	680 + 90
Ammonium acetate	22 + 1.9	500 + 70
Sodium acetate	24 + 2.1	750 + 120
P.C.A.	27 + 2.0	480 + 80

Values are expressed as nmoles/mg protein + S.E. for the GABA content
and as nmoles/mg prot/hr for the turnover.
Each value is the mean + S E of at least 5 animals.
Ammonium and sodium acetate were administered at a dose of 8 mmoles/
Kg; PCA was performed 4 weeks before the experiments.

CONCLUSIONS

The results here reported indicate that ammonium ions increase
the release and the formation of glutamic acid in the brain. The
resulting increased concentration of this amino acid in the extra-
cellular spaces may be one of the factors to be considered in the
pathogenesis of hepatic encephalopathy. In fact, it is now generally
accepted that GLU not only plays a key role in several metabolic
pathways, but it is also a major excitatory transmitter[31] with possible neurotoxic actions.[32-34] When relatively high doses of glutamic
acid are injected intracisternally they cause tremor, abnormal muscular excitability and convulsions.[35] Similarly rats receiving large
doses of ammonium salts die after periods of tremor and convulsions.
The same symptoms are observed in the course of hepatic coma in
man.[4,16]

Moreover, the systemic administration of the local application
of large doses of glutamate cause neuronal degeneration and gliosis.
[32-34] Relatively similar anatomopathological findings may be observed in rats bearing portocaval anastomosis[27,36] or in men who have
died after chronic liver failure.[37]

From our data it seems reasonable to suppose that drugs, able
to modify the interactions of GLU with its receptors, may be of some
value in the prevention and the treatment of hepatic encephalopathy.
In support of this concept it has been reported that α-methylglu-
tamic acid[38] and other esters of GLU[39,40] protect rats from ammonia
toxicity. The mechanism of action of these molecules is far from
being clear.[38] However, most of them have antagonistic properties
on the receptors for GLU.[41, 42] This finding is in agreement with
our experimental results.

We also found that the GABA blood concentration increases after
portocaval anastomosis. However, no changes were observed in the
GABA brain content or in the release and the turnover rate of this
inhibitory neurotransmitter. The cause and the origin of the increased GABA blood concentration are not explained by our experimental
data. In fact, the experiments reported herewith do not rule out
an increased GABA synthesis in the gut from bacterial sources. It
has been suggested that GABA may play a role in the encephalopathy
which occurs in acute hepatic failure.[43,44] However, a general
increase in the activity of the GABAergic system, as suggested by
these authors, should induce experimental and clinical pictures
similar to those observed when large doses of GABA agonists or of
drugs which facilitate the GABAergic neurotransmission (benzodiazepines or barbiturates)[45-47] are administered. A facilitation of
GABAergic transmission is expected to induce a coma characterized
by myorelaxation, hypotension, hypoventilation. Completely different
clinical pictures are observed during hepatic encephalopathy.[16]

In conclusion, our experimental results support the idea that
an increased concentration of ammonium ions in the plasma or in the
cerebrospinal fluid is associated with increased synthesis and
release of GLU. Preliminary results obtained in our laboratory indicate that other excitatory neurotoxins, provided with actions similar
to those of GLU and originating from the metabolism of tryptophan,
are also increased during chronic hepatic encephalopathy.

The described modifications of the excitatory transmitter
systems may have direct implications, not only for a better understanding, but also for the prevention and therapy of chronic hepatic
encephalopathy.

ACKNOWLEDGEMENTS: The research was supported by grants n.810029204,
800039404 from CNR and from the University of Firenze (M.P.I.). We
are grateful to Miss M. Baggiani for typing the manuscript.

REFERENCES
1. P. J. Roberts, J. Storm-Mathisen, and G.A.R. Johnston,"Gluta-
       mate: Transmitter in the Central Nervous System" 1-222, J.
       Wiley and Sons eds. Chichester (1981).
2. G. Di Chiara, G. L. Gessa, eds. 1981, "Glutamate as a neuro-
       transmitter", Adv. Biochem. Psychopharmacol. Vol. 27, Raven
       Press, New York.
3. J. T. Coyle, Neurotoxic amino acids in human degenerative
       disorders, Trends in Neurosciences, 5:287-288 (1982).
4. H. O. Conn and M. Lieberthal, "The Hepatic Coma Syndromes and
       the Lactulose" William and Wilkins, Baltimore (1979).
5. R. Schwartz, G. B. Philips, G. J. Gabudza Jr., and C. S. David-
       son, Blood ammonia and electrolytes in hepatic coma, J. Lab.

Clin. Med., 42:499-508 (1953).

6. S. P. Bessman, J. F. Fazekas ,and A. N. Bessman, Uptake of ammo-
    nia by the brain in hepatic coma, Proc. Soc. Exp. Biol. Med.,
    85: 66-67 (1954).

7. C. J. Fisher and W. W. Faloon, Blood ammonia levels in hepatic
    cirrhosis: their control by the oral administration of
    neomycin, N. Eng. J. Med., 256: 1030-1050 (1957).

8. H. F. Bradford and H. F. Ward, On glutaminase activity in mam-
    malian synaptosomes, Brain Research, 110:115-125 (1976).

9. M. H. Kyu and J. B. Cavanagh, Some effects of portocaval ana-
    stomosis in the male rat, Brit. J. Exp. Path., 51:217-227
    (1970).

10. M. Ehrlich, F. Plum, and T. E. Duffy, Blood and brain ammonia
    concentrations after portocaval anastomosis: effects of acute
    loading, J. Neurochem., 34:1538-1542 (1980).

11. B. Hindfelt, On mechanisms in hyperammonemic coma with parti-
    cular reference to hepatic encephalopathy, in: "Annals of
    New York Ac. of Sciences", Vol. 252, 116-123 (1975).

12. G. Zanchin, P. Rigotti, N. Dussini, P. Vassanelli and L. Bat-
    tistini, Cerebral amino acid levels and uptake in rats after
    portocaval anastomosis: regional studies "in vivo", J. Neu-
    roscience Research, 4:301-310 (1979).

13. S. Kamata, A. Okada, T. Watanabe, Y. Kawashima ,and S. Schenker,
    Hepatic encephalopathy, Gastroenterology, 76:184-195 (1979).

14. G. B. Philips, R. Schwartz, G. J. Gabuzda, and C. S. Davidson,
    The syndrome of impending hepatic coma in patients with
    cirrhosis of the liver, given certain nitrogenous substance,
    New Eng. J. Med.,247:239-243 (1952).

15. W. V. Mc Dermott and R. D. Adams, Episodic stupor associated
    with Eck fistula in the human with particular reference to
    the metabolism of ammonia, J. Clin. Invest., 33:1-9 (1954).

16. A. M. Hoyumpa, P. V. Desmono, G. R. Auant, R. K. Roberts, and
    S. Schenker, Hepatic encephalopathy, Gastroenterology, 76:
    184-195 (1979).

17. F. Vergara, F. Plum, and T. E. Duffy, α-ketoglutaramate: in
    creased concentrations in the cerebrospinal fluid of patients
    in hepatic coma, Science, 183:81-83 (1974).

18. M. H. Rosen, N. Yoshimura, J.M. Hodgman, and J.E. Fischer,Plasma
    amino acid patterns in hepatic encephalopathy of differing
    etiology, Gastroenterology, 72:483-487 (1977).

19. F. Moroni, R. Corradetti, F. Casamenti, G. Moneti,and G. Pepeu,
    The release of endogenous GABA and GLU from the cerebral
    cortex in the rat, Naunyn-Schmiedeberg's Arch. Pharmacol.,
    316:235-239 (1981).

20. F. Moroni, D. L. Cheney, E. Peralta, and E. Costa, Opiate re-
    ceptor agonists as modulators of GABA turnover in the nucleus
    caudatus, globus pallidus and substantia nigra of the rat,
    J. Pharmacol. Exp. Ther., 270:870-877 (1978).

21. F. Moroni, Turnover as a tool to explore the function of GABA
    ergic synapses: Physiological and pharmacological studies,

in: GABA: Biochemistry and CNS functions, "Advances in Experimental Medicine", P. Mandel and F.V. De Feudis eds., 123: 189-204, Plenum Press, New York (1979).

22. A. Guidotti, M. Baraldi, J. P. Schwartz, and E. Costa, Molecular mechanism regulating the interactions between the benzodiazemines and GABA receptors in the central nervous system, Pharmacol. Biochem. Behav., 10:803-807 (1979).

23. F. Moroni, G. Lombardi, G. Moneti, and C. Cortesini, The release and the neosynthesis of glutamic acid are increased in experimental models of hepatic encephalopathy, J. Neurochem., in press (1982).

24. L. Bertilsson, C. C. Mao, and E. Costa, Application of principles of steady-state kinetics to the estimation of GABA turnover rate in nuclei of rat brain, J. Pharmacol. Exp. Ther., 200:277-284 (1977).

25. S. H. Lee and B. Fisher, Portocaval shunt in the rat, Surgery, 50:668-672 (1961).

26. A. J. Zamora, J. B. Cavanagh, and M. H. Kyu, Ultrastructural responses of the astrocytes to portocaval anastomosis in the rat, J. Neural. Sci., 18:25-45 (1973).

27. M. D. Noremberg, A light and electron microscopic study of experimental portal-systemic (ammonia) encephalopathy, J. Lab. Investigation, 36:618-627 (1977).

28. M. D. Tricklebank, J. L. Smart, D. L. Bloxam and G. Curzon, Effects of chronic experimental liver dysfunction and L-tryptophan on behavior in the rat, Pharmacol. Biochem. and Behavior, 9:181-189 (1978).

29. G. Simert, A. Nobin, E. Rosengren,and J. Vang, Neurotransmitter changes in the rat brain after portocaval anastomosis, Eur. Surg. Res., 10:73-85 (1978).

30. G. S. Sarna, M. W. B. Bradbury, J. E. Cremer, J. C. K. Lai, and H. M. Teal, Brain metabolism and specific transport at the blood-brain barrier after portocaval anastomosis in the rat, Brain Res., 160:69-83 (1979).

31. K. Krnjevic, Chemical nature of synaptic transmission in vertebrates, Physiol. Rev., 54:418-540 (1974).

32. J. W. Olney, O. L. Ho, and V. Rhee, Cytotoxic effects of acidic and sulphur containing amino acids on the infant mouse central nervous system, Exp. Brain Res., 14:61-76 (1971).

33. A. Plaitakis, S. Berl, and D. M. Yahr, Abnormal glutamate metabolism in adult-onset degenerative neurological disorder, Science, 216:193-196 (1982).

34. R. Schwarcz, C. Kohler, R. M. Mangano,and A. N. Neophytides, Glutamate-induced neuronal degeneration: Studies on the role of glutamate re-uptake in "Glutamate as a Neurotransmitter", G. Di Chiara and G. L. Gessa, eds., 403-412, Raven Press, New York (1981).

35. H. Hennecke, P. Wiechert, Seizures and the dose of L-glutamic acid in rats, Epilepsia, 11:327-331 (1970).

36. J. B. Cavanagh, P. D. Lewis, W. F. Blakemore,and M. H. Kyu, Changes in cerebellar cortex in rats after portocaval anastomosis, J. Neurol. Sci., 15:13-26 (1972).

37. T. E. Starzl, L. J. Foep, C. G. Halgrimson, J. Hood, G. P. J. Schroter, F. N. Porter, and R. Weil, Fifteen years of clinical liver transplantation, Gastroenterology, 77:370-382 (1979).

38. C. Lamar, Ammonia toxicity in rats: protection by α-metylglutamic acid, Toxicology and Applied Pharmacology, 17:795-803 (1970).

39. L. Chiosa, V. Niculescu, C. Biociocat, and C. Stancu, The protective action of N-acetyl and N-carbamyl derivatives of glutamic and aspartic acids against ammonia intoxication, Biochem. Pharmacol., 14:1635-1643 (1965).

40. S. Kim, W. F. Paif, and P. Cohen, Ammonia intoxication in rats: protection by N-carbamyl-L-glutamate plus L-arginine, Proc. Natl. Acad. Sci., 69:3530-3533 (1972).

41. A. Nistri and A. Costanti, Pharmacological characterization of different types of GABA and glutamate receptors in vertebrates and invertebrates, Progress Neurobiology, 13:117-235 (1981).

42. E. Puil, S-glutamate: its interactions with spinal neurons, Brain Res., 228:229-322 (1981).

43. D. F. Shafer and E. A. Jones, Hepatic encephalopathy and the γ-aminobutyric acid neurotransmitter system. Lancet Jan., 18-20 (1982).

44. N. L. Zeneroli, E. Iuliano, G. Racagni, and M. Baraldi, Metabolism and brain uptake of γ-aminobutyric acid in galactosamine-induced hepatic encephalopathy in rats, J. Neurochem., 38:1219-1222 (1982).

45. A. Guidotti, D. I. Cheney, M. Trabucchi, M. Doteuchi, C. T. Wang,and R. A. Hawkins, Focussed microwave radiation: a technique to minimize post mortem changes of cyclic nucleotides, DOPA and choline and to preserve brain morphology, Neuropharmacology, 13: 1115-1122 (1974).

46. G. A. R. Johnston, Physiologic pharmacology of GABA and its antagonists in the vertebrate nervous system, in: "GABA in Nervous System Function", E. Roberts, T. N. Chase, and D. B. Tower, eds., 395-412, Raven Press, New York (1976).

47. R. A. Mac Donald and J. L. Barker, Anticonvulsant and anaesthetic barbiturates: Different postsynaptic actions in cultured mammalian spinal cord neurons: A common mode of anticonvulsant action, Brain Res., 167:323-336 (1979).

THE DEVELOPMENT OF THE FALSE NEUROTRANSMITTER CONCEPT

OF HEPATIC ENCEPHALOPATHY

J. E. Fischer

Department of Surgery, University of Cincinnati
Medical Center, Cincinnati, Ohio, U.S.A.

INTRODUCTION

A. The Concept of False Neurochemical Transmitters

The concept of weak, or false, neurochemical transmitters arose
in the early 60's to describe a series of potential neurotransmitters
which were similar in structure to true aminergic neurotransmitters,
norepinephrine and epinephrine, and which, when tested pharmacologically, manifested weak, or in some cases, almost absent pharmacological action.[1] According to this concept, the sympathetic nerve
or, by extension, the central nervous system, is unable to select
between amines presented to it, that is unable to detect or choose
between various aminergic neurotransmitters, provided they meet min-
imum structural requirements. In the case of the catecholamine and
aminergic nerves, these structural requirements include a phenolic
ring and a beta hydroxy group on a short carboxyl side change. It
is curious that the normal adrenergic nervous system is incapable
of distinguishing between these various potential neurotransmitters
and that the maintenance of normal neurotransmitter profiles within
the peripheral sympathetic nerve or the central nervous system is
apparently dependent on the regulating ability of the liver to regulate different metabolites, including the precursors of these
various adrenergic transmitters, namely the aromatic and heterocyclic amino acids.

B. The Concept of False Neurochemical Transmitters in Liver Disease
and Hepatic Encephalopathy

The concept of false neurochemical transmitters, which has subsequently been modified, proposes that under circumstances of dimi-

nished hepatic function or shunting of portal blood around the liver,
either anatomically, as in the post-surgical shunts, or physiologically, as in the failing liver, amines or their amino acid precursors
bypass the liver, flooding the central and peripheral nervous system
with an abnormal amino acid profile, which results in an abnormal
central and peripheral adrenergic neurotransmitter .[1] In the central
nervous system, where consciousness and the overall state of alert-
ness of the central nervous system is controlled, in part, at least,
by the midline primitive aminergic nervous system, the balance in
aminergic neurotransmitters is altered. These include increased
octopamine and other B-phenylethanolamines as well as decreased norepinephrine, decreased dopamine, and increased serotonin. The central aminergic system, although making up only 5% of the central
neurotransmitters, is unusual in that its anatomical arrangement is
such that a few neurons have extensive ramifications and connections
so that the locus caeruleus, for example, situated under the fourth
ventricle, a noradrenergic collection of neurons, with only 1500
cell bodies, has ramifications throughout the entire brain. The
synapses of the central aminergic system do not end in classical
endplate-neuron synaptic arrangements, but end free in the matrix,[12]
so that no neuron in the vicinity is more than 25-30 angstroms away
from the nerve ending, almost as if the release of such materials
into the matrix controls the function of other neurons in the vicinity. Thus the emphasis as to aminergic systems within the central
nervous system is a change in balance between serotonin, norepinephrine, and various beta-hydroxyphenylethylamines, in addition to
decreases in specific dopamine, that in the striatum.

In the periphery, noradrenergic neurons are primarily responsible for the maintenance of normal vascular tone. One may view the
body as consisting of two entirely separate sets of vascular systems
supplying either high priority or low priority organs. The high
priority organs, such as brain, heart and kidney, normally have a
low resting vascular tone, as flow is important and do not have an
excessive amount of noradrenergic control. The low priority organs,
such as skin, gut and muscle, tend to have a high resting vascular
tone with norepinephrine being, among other things, largely responsible for the maintenance of such tone. If one depletes norepinephrine within such nerve terminals, as occurs in terminal liver
failure,[3] the result is the opening of such shunts in peripheral
muscle, skin and splanchnic bed, leading to the vasodilated, high
cardiac output patient one usually sees with the failing liver.
Under such circumstances, if cardiac output remains the same, blood
pressure will be diminished, as is observed, and less of a fraction
of cardiac output will be delivered to the heart, brain and kidney.
Cardiac output will compensate and initially keeps pace. With respect
to the kidney, overall blood flow is at first maintained at normal
levels, but with a diminished fraction of the elevated cardiac output. When cardiac output can no longer keep pace, absolute output to
the kidney falls, and the Type II hepatorenal syndrome,[4] as we have

previously named it, (after Cohn) ensues.[5]

The initial false neurotransmitter hypothesis suggested that it
was either amines themselves or their amino acid precursors which
were responsible for the development of such symptomatology. It
became immediately clear, however, that the blood brain barrier at
least in animals with liver disease remained impervious to amines
themselves,[6] and thus we began to investigate the relationship
between such central nervous system amines, such as octopamine, and
their amino acid precursors, such as tyrosine and phenylalanine. It
quickly became apparent that if one used a simple measure of liver
disease, such as percentage of at least liver weight over body weight,
in which normal animals have liver weight of 3.2 g/100 g of rat,
that there was an excellent correlation between decrease in liver
weight per 100 g of rat and increased plasma and brain tyrosine, in
turn, related to increased brain octopamine.[7] The correlation between
brain tyrosine and brain octopamine was excellent, suggesting that
at least in animals with liver disease, the two were directly related.

C. Relationship between Central Amines and Peripheral and Central Amino Acids

We then turned our attention to the relationship between peripheral and central nervous system amino acids. In the plasma, it had
been known for some time that an abnormal plasma amino acid pattern
was present in patients with liver disease. Increased aromatic and
heterocyclic amino acids, such as phenylalanine, tyrosine, free but
not necessarily total tryptophan, and decreased branched-chain amino
acids (valine, leucine, and isoleucine) were present. These six
amino acids competed with the remaining neutral amino acids (methionine, histidine, tyrosine), for entry via a single system, system L
across the blood barrier.[8] It soon became apparent that one could
not explain the increased concentrations of these amino acids on
the basis of plasma competition alone, and that some alteration, or
increased transport, across the blood brain barrier was necessary.[6]
These changes will be discussed separately by Howard James in another
presentation.

SPECIFIC ASPECTS OF THE FALSE NEUROTRANSMITTER HYPOTHESIS

A. Introduction

I would next like to discuss three separate aspects of the amino
acid neurotransmitter hypothesis, which bear on the etiology. It has
already been confirmed by several laboratories that the relationship
between brain norepinephrine and brain dopamine with hepatic coma is
such that, as animals go into experimental hepatic coma, brain norepinephrine decreases.[9] While others have related the etiologic agent
of this decrease to increased brain tyramine secondary to decarboxylation of tyrosine, it should be pointed out that tyramine is not a

unique product, but just one of a series of phenylethylamines and
aminergic products of the aromatic amino acids. One of such products,
phenylethylamine, transverses the blood brain barrier; beta-hydroxy-
phenylethanolamine, tyramine and octopamine do not.

B. Correlations between Plasma Octopamine and Hepatic Coma

Nespoli and his collaborators, in a very interesting paper,
have pointed out relationships between stage of coma and plasma
levels of amino acid such as phenylalanine, tyrosine, free tryptophan,
as well as amines such as octopamine.[10] Furthermore, and more importantly, they have pointed out the relationship between octopamine
and the high output, decreased peripheral vascular resistant hemo-
dynamic state, which is so common in hepatic failure. This, in fact,
can be taken as a verification of one of the hypothetical points of
the false neurotransmitter hypothesis.

C. Reproduction of Hepatic Coma in Normal Animals

Several individual points come up for discussion with relation
to the amino acid false neurotransmitter hypothesis. They are:

1. If excesses of aromatic amino acids, notably, phenylalanine,
   tyrosine and tryptophan, are directly or indirectly responsible
   for metabolic encephalopathy, known as hepatic coma, it should
   be possible to reproduce such findings in normal animals by
   infusion of such amino acids.

2. If octopamine, although but one of a variety of central amines
   and depletion of norepinephrine, as well as accumulation of serotonin, is responsible for some of the symptoms of hepatic encephalopathy, it should be possible to detect some form of neurological depression by injecting large amounts of octopamine.

3. It is still not clear whether the toxicity of ammonia is direct
   or indirect. If, as the amino acid neurotransmitter hypothesis
   infers, toxicity of ammonia is indirect, it should be possible
   to protect animals from the toxicity of ammonia by infusion of
   branched-chain amino acids.

4. An outgrowth of the amino acid neurotransmitter hypothesis is
   that, if the derangements in central neurotransmitters are secondary to the derangements in central aromatic amino acids, it
   should be possible to protect experimental animals and patients
   from hepatic encephalopathy by the infusion of branched-chain
   amino acids, which would compete with the excessive aromatic
   amino acids within the plasma across system L.

All of these points will be discussed in this manuscript, except
for the fourth, which is a subject of a separate round table of this

symposium.

D. The Ability to Cause Coma by Infusion of Aromatic Amino Acids in Normal Dogs

We have previously remarked that the precursors of the central amines, octopamine, are either phenylalaline or tyrosine, and that of excessive serotonin, tryptophan. Since the amines themselves do not traverse the blood brain barrier, which remains relatively normal, even in fulminant hepatic coma, until the last stages of the disease are reached, it should be possible to cause a readily reversible metabolic coma-like state by infusion of amino acids, such as phenylalanine and tryptophan, in normal animals. One cannot infuse tyrosine, since tyrosine is not soluble in sufficient amount to increase plasma levels.

In the following experiment, carotid loops, a procedure by which carotid arteries are exteriorized in subcutaneous pouches, were prepared in normal animals, most of which had been prepared with ind-welling lateral ventricular CNS cannulas. This enabled the experi-mentor to, under local anesthesia, infuse various materials directly into the carotid arteries. A variety of combinations of amino acids in solution were infused into such animals, including methionine alone, phenylalanine alone, tryptophan alone, and valine alone. We have re ntly reported that a combination of 1% phenylalanine + 1% tryptopl n, or 1.5% phenylalanine + 0.5% tryptophan, was sufficient to rende these animals comatose. The addition of a relatively small amount o branched-chain amino acids to the infusate, was protective of the a mals and they did not go into coma, even after 7 hours of infusion.[1]

Anal is of CSF in such animals reveals that the necessity for productio of coma in such animals is a CSF level of phenylalanine of approxi ately 10% normal, and that of tryptophan, presumably as a precurso of serotonin, of 29x normal. The levels of phenylalanine in the CSF re somewhat higher than seen in experimental hepatic coma, seco ary to portacaval shunt, but of the same order of mag-nitude. The concentrations of tryptophan are considerably higher. Of course, e relationships of the concentrations in CSF and brain levels are t clear from these experiments.

E. Can Octop nine Itself Cause Neurological Depression?

An oft- oted argument against the amino acid neurotransmitter hypothesis is that large amounts of octopamine, given intraventri-cularly to ra ;, profoundly depletes norepinephrine, and yet does not cause com In that study, reported by Zieve and Olsen,[12] the animals were rely inspected, and no measurements of neurological function were rried out. Secondly, large amounts of octopamine will deplete t ptophan as well, and since coma appears to be the result of both the products of phenylalanine as well as tryptophan,[11] coma would not be expected to result. Finally, the rat is a very resistant animal to coma, probably not a good choice for an experimental model; thus the necessity for a neurological examination.

My colleagues Plinio Bernardini and Bill Chance, have devised a rat neurological examination in which 17 different points are examined with a point value for each.[13] Octopamine was infused as described by Zieve and Olsen, and the rats examined neurologically. Regardless of whether animals were normal or shunted, octopamine in and of itself produced profound neurological depression with resistance and response to pain being most protected.[13] The addition of tryptophan in the infusion, added to the depression, but most of the neurological depression appeared to result from the infusion of octopamine and after the first dose.

It should be pointed out that octopamine is only one of the series of phenylethylamines which we have implicated in the etiology of hepatic encephalopathy. The production of profound neurological depression by such a gross technique of intraventricular injection with its irregular diffusion suggests that the presence of such large amounts of amines normally present in trace concentrations may, in fact, be causative in hepatic encephalopathy.

F. Is Ammonia Directly Toxic, or does it Operate Via Influx of Aromatic Amino Acids?

In a previous series of articles, James and coworkers have argued that ammonia and its intracerebral product, glutamine, are primarily involved in the increased exchange of aromatic amino acids across the blood brain barrier.[14,15] If this is the case, and ammonia is not directly toxic (a mechanism of toxicity is still not proposed after five decades), it should be possible to protect against the toxic effects of ammonia in normal animals by the administration of branched-chain amino acids. In the following experiments, normal rats were infused with either saline (as a control) 0.4 M ammonia, or 0.4 M ammonia and branched-chain amino acids. Neurological examinations were undertaken as previously described. In the initial experiment, profound neurological depression was seen after 0.4 M ammonia with survival of only about 6 hours. The infusion of branched-chain amino acids with ammonia was sufficient to protect the animal against neurological depression , doubling the time for survival and slowing the appearance of neurological symptoms. These results were unchanged with the administration of glucose to protect the animals against hypoglycemia.

The results suggest that the toxicity of ammonia is perhaps mediated by exchange of amino acids crossed by blood brain barrier. One possible flaw in this experiment is that the administration of the branched-chain amino acids may accelerate to aid the metabolism of ammonia, possibly by the production of glutamine or alanine from the muscle and enabling metabolism of ammonia via muscle. Experiments are currently underway in which identical levels of ammonia are present within the plasma in the ammonia and branched-chain amino acids.

G. The Use of Branched-Chain Amino Acids as Therapy in Hepatic Encephalopathy

Although not discussed in this manuscript, but elsewhere in this symposium, it is now becoming abundantly clear through the results of a variety of studies that the administration of branched-chain amino acids, either alone or in combination with other amino acids in the presence of hypertonic dextrose, is efficacious in the treatment of hepatic encephalopathy.

Taken together, all of these findings suggest that the amino acid neurotransmitter hypothesis is extremely relevant to the etiology of hepatic encephalopathy and may, in fact, be at least part of the mechanism by which hepatic coma supervenes.

REFERENCES

1. J. E. Fischer and R. J. Baldessarini, False neurotransmitters and hepatic failure, Lancet ii: 75 (1981).
2. K. Dismukes, A new look at the aminergic nervous system, Nature 269: 557 (1977).
3. M. L. Mashford, W. A. Mahon, and T. C. Chalmers, Studies of the cardiovascular system in the hypotension of liver failure, N. Engl. J. Med. 267: 1071 (1962).
4. J. E. Fischer and R. H. Bower, Amino acid in liverdisease, in: "The Kidney in Liver Disease," M. Epstein ed., Elsevier Publishing New York, 2nd edition, pp. 515-534 (1982).
5. F. E. Tristani and J. J. Cohn. Systemic and renal demodynamics in organic hepatic failure: Effect of volume expansion, J. Clin. Invest. 46: 1894 (1967).
6. J. H. James, J. Escourrou,and J. E. Fischer, Blood brain neutral amino acid transport activity is increased after portacaval anastomosis, Science 200: 1395 (1978).
7. J. H. James, J. M. Hodgman, J. M. Funovics, and J. E. Fischer Alterations in brain octopamine and brain tyrosine following portacaval anastomosis in rats, J. Neurochem. 27: 223 (1967).
8. W. K. Oldendorf, Brain uptake of radiolabelled amino acids, amines and hexoses after arterial injection, Amer. J. Phys. 221: 1629 (1971).
9. B. A. Faraj, V. M. Camp, J. E. Ansley, J. Scott, F. M. Ali, and E. J. Malveaux, Evidence of central hypertyraminemia in hepatic encephalopathy, J. Clin. Invest. 67: 395 (1981).
10. A. Nespoli, G. Bevilacqua, G. Staudacher, N. Rossi, E. Salerno, and M. R. Castelli, The role of false neurotransmitters in the pathogenesis of hepatic encephalopathy and hyperdinamic

syndrome in cirrhosis, Arch. Surg. 116: 1129 (1981).

11. F. Rossi-Fanelli, F. H. Freund, R. Krause, A. R. Smith, J. H. James, S. Castorina-Ziparo,and J. E. Fischer, Induction of coma in normal dogs by infusion of aromatic amino acids and prevention by addition of branched chain amino acids, Gastroenterology 83: 664 (1982).

12. L. Zieve and R. L. Olsen, Can hepatic coma be caused by a reduction in brain noradrenaline or dopamine? Gut 18:688(1977).

13. W. T. Chance, A. P. Bernadini, J. H. James, L. L. Edwards, K. Minnema, and J.E. Fischer, Behavioral depression following intraventricular infusion of octopamine in rats. Submitted for publication.

14. J. H. James, V. Ziparo, B. Jeppson,and J. E. Fischer Hyperammonaemia, plasma amino acid imbalance, and blood-brain amino acid transport: A unified theory of portal systemic encephalopathy, Lancet ii: 772 (1979).

15. J. H. James and J. E. Fischer, The transport of neutral amino acids at the blood-brain barrier, Pharmacology 22: 1 (1980).

STUDIES RELATING TO A THEORETICAL UNDERSTANDING OF ALTERED

BLOOD-BRAIN BARRIER TRANSPORT IN LIVER DISEASE

H. J. James, B. Jeppsson, T. Jonung,
P. Rigotti And J. E. Fischer

Department of Surgery, University of Cincinnati
Medical Center, Cincinnati, Ohio, U.S.A.

INTRODUCTION

Evidence from several sources suggests that blood-brain transport of the large neutral amino acids (NAA) is abnormal in animals with a portacaval anastomosis (PCA) and in patients with liver cirrhosis and portalsystemic shunting. The concentrations in brain of the neutral amino acids methionine, phenylalanine, tyrosine, tryptophan and histidine are markedly elevated in rats after PCA.[1-3] The concentrations of many large NAA are elevated several-fold in the cerebrospinal fluid of dogs after PCA and of patients with liver cirrhosis.[4,5]

High concentrations of NAA in the brain cannot be completely explained by the changes in plasma NAA concentrations which accompany portal-systemic shunting. After PCA in rats, the rise in brain tyrosine exceeds either the rise in plasma tyrosine or the increase in the plasma ratio of tyrosine to the other NAA competing for blood-brain transport.[2,6] The uptake of radiolabeled NAA by brain slices of rats with PCA is no greater than that by brain slices from normal rats.[7] In contrast, higher uptake of NAA by brain from blood after PCA has been demonstrated.[1,3,7]

Increased blood-brain transport after PCA has been shown only for the NAA, whereas brain uptake of basic amino acids, pyruvate, butyrate, glucose and sodium after PCA has been described as either decreased or unchanged.[1,3,9,10] After PCA, competition among circulating NAA for blood-brain transport can be readily demonstrated; administration of leucine, isoleucine and valine lowers brain tryptophan levels both in control rats and in rats with PCA.[11] In dogs after PCA, intravenous infusion of solutions rich in leucine, isoleucine

61

and valine rapidly lowers the concentrations of other large NAA in
the cisternal cerebrospinal fluid.[4]

These observations suggest that in human liver disease or after
PCA the activity of the barrier NAA transport system increases, per-
mitting brain to concentrate several NAA to levels higher than those
in the plasma. In liver disease or after PCA, the concentration of
glutamine in brain is markedly increased,[12] and the rate of efflux
of glutamine from brain is also apparently increased.[13] Glutamine
is thought to be a weakly competing substrate for the blood-brain
NAA transport system and, therefore, the efflux of glutamine from
brain is probably mediated in some part by the large NAA transport
system. High brain concentrations of glutamine after PCA could either
raise the influx of NAA from blood by accelerating exchange transport
via the NAA transport system or inhibit the efflux of NAA from brain
by competing for transport at the antiluminal membranes of the cerebral capillaries. The following observations gathered in experiments in vivo support the concept of a role for glutamine in altered
blood-brain neutral amino acid transport in hyperammonemic states.

MATERIALS AND METHODS

Animals with Portacaval Shunts

Male Sprague-Dawley rats (250-300 g) underwent surgical creation
of a portacaval anastomosis under ether anesthesia. The rats were
fed with Purina rat chow ad lib. and water was available at all
times. A total of 61 rats with PCA were studied. Rats were killed
by decapitation at various times from 13-74 days after PCA.

Animals receiving Ammonia Infusions

Male Sprague-Dawley rats (350-400 g) received a silastic catheter
in the jugular vein under ether anesthesia. The catheter was protected
by a flexible metal sheath attached to a swivel. Rats were infused
with a mixture of 0.4 M ammonium salts (0.2 M ammonium acetate +
0.2 M ammonium bicarbonate, pH 7.4) at a rate of 2.5 ml/h for 24 h.
Rats were decapitated 24 h later for amino acid analyses or for
blood-brain transport studies. In parallel studies rats received
methionine sulfoximine (150 mg/kg) i.p. 2h before ammonia infusions
were begun. Methionine sulfoximine (MSO) is an irreversible inhibitor
of glutamine synthetase.

Amino Acid Analysis

Free amino acids of plasma and brain were analyzed using a
Beckman 121-MB automatic amino acid analyzer and litium citrate
buffers which separate glutamic acid, glutamine and asparagine.
Plasma was deproteinized by mixing with an equal volume of 7.5%(wt/
vol) sulfosalicylic acid pH 1.7, containing an internal standard.

Brain tissue was homogenized in three volumes (3 x weight) of 5% (wt/vol), sulfosalicylic acid, pH 1.4, containing an internal standard.

Special precautions were taken to prevent loss of glutamine in samples. We determined that glutamine solutions were stable for at least 3 weeks frozen and at least 1 week refrigerated. Therefore all steps in the preparation of brain samples were performed in the cold and samples were analyzed within two weeks after killing.

Kinetics of the Inhibition by Glutamine of Blood-Brain Uptake of Phenylalanine in Normal Rats

In order to obtain an estimate of the Michaelis constant, Km, of glutamine for the NAA transport system of the blood-brain barrier, we studied the effect of various concentration of L-glutamine on the in vivo brain uptake of radiolabeled L-phenylalanine using the Oldendorf carotid injection technique.[14] Pardridge[15] has shown that the Ki of transport of one NAA for another, i.e., the concentration at which 50% inhibition of the saturable component of uptake occurs, is close to the Km of transport determined by self-competition for uptake. The following studies were performed only in unoperated male Sprague-Dawley rats (250-300 g).

Carotid injection solutions contained in 0.2 ml, 0.2 μCi (L-^{14}C) phenylalanine (2 μM, New England Nuclear, Boston MA), and 1.0 μCi (^{3}H) water as diffusible reference in Ringer's solution buffered to pH 7.4 with 10 mM Hepes buffer. Solutions containing unlabeled glutamine were prepared as above but containing 2, 8, 10, 20 or 40 mM L-glutamine. Test solutions were rapidly injected into the right common carotid artery of rats under pentobarbital anesthesia (45 mg/kg). Rats were decapitated 15 seconds later and the brain were immediately removed. A sample of brain tissue ipsilateral to the injection and rostral to the mid-brain was extruded through a 20-gauge needle into 1.0 ml NCS tissue solubilizer. Radioactivity in the brain tissue samples and the injection solution was analyzed by double-isotope liquid scintillation counting using standard techniques. The brain uptake index (BUI) was calculated from the ratio of dpm of ^{14}C to ^{3}H in brain tissue divided by the same ratio in the injection solution multiplied by 100. The calculation of Ki of glutamine of phenylalanine uptake from a double reciprocal transformation of the data was performed as described by Pardridge.[15]

Kinetics of Blood-Brain Transport in Ammonia-Infused Rats

Kinetic analysis of the uptake of phenylalanine and leucine in the brain cortex of rats was performed essentially as described by Pardridge et al.[16] Blood flow was first determined in ammonia infused rats and in controls by BuOH washout rate. Carotid injections were performed exactly as above but containing radiolabeled amino acid,

^3H_2O and various concentrations of unlabeldd amino acid. Transport parameters were calculated by nonlinear least-squares regression as reported by Pardridge et al.[16]

Correlation Analysis

Analysis of Pearson product-moment correlation coefficients was perfomed to determine the relationship between the brain glutamine concentration and the brain NAA concentrations in control rats and in rats with PCA.

RESULTS

Kinetics of the Inhibition of Brain Uptake of Phenylalanine by Glutamine

Addition of increasing concentrations of glutamine to the carotid injection solution reduced in a concentration-dependent manner the brain uptake of ^{14}C-phenylalanine by normal rats. If it is assumed that this represents competitive inhibition for blood-brain transport, the Ki (8.5 ± 1.1 mM) obtained by double-reciprocal transformation of the data may be taken as a reasonable approximation of the Km of transport of glutamine. Table 1 compares this Km value for glutamine with Km values for other neutral amino acids from Pardridge and Mietus.[17]

Correlation Analysis in Rats with PCA

In control rats, no significant positive correlation was found between brain glutamine concentrations and brain NAA concentrations (Table 2). In rats with PCA, the brain concentrations of Tyr, Phe, Thr, Met and His (Table 2) correlated significantly with the brain glutamine concentration. Including both control and PCA rats together in this correlation tended to yield higher values of r than when only the PCA group was considered alone.

Effect of Ammonia Infusion and MSO on Brain Amino Acid Levels

Table 3 shows that rats infused with ammonia only had high brain levels of neutral amino acids and of glutamine, whereas rats pretreated with MSO had low brain levels of glutamine and normal brain levels of other neutral amino acids.

Effect of Ammonia Infusion on Kinetics of Brain uptake of Phenylalanine and Leucine

Ammonia infusion significantly increased the Vmax of uptake of phenylalanine into brain cortex (43 ± 5 nmol/g/min, NH_3 vs 21 ± 3, control), but had no significant effect on the Km of uptake (132 ± 16 μM, NH_3 vs 90 ± 14 μM, control). Ammonia infusion also signif-

Table 1.

NAA	Uncompeted Transport Km (mM)	Relative Affinity
Leucine	.10	100%
Phenylalanine	.11	91%
Tyrosine	.15	67%
Tryptophan	.16	63%
Methionine	.18	56%
Histidine	.24	42%
Isoleucine	.28	36%
Valine	.51	20%
Threonine	.73	14%
Glutamine	8.50	1.2%

Table 2. Correlation between Brain NAA Concentrations and the Brain Glutamine Concentration

		Thr	Val	Met	Ile	Leu	Tyr	Phe	His
Control (7)									
	r =	.588	-.859	.075	.013	-.228	.248	.253	.321
	$P <$	ns	.02	ns	ns	ns	ns	ns	ns
PCA (61)	r =	.419	-.158	.589	-.228	.101	.922	.960	.941
	$P <$	.001	ns	.001	ns	ns	.001	.001	.001
PCA + Control (N=68)									
	r =	.414	-.169	.668	-.139	.200	.932	.964	.950
	$P <$	.001	ns	.001	ns	ns	.001	.001	.001

icantly increased the constant of nonsaturable uptake (K_d = 0.071, NH_3 vs 0.033 ml/min/g). The Vmax of uptake of leucine was significantly increased by ammonia infusion (108 $\pm$ 23 nmol/g/min vs 32+4, control) as was the Km of uptake (346 $\pm$ 79 μM vs 185 $\pm$ 24, control). Ammonia infusion also significantly increased the K_d of leucine uptake (0.021 ml/min/g) vs 0.013, control).

DISCUSSION

The brain uptake of trace quantities (< 0.1 Km) of various NAA as measured using the carotid artery, single-injection technique of Oldendorf is markedly higher in rats with PCA than in controls.[1-3] Mans et al.,[8] using an autoradiographic technique, studied the effect of PCA on the distribution of radioactivity in brain after a brief (1.5 min) infusion of ^{14}C-labeled Phe, tryptophan and Leu. The latter authors reported that PCA resulted in enhanced influx of all three neutral amino acids but that the increase in Leu influx was much less than the increase in influx of the others. Determining whether the activity of blood-brain barrier neutral amino acid transport is enhanced for all amino acids equally after PCA or whether this enhancement is selective is clearly important for under-standing the mechanism underlying the effect of liver disease and hyperammonemia on brain amino acid uptake.

One mechanism[6] which has been proposed to account for the increased influx of neutral NAA after PCA involves the accumulation in brain of glutamine, a by-product of cerebral detoxification of ammonia and a weak competitor for the blood-brain neutral amino acid transport system. High brain levels of glutamine, it was proposed, might increase brain uptake of NAA by acceleration of exchange transport or by competing with other NAA in brain for efflux. In support of this hypothesis, Gimmon et al.[18] demonstrated that several NAA accumulate to high levels in brains of normal rats infused for 24 hr with ammonium salts. The present studies, including measure-ments of transport per se, show that the accumulation of various NAA in brain after PCA is proportional to the accumulation of glu-tamine in brain. Moreover, in rats infused with ammonia, accumulation of amino acids did not occur when glutamine synthesis was blocked.

The observed increase in Vmax of phenylalanine and leucine uptake in ammonia-infused rats is consistent with an increased rate of exchange transport, and hence of carrier availability, on the luminal side of the blood-brain barrier. The possibility that this increase also may represent an increase in number of carriers seems to be small in rats only exposed to ammonia for 24 hr. One would expect enhanced carrier synthesis to require a longer time for induction, although this is only speculation.

The differential effects of ammonia infusion on Km of transport are more difficult to explain. Leucine is rapidly metabolized in brain, while phenylalanine is not. In theory, the Km represents a measure of affinity of the carrier for the amino acid, presumably a structural property of the carrier. However, it should be recalled that it is not only transport alone that was measured in the kinetic studies, but also retention of the labeled carbon atoms of the amino acid in the brain until decapitation. Rapid conversion of amino acid carbon in leucine to $^{14}CO_2$ and removal of CO_2 to the blood would thus

Table 3. Effect of NH_3 and MSO Treatments on Brain Amino Acid
Levels in Normal Rats

Treatments	MSO + NH_3	Sal. + NH_3
Glutamine	2500± 15	27,000±1500
Phenylalanine	70± 3	245± 18
Tyrosine	46± 5	167± 8
Methionine	51± 8	97± 12
Histidine	83± 7	213± 18

lead to underestimation of the amount of leucine taken up. This loss
of transported label would presumably be more severe at lower concentrations and perhaps lead to a shift in the observed Km. In this
case, if the metabolism of leucine were inhibited, for example, by
cycloserine, then ammonia infusion should only alter the Vmax and
not the Km of leucine.

In summary, the studies reported here continue to support the
hypothesis that high blood ammonia results secondarily in high brain
levels of various neutral amino acids. The obligatory intermediate
in this effect seems to be synthesis of glutamine. Glutamine probably reduces the efflux of other neutral amino acids in brain by
competition for efflux on the neutral amino acid carrier. High brain
levels of all neutral amino acids raise the rate of carrier mediated
exchange as revealed in kinetic studies. If it is desired to lower
the brain levels of some neutral amino acids, then two routes are
available: 1) reduction of circulating ammonia levels, and 2) increasing the competition for blood-brain transport in the blood
compartment using branched-chain amino acids. These latter amino
acids will not accumulate in brain due to their rapid metabolism and
provide significant inhibition of transport with the other neutral
amino acids in blood.

ACKNOWLEDGEMENT

Supported in part by USPHS Grant # AM25347.

REFERENCES

1. J. H. James, J. Escourrou, and J. E. Fischer, Blood-brain neutral
amino acid transport activity is increased after portacaval
anastomosis, Science 200: 1385 (1978).
2. D. L. Blowam and G. Curzon, A study of proposed determinants of

brain tryptophan concentration in rats after portacaval anastomosis or sham operation, J. Neurochem. 31: 1255 (1978).

3.   G. Zanchin, P. Rigotti, N. Dussini, P. Vassanelli, and L. Batti-
     stin, Cerebral amino acid levels and uptake in rats after
     portacaval anastomosis, I. J. Neurosci. Res. 4: 301 (1979).

4.   A. R. Smith, F. Rossi-Fanelli, V. Ziparo, J. H. James, B. A.
     Perelle, and J. E. Fischer, Alterations in plasma and in CSF
     amino acids, amines and metabolites in hepatic coma, Ann.
     Surg. 187: 343 (1978).

5.   J. Ono, D. G. Hutson, R. S. Dombro, J. U. Levi, A. Livingstone,
     and R. Zeppa, Tryptophan and hepatic coma, Gastroenterology
     74: 196 (1978).

6   J. H. James, B. Jeppsson, V. Ziparo, and J. E. Fischer, Hyperam-
     monemia, plasma amino acid imbalance and blood-brain amino
     acid transport: a unified theory of portal-systemic encepha-
     lopathy, Lancet ii: 772 (1979).

7.   G. Zanchin, P. Rigotti, F. Bettineschi, P. Vassanelli, and L.
     Battistin, Cerebral amino acid levels and uptake in rats
     after portacaval anastomosis, I. J. Neurosci. Res. 4: 291
     (1979).

8.   A. M. Mans, J. F. Biebuyck, K. Shelly, and R. A. Hawkins Regio-
     nal blood-brain barrier permeability to amino acids after
     portacaval anastomosis, J. Neurochem. 38: 705 (1982).

9.   J. E. Cremer, J. C. Lal, and G. S. Sarna Rapid blood-brain
     transport and metabolism of butyrate and pyruvate in the
     rat after portacaval anastomosis, J. Physiol. (Lond) 266:
     70P (1977).

10. G. S. Sarna, M. W. B. Bradbury, and J. Cavanaugh, Permeability
     of the blood-brain barrier after portacaval anastomosis in
     the rat, Brain Res. 138: 550 (1977).

11. M. G. Cummings, P. B. Soeters, J. H. James, J. K. Kane, and J.
     E. Fischer, Regional brain indoleamine metabolism following
     chronic portacaval anastomosis in the rat, J. Neurochem.
     27: 501 (1975).

12. A. M. Williams, M. T. Kyu, J. C. B. Fenton, and J. B. Cavanagh
     The glutamate and the glutamine content of rat brain after
     portacaval anastomosis, J. Neurochem. 19: 1073 (1962).

13. A. Gjedde, A. H. Lockwood, T. E. Duffy, and F. Plum, Cerebral
     blood flow and metabolism in chronically hyperammonemic
     rats: effect of an acute ammonia challenge, Ann. Neurol. 3:
     325 (1978).

14. W. H. Oldendorf, Measurement of brain uptake of radiolabelled
     substances using a tritiated water internal standard, Brain
     Res. 24: 372 (1970).

15. W. M. Pardridge, Kinetics of competitive inhibition of neutral
     aminoacid transport across the blood-brain barrier, J.
     Neurochem. 28: 103 (1977).

16. W. M. Pardridge, P. D. Crane, L. J. Mietus, and W. H. Oldendorf,
     Kinetics of regional blood-brain barrier transport and brain
     phosphorylation of glucose and 2-deoxyglucose in the barbi-

turate-anesthetized rat, J. Neurochem. 38: 560 (1982).

17. W. M. Pardridge and L. J. Mietos, Kinetics of neutral amino acid transport through the blood-brain barrier of the newborn rabbit, J. Neurochem. 38: 955 (1982).

18. Z. Gimmon, J. H. James, M. von Mayenfeldt, and J. E. Fischer, Opposing Effects of Prolonged Ammonia and Branched-Chain Amino Acid Infusions on the Accumulation of Aromatic Amino Acids by Brain, in:"Metabolism and Clinical Implications of Branched-Chain Amino and Ketoacids" M. Walser and J. R. Williamson, eds. , Elsevier North Holland, New York, pp. 487-492 (1981).

AMINO ACID TRANSPORT IN ISOLATED BRAIN CAPILLARIES

P. Cardelli-Cangiano,[*] C. Cangiano,[**] A. Fiori[*] and
R. Strom[*]

[*]Department of Biochemistry, University of Rome, P.le
Aldo Moro, 00185 Rome, Italy, [**]3rd Department of
Internal Medicine, University of Rome, Viale dell'Uni-
versità 37, 00161, Rome, Italy

INTRODUCTION

In patients and in experimental animals with severe hepatic
failure and/or portal systemic shunting of the circulation, pathologic changes have been described in the transport capacity for
neutral amino acids at the level of the blood-brain barrier.

The concentration, in cerebrospinal fluid and brain, of aromatic amino acids is thus considerably increased.[1-5] The factors
involved in this alteration of transport capacity deserve however
a more detailed investigation. In Table 1 are summarized some
features of the main transport systems known to exist, in mammalian
cells, for neutral and cationic amino acids, the various systems
being characterized not only by their active transport or exchanging
properties and by their substrate specificity, but also by their
dependence on pH, Na^+ ions, membrane potential, and on hormonal
and nutritional factors.[6-8]

In the endothelial cells of brain capillaries which are the
anatomical counterpart of the blood-brain barrier,[9-11] the ASC
system has been reported to be present only in the early neonatal
stage.[12] In the adult, therefore, the neutral amino acids are transported essentially by the Na^+-dependent concentrative A-system,
specific for amino acids with a short polar side chain, and/or by
the Na^+-independent exchanging L-system, preferred by amino acids
with a bulky apolar side chain.

Betz et al.[10] from a comparison of the in vivo and in vitro

71

Table 1. Main transport systems for neutral and cationic amino acids (from ref. 6,8,12)

Name		Capability of		Sensitivity to					Amino acid specificity
		Concentration	Exchange	pH	Na$^+$	ΔV	Hormone (insulin, glucagon, somatotropine, cate cholamine)	Nutritional deficiencies	
Neutral amino acid	A	+	−	+	+	+	+	+	Gly, Pro, Ala, Ser, His, Met, (Val, Leu, Ileu, Phe, Tyr, Trp).
	ASC	+	+−	−	+	?	−	−	Ala, Ser, Thr, Cys
	L	(+̄)	+	−	−	−	−	−	Val, Leu, Ileu, Met, His, Phe, Tyr, Trp, (Ala, Ser, Thr, Cys)
Cationic amino acid	Ly$^+$	−	+	(−)	−	−	−	−	Lys, Arg, (His–Na$^+$, Phe–Na$^+$, Tyr–Na$^+$, Trp–Na$^+$).

permeability properties of brain microvessels, proposed an asymmetric location, in the endothelial cells of the blood-brain barrier, of the amino acid transport systems, the A-system being present only on the abluminal side of the microvessels, while the L-system is active on both luminal and abluminal sides.

The involvement of an increased activity of the L-system in some pathological conditions (such as hyperammonemia and porto-systemic shunting) has recently been suggested.[2,13] In this hypothesis, an increase of glutamine content in the brain would result in an accelerated exchange, through the L-system, of aromatic amino acids, as visualized e.g. by Figure 1.

The present report describes in vitro experiments performed with the aim of validating this hypothesis and of clarifying the various aspects of regulation of amino acids transport in brain microvessels. Figure 2 shows the appearance, in the scanning electron microscope, of a typical preparation of brain microvessels from adult bovine gray matter. Although the polarity of the blood-brain barrier is lost in this in vitro system, such preparations allow, in well-defined experimental conditions, a detailed and reproducible kinetic study of amino acid uptake in brain microvessels.

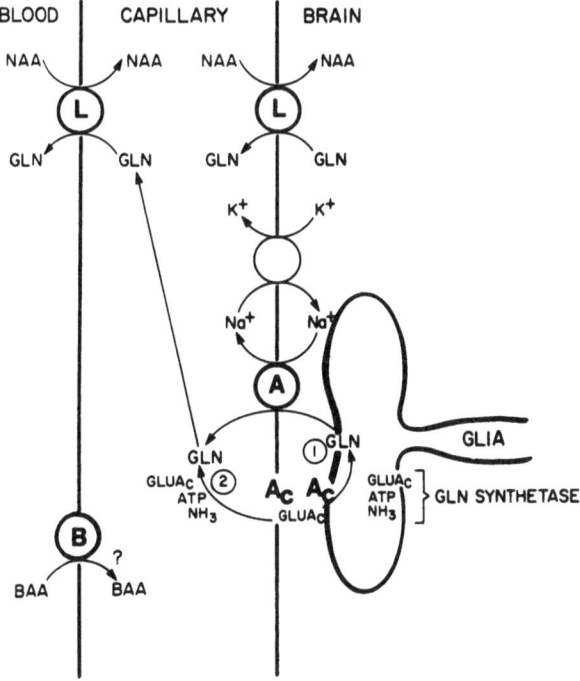

Fig. 1. Proposed distribution of the amino acid transport systems in a hypothetic section of a brain capillary endothelial cell. For details see text.

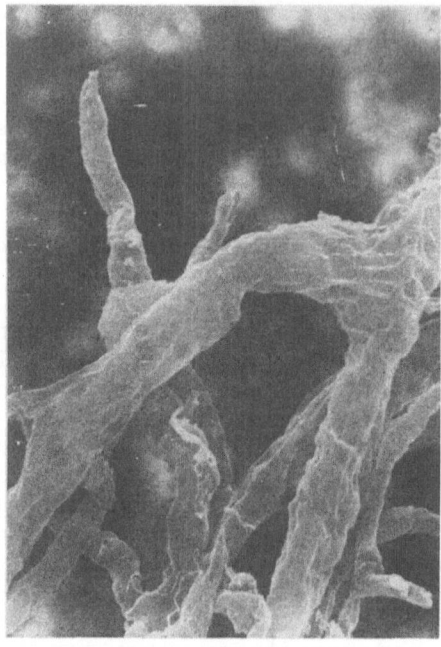

├────────┤ 10 µm

Fig. 2.   Scanning electron microscope of isolated brain microvessels.
          There is no gross damage of the microvessels nor contami-
          nation by nerve cells or by glia.

Characterization of the Transport Systems for Neutral Amino Acids
Existing in Brain Microvessels

        By examining the effect of substrate concentration on the
initial rate of uptake, it could be shown[13] that, in our preparations of brain microvessels, the uptake of neutral amino acids has
at least two components: a diffusional one, which is strictly proportional to the substrate concentration, and a mediated transport,
which follows a Michaelis-Menten kinetics. The latter could be
assigned, for the various amino acids, to the A- or to the L-system
according to the sensitivity to inhibition by methylamino-isobutyric
acid or by β-2-aminobicyclo-heptane carboxylic acid (BCH), respectively, and on the basis of the Na^+ dependence.

        Digestion with Clostridium histolyticum collagenase proved,

moreover, to solubilize preferentially, together with some enzymes and other proteins, the A-system, the specific activity of which decreased therefore in the particular function, while that of the L-system underwent a cospicuous increase (see also Table 6).

The following results were found to substantiate the hypo-thesis[2,13] that NH_4^+ ions act by inducing the intracellular formation of glutamine, which is then used in a L-system-mediated exchange, leading to an increased uptake of the hydrophobic amino acids:

a) Preincubation with 0.25 mM NH_4^+ results in increased levels of glutamine (Table 2).

b) The stimulation, by 0.25 mM NH_4^+, of hydrophobic amino acid uptake is abolished, as shown in Table 3, by the presence of methionine sulfoximine, a well-known inhibitor of glutamine synthetase which indeed prevents the NH_4^+-dependent increase of intracellular glu-tamine.[15]

c) Pre-loading with glutamine (in the presence of Na^+ ions) results in an increased rate of uptake of hydrophobic amino acids.[15] The increased rate of uptake declines to basal levels with a time course similar to that of glutamine efflux (Table 4). The rate of glutamine efflux is higher in the presence, in the extracell-ular fluid, of hydrophobic amino acids (Fig. 3).

d) Both incubation with NH_4^+ ions and preloading with glutamine increase specifically the V_{max} of uptake of hydrophobic amino acids; no effect on K_m, on passive diffusion rate, nor on the uptake of polar amino acids (Table 5).

e) Digestion with collagenase, which removes (together with other proteins) the A-system but not the L-system nor glutamine syn-thetase, abolishes the stimulating effect of glutamine pre-loading, but results in a more evident stimulating effect of NH_4^+ ions (Table 6).

Can a Similar Mechanism be Extended to Other Substances Having a Pathogenic Role in Hepatic Encephalopathy?

The ability to enter the endothelial cells via the concentra-tive A-system and to induce thereafter, through an accelerated exchange mechanism, an increased rate of uptake of hydrophobic neutral amino acids via the L-system, is not unique of glutamine, but is shared by other long-chain neutral amino acids, viz. methionine (Figure 4), which can be transported by both the A- and the L-system. In fact, the stimulating effect of preloading with methionine on the uptake of tyrosine by brain microvessels is even larger than that of glutamine. This finding can not only be of some

Table 2. Effect of NH_4^+ ions on amino acid uptake by brain microvessels. The uptake was measured after 5 min incubation at 37°C, in the presence of ^{14}C-labeled neutral amino acid (0.67 μCi/ml) of the isolated microvessels, in the presence or in the absence of 0.25 mM NH_4^+ ions. The data, expressed as dpm.mg protein^{-1}, are the average ($\pm$ SD) of three different determinations.

Amino acid	A control (no NH_4^+)	B 0.25 mM NH_4^+ (as NH_4HCO_3)[4]	B/A ratio
leucine (spec. radioact. 345 mCi/mmols)	5935±443	11871±177*	2.00
phenylalanine (spec. radioact. 501 mCi/mmols)	7918±883	12828±405*	1.70
cycloleucine (spec. radioact. 55 mCi/mmols)	4157±165	5001±315*	1.20
β-2-aminobicycloheptane carboxylic acid (spec. radioact. 5 mCi/mmols)	6550±165	11340±320*	1.70
α-methylamino-isobutyric acid (spec. radioact. 25 mCi/mmols)	4265±189	4337±180	1.01

$P \leq 0.05$ *

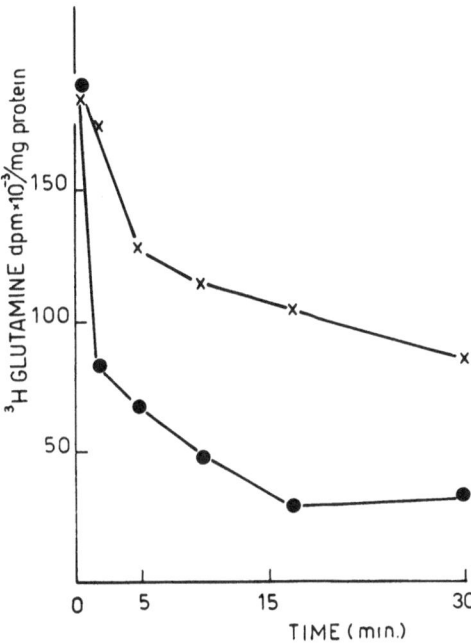

Fig. 3.   Glutamine efflux from brain microvessels. Microvessels were
preloaded with ^{3}H-glutamine (specific activity 3.37 Ci/mmole)
for 20 min at 37°C, rapidly washed and resuspended gluta-
mine-free buffer. The ^{3}H-glutamine e-flux was followed in
the absence (x) or in the presence (o) of 1 mM cold leucine
in the extracellular fluid.

interest in view of the high plasma and liquor levels of methionine,[1]
but can also be a basis for the well known pathogenic effect
exerted by methanethiol.[16] This mercaptan by itself was found, in
our experimental system, to be ineffective on any of the amino acid
transport systems; if however the microvessels were preloaded simultaneously with cystine (or cysteine) plus methanethiol, there was a
marked enhancement of the L-system mediated uptake fo hydrophobic
neutral amino acids (Figure 4). Cystine or cysteine alone were
ineffective, nor could they be replaced by alanine, serine or other
non-sulphur-containing amino acids. The stimulation of the L-system
can be attributed to the formation of the mixed disulfide methyl-
thiocysteine (Figure 5), whose chemical structure is very similar
to that of methionine; in aqueous mixtures of methanethiol and
cystine a compound is indeed formed, which on the amino acid analyzer
is barely distinguishable from methionine.

DISCUSSION

The brain microvessel preparations used in these experiments

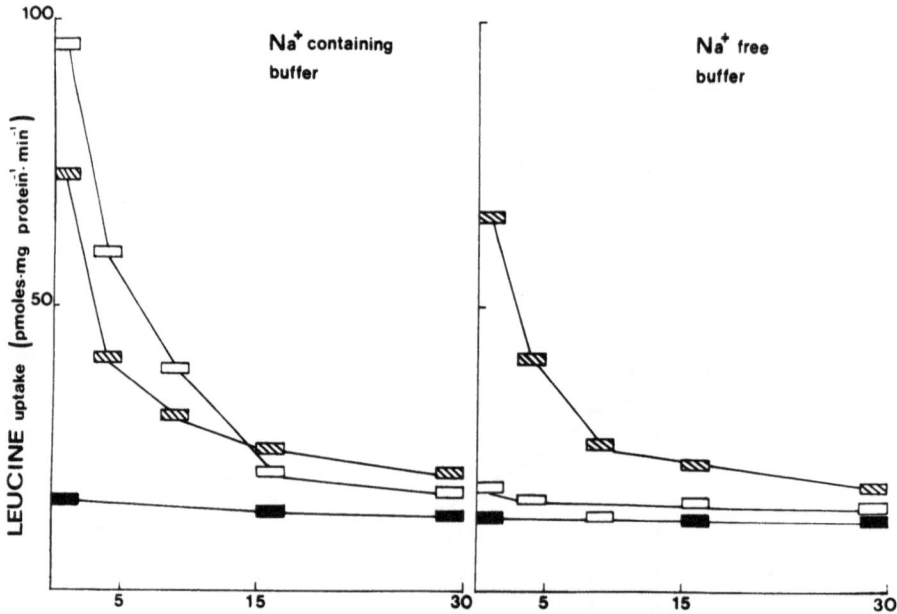

Fig. 4.   Leucine uptake measured (as initial rate) at fixed intervals
          after 20 min preloading with 20 mM methionine (open bars) or
          with 20 mM cysteine plus an equimolar concentration of
          CH_3SH (dashed bars). After the preloading step (effected
          in the presence or in the absence of Na^+ ions), the micro-
          vessels were washed and resuspended in Na^+-containing or
          in Na^+-free buffer. Closed bars represent control micro-
          vessels in which the preloading step was performed in the
          absence of either methionine or S-methylthiocysteine.

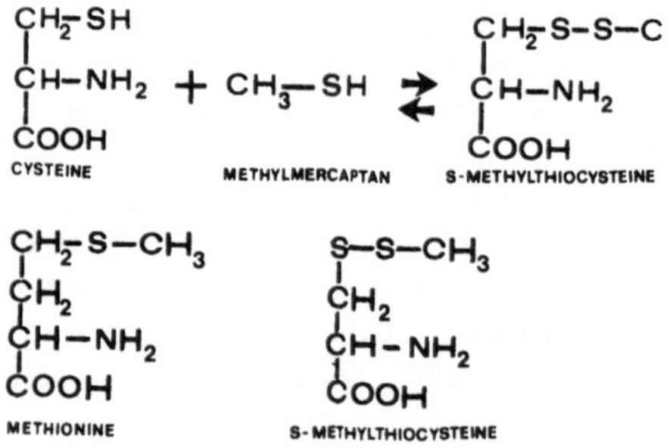

Fig. 5.   Chemical reaction indicating the formation of the mixed
          disulfide S-methylthiocysteine.

Table 3. Effect, on the intracellular glutamine levels and on a 5 min uptake of ^{14}C leucine (0.04 mCi/mmole), of 20 min preincubation of brain microvessels in buffer with or without 0.25 mM NH_4HCO_3 in the presence or absence of 5 mM methionine sulfoximine. Data are the mean $\pm$ S.D.

NH_4HCO_3 (mM)	Methionine sulfoximine (mM)	Glutamine content (nmoles/gr cells)	5 min uptake of ^{14}C-leucine (dpm/mg protein)
0	0	99 + 11	3585 + 374
0.25	0	137 + 16	6394 + 400
0	5	59 + 10	3670 + 310
0.25	5	51 + 14	3595 + 275

$P \leq 0.01$

Table 4. Effect of glutamine preload on the subsequent amino acid uptake.
The initial rate of amino acid uptake was measured at various time intervals following preloading of the microvessels with 20 mM glutamine for 20 min at 37°C. Data shown are expressed as pmoles.min^{-1}.mg protein^{-1} and are the mean + SD of three experiments. Each measurement of amino acid uptake required approximately 2 minutes, this being therefore the uncertainty in the evaluation of the time interval elapsed after the preloading step. Microvessels preincubated in the absence of glutamine had a constant rate of amino acid uptake, the mean being 21+3 over the 30 min interval.

^{14}C labeled amino acid	Time intervals, in minutes between end of preloading and uptake				
	0-2	3-5	8-10	15-17	28-30
tyrosine	73+4	45+2	27+3	26+4	28+6
leucine	78+3	65+1	32+2	27+3	25+5
methylamino isobutyric acid	22+4	24+2	20+3	24+2	23+2

Table 5. Values of the steady state kinetic parameters for tyrosine or for leucine uptake by brain microvessels either preloaded with 20 mM glutamine or in the presence of 0.25 mM NH_4 ions

		K_d (min^{-1})	V_{max} ($nmoles.min^{-1}.mg\ prot.^{-1}$)	K_m (μM)
leucine uptake	no addition	0.76	300	145
	plus 0.25 mM NH_4 ions	0.81	418	146
	after 20 min preincubation in the absence of glutamine	0.90	230	171
tyrosine uptake	after 20 min preincubation with 20 mM glutamine	0.86	410	180

Table 6. Effect of collagenase digestion of mechanically isolated brain microvessels on amino acid uptake.

In some experiments the isolated microvessels (approximately 2 mg/ml) were preincubated with 0.6 mg/ml of crude collagenase (from clostridium histolyticum) for 20 min at 37°C, being then washed and resuspended in a collagenase-free buffer. The uptake of ^{14}C labeled amino acids was then measured for 5 min at 37°C. Control microvessels followed the same procedure, except for the absence of collagenase during the preincubation step. Data are expressed as the mean $\pm$ SD from three different experiments.

Labeled amino acid	15 min uptake of label (as dpm.mg protein^{-1}) by			
	untreated microvessels		collagenase treated microvessels	
	NH_4^+ free buffer	plus NH_4^+ 0.25 mM	NH_4^+ free buffer	plus NH_4^+ 0.25 mM
methylamino-isobutyric-acid	4265+189	4337+180	1250+103	---
leucine	5935+443	11871+177	15170+710	28645+301
β-aminobicyclo-heptanecarboxylic acid	6560+165	11340+320	18531+1301	29245+277

Table 7. Effect of 20 min incubation with 4 U/ml of insulin
or with 0.5 mg/ml of polilysine (MW 3000) on the
uptake of methylamino-isobutyric acid by brain microvessels. The hormone or the cationic peptide were
present throughout the experiment. The labeled amino
acid was added at the end of the preincubation step,
and the uptake measured after 15 min at 37°C.
Data are expressed as dpm.mg protein^{-1} and are the
mean $\pm$ SD of three different determinations.

	15 min uptake
Control	5245 ± 167
+ insulin	9042 ± 187
+ polilysine	7081 ± 167

have allowed the experimental verification of several consequences
of the NH_4^+-glutamine hypothesis of the pathogenesis of the brain
amino acid imbalance in hepatic encephalopathy, and appears moreover
to lead to a methanethiol-methylthiocysteine extension of this
hypothesis.

A most interesting aspect of these results is the finding
that in brain microvessels there is often a coordination between
A- and L-transport systems, the exchanging properties of the latter
being stimulated by the concentrative ability of the former one.
In this respect, the asymmetric location of the A-system can be
expected to lead to an unidirectional stimulation from blood to
brain, of the transport of the hydrophobic amino acids.

Thanks to this coordination moreover, the regulation of the
A-system by pH, concentration of Na^+ ions, potential differences,
nutritional deficiencies, and/or by hormones (Table 1) is also
reflected on the L-system-mediated transport. The sensitivity to
insulin and to cationic peptides of the brain microvessels A-
transport system (Table 7) can thus presumably be extended also
to the uptake of hydrophobic amino acids. On the other hand, the
intracellular formation of glutamine and/or of S-methylthiocystine
can directly lead to a stimulation of the L-system by an alternative pathway which is independent from the functioning of the A-
system but is regulated by intracellular metabolic events.

REFERENCES

1. A. Cascino, C. Cangiano, F. Fiaccadori, F. Ghinelli, M. Merli,
    G. Pelosi, O. Riggio, F. Rossi-Fanelli, D. Sacchini, M. Stor-
    toni, and L. Capocaccia, Plasma and cerebrospinal fluid amino
    acid patterns in hepatic encephalopathy, Dig. Dis. Sci.27:
    828 (1982).
2. J. H. James, V. Ziparo, B. Jeppsson, and J. E. Fischer, Hyper-
    ammonemia, plasma aminoacid imbalance, and blood-brain ami-
    noacid transport: a unified theory of portal-systemic ence-
    phalopathy, Lancet ii: 772 (1979).
3. J. Ono, D. G. Huston, R. S. Dombro, J. U. Levy, A. Livingstone,
    and R. Zeppa, Tryptophan and hepatic coma, Gastroenterology
    74: 196 (1978).
4. A. R. Smith, F. Rossi-Fanelli, V. Ziparo, J. H. James, B. A.
    Perrelle, and J. E. Fischer, Alterations in plasma and CSF
    amino acids,amines and metabolites in hepatic coma, Annals
    Surg. 187: 343 (1978).
5. F. Rossi-Fanelli, H. Freund, R. Krause, A. R. Smith, J. H. James,
    S. Castorina-Ziparo, and J. E. Fischer, Induction of coma in
    normal dogs by the infusion of aromatic amino acids and its
    prevention by the addition of branched-chain amino acids,
    Gastroenterology 83: 664 (1982).
6. H. N. Christensen, M. Liang, and E. G. Archer, A distinct Na^+-
    -requiring transport system for alanine, serine, cysteine
    and similar amino acids, J. Biol. Chem. 242: 5237 (1967).
7. M. S. Kilberg, M. E. Handlogten, and H. N. Christensen, Charac-
    teristics of amino acid transport system in rat liver for
    glutamine, asparagine, histidine, and closely related ana-
    logs, J. Biol. Chem.255(9): 4011 (1980).
8. G. C. Gazzola, V. Dall'Asta,and G. Guidotti, Adaptive regulation
    of amino acid transport in cultured human fibroblasts, J.
    Biol. Chem. 256(7): 3191 (1981).
9. G. Sessa, M. Orlowsky, and J. P. Green, γ-Glutamyl-transpepti-
    dase in brain capillaries: possible site of a blood-brain
    barrier for amino acids, Science 184: 66 (1974).
10. A. L. Betz and G. W. Goldstein, Polarity of the blood-brain
    barrier: neutral amino acid transport into isolated brain
    capillaries, Science 202: 225 (1978).
11. A. L. Betz, J. Csejtey, and G. W. Goldstein, Hexsose transport
    and phosphorylation by capillaries isolated from rat brain,
    Am. J. Physiol. 236: C 96 (1979).
12. H. N. Christensen, On the development of amino acid transport
    system, Fed. Proc. 32(1): 19 (1973).
13. P. Cardelli-Cangiano, C. Cangiano, J. H. James, B. Jeppsson,
    W. Brenner, and J. E. Fischer, Uptake of amino acids by brain
    microvessels isolated from rat after portacaval anastomosis,
    J. Neurochem. 36: 627 (1981).
14. C. Cangiano, P. Cardelli-Cangiano, J. H. James, and J. E. Fischer,
    Ammonia stimulates amino acid uptake by isolated bovine

brain microvessels, Gastroenterology 78: 1308 (1980).

15. C. Cangiano, P. Cardelli-Cangiano, J. H. James, F. Rossi-Fanelli, M. A. Patrizi, K. A. Brackett, R. Strom, and J. E. Fischer, Brain microvessels take up large neutral amino acids in exchange for glutamine. Cooperative role of Na-dependent and Na-independent systems, J. Biol. Chem. (accepted for publication (1983).

16. L. Zieve and W. M. Doizaki, Brain and blood methanethiol and ammonia concentrations in experimental hepatic coma and coma due to injections of various combinations of these substances, Gastroenterology 79: 2 (1976).

CEREBRO-SPINAL FLUID AMINO ACID PATTERN IN HEPATIC ENCEPHALOPATHY

C. Cangiano, A. Cascino, S. Del Signore, F. Fiaccadori,[*]
F. Ghinelli,[*] M. Muscaritoli, G. Pelosi,[*] D. Sacchini,[*]
and F. Rossi Fanelli

3rd Department of Internal Medicine, University of Rome
[*]Division of Infectious Diseases, Ospedali Riuniti, Parma,
Italy

INTRODUCTION

The altered plasma amino acid pattern (i.e. increased levels
of aromatic amino acids and decreased levels of branched-chain
amino acids) which is likely to be involved in the profound derange-
ment of the neurotransmission observed in hepatic encephalopathy
(HE) is a characteristic feature of cirrhotic patients. However
previous studies from this[1] as well as from other laboratories[2-4]
have failed to demonstrate any correlation between HE and plasma
amino acid imbalance.

We have recently demonstrated that unlike in plasma, cerebrospinal fluid (CSF) amino acid patterns closely parallel the mental
state of patients with chronic liver disease.[5,6] These studies have
also demonstrated that in patients in grade 0 HE, CSF levels of
almost all amino acids are significantly higher than in controls,
showing a nearly two fold increase of CSF/plasma ratio of different
categories of neutral amino acids. In particular, comparable increases were observed not only of aromatic amino acids, which were
already increased in plasma, but also of branched-chain amino acids,
which in plasma were consistently decreased. Among neutral amino
acids, glycine, alanine, serine and threonine, which are known not
to easily cross the blood-brain barrier (BBB) and have consequently
been called "low uptake" amino acids[7] showed a similar two fold
rise of the CSF/plasma ratio, despite their normal plasma levels.
In grade 3-4 HE CSF amino acid pattern was characterized by a
further significant increase of only phenylalanine, tyrosine, tryptophan, methionine and glutamine. Interestingly, the plasma levels

87

of these amino acids were unchanged. These findings led us to hypothesize that BBB's behaviour in chronic liver failure without encephalopathy may be quite different from that in HE. We suggested that BBB
permeability is not-specifically altered in chronic liver failure
without encephalopathy, whereas when HE supervenes a selective
stimulation of neutral amino acid transport system across the BBB
seems to take place.[5,6] This hypothesis was put forward considering
the physiological role played by the BBB in the blood-brain amino
acid transport.

BLOOD-BRAIN BARRIER AMINO ACID TRANSPORT

     Circulating amino acids are transported across the BBB by one
of the three individual transport systems that have an affinity for
either neutral, basic or acidic amino acids.[8] As for neutral amino
acids, blood-brain transport seems to be regulated by a saturable
system called L-system which follows the rules of a competitive
exchange system. In addition to the saturable component of the
blood-brain transport of neutral amino acids, data obtained in vivo
and in vitro[8,9] suggest the presence of a non-saturable component
(probably diffusion) which under physiological conditions do not
significantly influence the brain levels of neutral amino acids.
Thus the brain levels of any particular neutral amino acid seem to
depend upon different factors: (i) The affinity for the carrier
system. Experimental data suggest that neutral amino acids are
transported into the brain owing to their affinity for the L-system
which is expressed by the value of the apparent Km. Since individual
Km values of most of the amino acids approximate their plasma levels,
the barrier transport, in the absence of competition, would be expected
to be exquisitely sensitive to changes in blood amino acid levels.
(ii) Competition in plasma with other neutral amino acids. Since
multiple amino acids compete for a common binding site, the net
affinity of the carrier system for a given amino acid varies depending upon the plasma concentration of competing amino acids. Upon
physiological conditions brain entry of a given amino acid will in
fact closely reflect the ratio in plasma between its concentration
and the sum of the competing amino acids. (iii) The activity of the
L-System. Under physiological conditions the L-system activity can
be considered constant. However, the L-system follows the properties
of all the exchange systems, on that its transport activity may be
increased by high internal concentrations of one or more transported
compounds. It is therefore conceivable that high concentrations of
one or more neutral amino acids in the brain side of the BBB can
accelerate the blood to brain transport of other neutral amino
acids. This led James et al.[10] to hypothesize that the increased
blood-brain neutral amino acid transport found in animals with PCA
and hyperammonemia[11] might be linked to brain glutamine accumulation.
According to this hypothesis hyperammonemia and the consequent rise
in brain glutamine would increase the efflux from the brain via the
L-system and in turn stimulate the blood-brain entry of neutral

amino acids. This hypothesis has recently been confirmed in vitro
on isolated brain microvessels (i.e. BBB).[12,13] A significant
correlation in fact was found between glutamine content and labeled
neutral amino acid uptake by microvessels.

RELATIONSHIP BETWEEN BLOOD AND BRAIN AMINO ACID PATTERNS IN
HEPATIC ENCEPHALOPATHY

To further test this hypothesis we decided to investigate in
human HE the possible relationship between CSF glutamine and plasma
and CSF neutral amino acids. For this purpose a·multiple regression
model was used (Figure 1). In this model CSF level of the given
Amino Acid was considered as the independent variable, whereas
either CSF glutamine or the plasma ratio Amino Acid/Competitors
were considered as independent variables. The significant correlation between these three variables has been statistically evaluated
in a series of patients in whom plasma and CSF samples were obtained
at two different moments during the evolution of HE. The first
sample was drawn upon admission at the Hospital (i.e. when patients
were in grade 3-4 HE) whereas the second sample was taken at least
ten days after complete mental recovery from HE (i.e. grade 0 HE).
Multiple regression analyses were then performed in 19 patients in
grade 3-4 HE and in 12 patients in grade 0 HE.

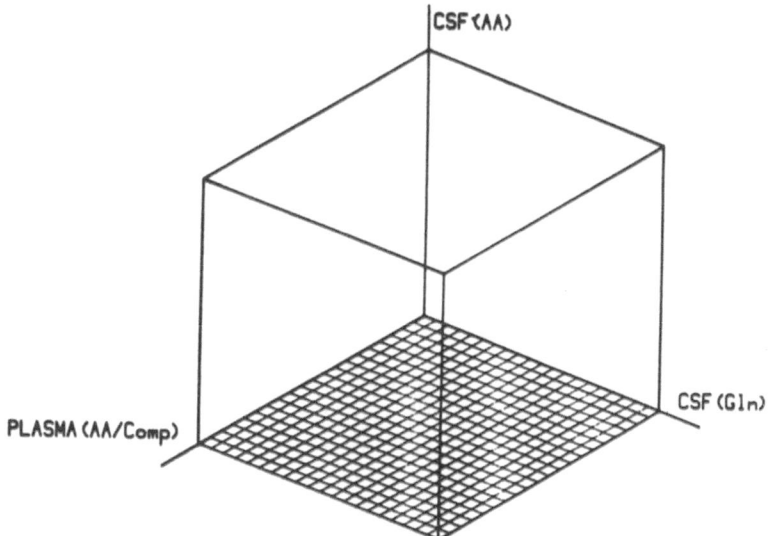

Fig. 1.   Multiple regression model used to assess statistical
          correlations among: (i) the CSF level of a given neutral
          amino acid [CSF(AA)], (ii) the CSF level of glutamine
          [CSF(Gln)], and (iii) the ratio in plasma between the
          given neutral amino acid and all the other competing
          neutral amino acids [Plasma(AA/Comp)].

    In grade 3-4 HE (Figure 2) CSF phenylalanine levels were closely
related either to CSF glutamine or to the ratio between plasma
phenylalanine and the sum of competing neutral amino acids (i.e.:
tyrosine, free tryptophan, valine, leucine, isoleucine and methionine). Conversely, when the same patients were in grade O HE such
a correlation could not be demonstrated (Figure 3). This suggests
that in grade O HE, factors different from those considered may
regulate CSF phenylalanine levels. In these patients linear regression analyses were then performed between the CSF levels of a given
neutral Amino Acid and each of the following: (i) CSF glutamine,
(ii) plasma Amino Acid level and (iii) the ratio in plasma with
competing amino acids. As shown in Table 1, the results obtained
for phenylalanine, leucine and alanine, a "low uptake" amino acid,
were quite similar. The best correlation was always found between
plasma and CSF levels of each of the amino acids considered. No
statistical correlations were found between CSF Amino Acid levels
and either CSF glutamine or the ratio in plasma Amino Acid/Compet-
itors.

    It can be thus hypothesized that in patients with liver
cirrhosis without HE the brain entry of a given neutral amino acid
is independent from the competition for the common carrier system
by other neutral amino acids. These observations together with the
significant correlation found between plasma and CSF amino acid
levels suggest that the major route for amino acid brain entry follow
the rules of a non-saturable transport system more than those of a
saturable one. Similar results were found for other groups of Amino
Acids.

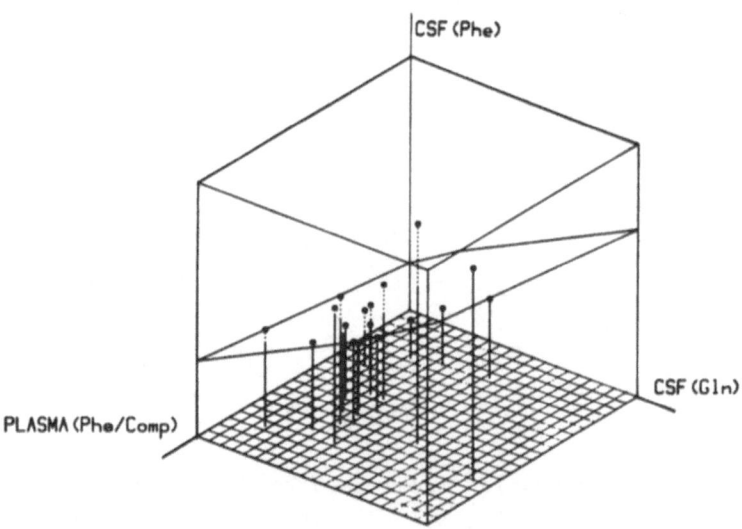

Fig. 2.   Multiple regression analysis using phenylalanine as test
          neutral amino acid in 19 patients in grade 3-4 HE.
          (r^2 = .7771, P < 0.001)

Table 1. Linear regression analyses between plasma and CSF
levels of different neutral amino acids in 12
cirrhotic patients in grade 0 HE.

	CSF Gln	Plasma Phe	Plasma Phe/comp
CSF Phe	r=0.33	r=0.63*	r=0.45
	CSF Gln	Plasma Leu	Plasma Leu/comp
CSF Leu	r=0.19	r=0.77**	r=0.55
	CSF Gln	Plasma Ala	Plasma Ala/comp
CSF Ala	r=0.29	r=0.77*	r=0.17

*
 P < 0.05
**
 P < 0.01

As shown in Figure 4, basic amino acids, which usually cross
the BBB via a specific transport system different from the L-system,
are increased in the CSF of patients in grade 0 HE despite their
normal plasma levels. In grade 3-4 HE no further increase of basic
amino acids could be demonstrated.

CONCLUSIONS

Experimental data obtained either in patients or in animals
seem to confirm the key role played by the BBB in the pathogenesis
of HE. In patients with chronic liver failure the BBB shows two
distinct behaviours depending upon the presence of HE. In cirrhotics
without signs of HE the significant increase of almost all CSF
amino acids could be attributed to a decreased selectivity of the
BBB amino acid transport which can be ascribed to the prevalence
of the non-saturable component of the blood-brain transport. In
grade 3-4 HE, the significant increase of only aromatic amino
acids and methionite suggests the presence of a selective stimulation of the L-system activity, probably consequent to the rise of
brain glutamine. Furthermore, the possibility of improving the
mental state of cirrhotic patients by appropriate treatment[14,15]
seems to confirm that a reversible change of the BBB activity may
play a role in the pathogenesis of HE.

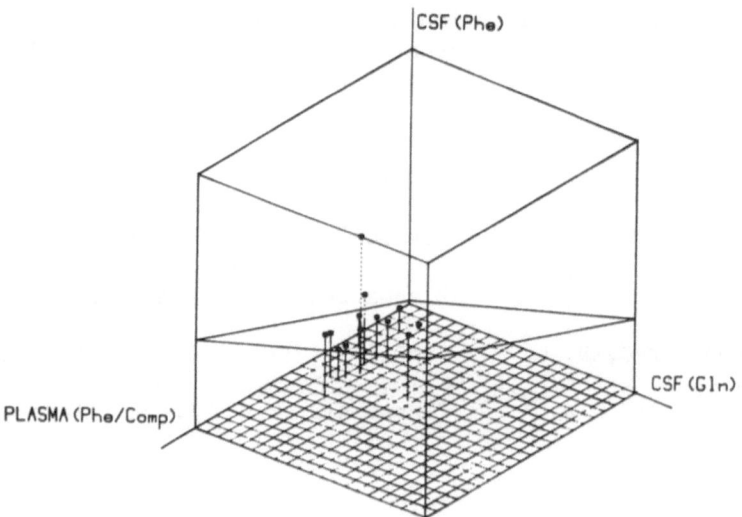

Fig. 3. Multiple regression analysis using phenylalanine as test neutral amino acid in 12 patients in grade O HE. (r^2=.2343, n.s.).

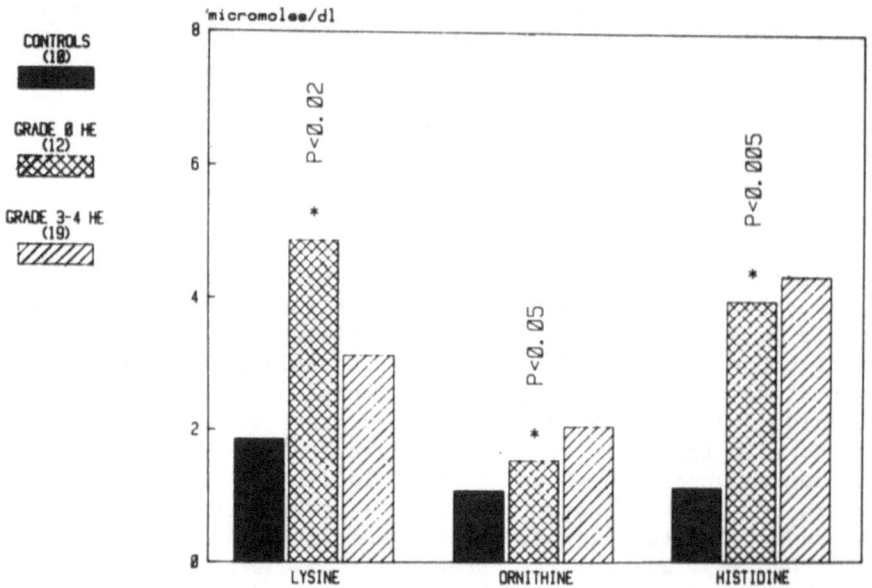

Fig. 4. CSF basic amino acid levels in 10 healthy controls, in 19 patients in grade 3-4 HE, and in 12 patients who completely regained their consciousness (i.e., grade O HE).

REFERENCES

1. A. Cascino, C. Cangiano, V. Calcaterra, F. Rossi-Fanelli,and L. Capocaccia, Plasma amino acid imbalance in patients with liver disease, Am. J. Dig. Dis. 23: 591 (1978).
2. M. Y. Morgan, J. P. Milsom, and S. Sherlock, Plasma ratio of valine, leucine and isoleucine to phenylalanine and tyrosine in liver disease, Gut 19: 1068 (1978).
3. D. G. Hutson, J. Ono, R. S. Dombro, V. J. Levi, A.Livingstone,and R. Zeppa, A longitudinal study of tryptophan involvement in hepatic coma, Am. J. Surg. 137: 235 (1979).
4. G. Marchesini, M. Zoli, C. Bondi, L. Cecchini, F. P. Bianchi,and E. Pisi, Prevalence of subclinical hepatic encephalopathy in cirrhotics and relationship to plasma amino acid imbalance, Dig. Dis. Sci. 25: 235 (1980).
5. C. Cangiano, A. Cascino, F. Fiaccadori, O. Riggio, F.Rossi-Fanelli, and L. Capocaccia, Is the blood-brain barrier really intact in portal-systemic encephalopathy? Lancet i: 1367 (1981).
6. A. Cascino, C. Cangiano, F. Fiaccadori, F. Ghinelli, M. Merli, G. Pelosi, O. Riggio, F. Rossi-Fanelli, D. Sacchini, M. Stortoni,and L. Capocaccia, Plasma and cerebrospinal fluid amino acid patterns in hepatic encephalopathy, Dig. Dis.Sci. 27: 828 (1982).
7. W. H. Oldendorf and J. Szabo, Amino acid assignment to one of the three blood-brain barrier amino acid carriers, Am. J. Physiol. 230: 94 (1976).
8. W. M. Pardridge, Regulation of amino acid availability to the brain in: "Nutrition and the Brain" Vol. 1 R. J. Wurtman, J. J. Wurtman, eds., Raven Press, New York (1979).
9. P. Cardelli-Cangiano, C. Cangiano, J. H. James, B. Jeppsson,W. Brenner,and J. E. Fischer, Uptake of amino acids by brain microvessels isolated from rats after portacaval anastomosis, J. Neurochem. 36: 627 (1981).
10. J. H. James, V. Ziparo, B. Jeppsson, and J. E. Fischer, Hyperammonemia, plasma amino acid imbalance and blood brain amino acid transport: A unified theory of portal-systemic encephalopathy, Lancet ii: 772 (1979).
11. J. H. James, J. Escourrou, and J.E. Fischer, Blood-brain neutral amino acid transport activity is increased after porta-caval anastomosis, Science 200: 1395 (1978).
12. C. Cangiano, P. Cardelli-Cangiano, J.H. James, and J.E. Fischer, Ammonia stimulates amino acid uptake by bovine isolated brain microvessels, Gastroenterology 78: 1302, (1980).
13. C. Cangiano, P. Cardelli-Cangiano, J. H. James, F. Rossi-Fanelli, M. A. Patrizi, K. A. Brackett, R. Strom, and J.E. Fischer, Brain microvessels take up large neutral amino acids in exchange for glutamine. Cooperative role of Na-dependent and Na-independent systems, J. Biol. Chem. (submitted for publication).

14. F. Fiaccadori, F. Ghinelli, G. Pelosi, D. Sacchini, G. L. Vaona,
     M. L. Zeneroli, E. Rocchi, V. Santunione, P. Gibertini, and E.
     Ventura, Selective amino acid solutions in hepatic encepha-
     lopathy, La Ricerca 10: 411 (1980).
15. F. Rossi-Fanelli, O. Riggio, C. Cangiano, A. Cascino, D. De
     Conciliis, M. Merli, M. Stortoni and G. Giunchi (Coordinator
     L. Capocaccia), Branched-chain amino acids vs. lactulose in
     the treatment of hepatic coma, Dig. Dis. Sci. 27: 929 (198").

ALTERATIONS OF PLASMA AND BRAIN TRYPTOPHAN IN HEPATIC ENCEPHALOPATHY:

A STUDY IN HUMANS AND IN EXPERIMENTAL ANIMALS

F. Salerno, M. Dell'Oca, P. Incerti, F. Uggeri°, and
E. Beretta°

Clinica Medica III and °Clinica Chirurgica V, Università
di Milano, Milano, Italy

SUMMARY

The role of tryptophan in the pathogenesis of hepatic encephalopathy has been investigated both in humans and in experimental
animals with a model of chronic liver failure. In a group of 149
patients with liver cirrhosis, it was shown that plasma free tryptophan (the amino acid not bound to albumin) significantly rose when
liver function was impaired. This increase was well correlated to
the grade of hepatic encephalopathy. The ratio free tryptophan/neutral
amino acids showed a comparable behavior. Additionally, free tryptophan markedly decreased in patients recovered from encephalopathy
after infusion of an amino acid solution rich in branched chain amino
acids. In rats with porto-caval anastomosis brain tryptophan significantly increased to a much larger extent than plasma free tryptophan did. An enhanced activity of the transport system specific for
neutral amino acids through the blood brain barrier was confirmed
and, at least partly, ascribed to the hyperinsulinemia present after
portocaval anastomosis. Serotonin brain levels showed a relatively
small increase compared to tryptophan and 5-hydroxyindolacetic acid,
implying that tryptophan-hydroxylase could be proportionately inhibited in such experimental model of chronic liver disease.

INTRODUCTION

Tryptophan is involved in the amino acid imbalance present in
patients with advanced liver cirrhosis.[1,2,3] In such patients plasma
free tryptophan, phenylalanine and tyrosine are all increased in
contrast to normal or decreased branched chain amino acids (BCAA).
This peripheral change would lead aromatic amino acids (AAA) to
accumulate in central nervous system (CNS), because all neutral

95

amino acids (BCAA + AAA) compete for transport across the blood brain barrier (BBB) through a common transport system.[4,5,6] The hypothesis that tryptophan is implicated in the pathogenesis of hepatic encephalopathy arose from the knowledge that brain tryptophan is the precursor of serotonin (5-HT), an aminergic neurotransmitter which exerts profound effects both on consciousness and on behavior of man and animals.[7,8] Moreover, it has been shown that the administration of L-tryptophan is comagenic in normal subjects,[9] in patients with liver disease[10,11] and in normal dogs when infused with phenylalanine.[12] However, as for other substances implicated in the pathogenesis of hepatic coma, a relationship of cause and effect with the neurological signs of coma is difficult to demonstrate.

In the present study, the behavior of tryptophan in severe liver disease and its possible involvement in the pathogenesis of portal systemic encephalopathy (PSE) has been evaluated both in humans and in experimental animals. Patients with chronic liver disease were investigated to determine the relationship between plasma tryptophan concentrations and the presence or the deepness of encephalopathy. Brain concentrations of tryptophan, 5-HT and 5-hydroxyindolacetic acid (5-HIAA), as well as the activity of the NAA transport system through the BBB, were measured in rats with PCA.

MATERIALS AND METHODS

Human Study

This study was carried out on 38 normal subjects (28 males and 10 females) and 149 cirrhotic patients (117 males and 32 females) defined by clinical, biochemical and (68% of cases) histological criteria (43 alcoholic, 45 postnecrotic, 55 cryptogenic and 6 primary biliary cirrhosis).

According to the neurological state assessed by the criteria of Adams and Foley[13] all patients were classified in three further groups: coma 0, coma 1-2 and coma 3-4. Nine patients with deep encephalopathy were studied before and after 5 days of treatment with total parenteral nutrition employing a glucose-amino acid solution rich in BCAA (BS666, Boehringer Biochemia Robin, Milan), the composition of which is the same as the FO80 first used by Fischer.[14] These patients were compared with 8 encephalopathic patients treated with lactulose enemas and oral protein intake restriction (less than 40 grams daily). Blood was collected into heparinized tubes on the morning after an overnight fasting. In all subjects plasma total and free tryptophan, the whole amino acid pattern, albumin, FFA, bilirubin, ammonia and glucose were evaluated.

Plasma total and free tryptophan were assayed by the method of Denkla and Dewey[15] as modified by Tagliamonte[16] after separation

of unbound tryptophan according to Stefanini.[17] Amino acid pattern
was determined in the supernatants of plasma samples deproteinized
with sulphosalicylic acid (50 mg/ml) by cation exchange chromatography with a Carlo Erba 3A28M amino acid analyzer (Carlo Erba, Rodano
Milan). FFA and ammonia were measured by colorimetric methods.[18,19]

Animal Study

Thirty-six male Sprague-Dawley rats (180-200 grams) were submitted to PCA according to the method of Funovics.[20] Twenty-eight
weight-matched animals were sham-operated as controls. In 8 PCA and
8 sham-operated animals diabetes was induced 4 days before the
sacrifice by injection of streptozotocin intraperitoneally (65 mg/kg,
Upjohn Ltd, dissolved in 0.07 M-sodium citrate buffer pH 4.5). Animals
were studied 28-32 days after PCA had been performed. In 16 PCA and
8 sham-operated rats blood was taken from the abdominal aorta just
before sacrifice, then animals were killed by decapitation and brain
rapidly removed, divided sagittally and immediately frozen on dry
ice. In these animals plasma and brain amino acids, 5-HT and 5-HIAA
were determined. In 12 PCA rats, 12 sham-operated controls and in
animals with streptozotocin-induced diabetes (8 PCA and 8 controls)
brain uptake of either tryptophan or leucine or ornithine was measured in vivo by the single injection dual isotope label technique of
Oldendorf[6] and expressed as brain uptake index (BUI), that is the
percent of amino acid uptaken in respect of free diffusable water.
Brain tryptophan, 5-HT and 5-HIAA were determined fluorimetrically
in acidified butanol extracts of one hemisphere according to the
method of Denkla and Dewey[15] and to that of Curzon and Green[21]
respectively. Brain amino acids were measured with an amino acid analyzer using hemispheres homogenized in a solution of sulphosalicylic
acid (30% in saline). Statistical analysis were performed with
Student's test for paired and unpaired data as appropriate.

RESULTS

Human Study

Table 1 reports the results obtained from the study of three
subgroups of cirrhotic patients compared to a group of normal
controls. Total tryptophan mean level was normal in patients without
any neurological symptoms (60.89 + 3.38 nmol/ml), but significantly
lower in patients with slight or deep coma (43.22 + 3.63 and 41.46
+ 5.63 nmol/ml respectively, P < 0.001 vs controls). Free tryptophan
mean levels were greatly increased in all groups of cirrhotic
patients, being 10.96 + 0.69 nmol/ml in patients with coma 0 (P < 0.01
vs controls), 15.57 + 1.26 noml/ml in patients with coma 1-2
(P < 0.01 vs coma 0) and 19.82 + 3.54 nmol/ml in patients with coma
3-4 (NS vs coma 1-2). Considering the factors which are known (or
suggested) to interfere with the binding of tryptophan on serum
albumin, it was found that: a) serum albumin was markedly decreased

Table 1. Concentration of plasma tryptophan and other plasma
substances interfering with their binding to albumin
in normal controls and in patients with liver cirrhosis

	controls (32)	coma 0 (80)	coma 1-2 (53)	coma 3-4 (16)
Total try (nmol/ml)	64.2+2.5	60.8+3.3	43.2+3.6	41.4+5.6
Free try (nmol/ml)	2.9+0.2	10.9+0.7	15.5+1.2	19.8+3.5
Albumin (g/dl)	4.4+0.3	3.34+0.08	2.94+0.08	2.77+0.15
Unconjugated bilirubin (mg/dl)	0.5+0.1	1.6+0.2	2.55+0.38	3.28+0.68
FFA (mEq)	0.35+0.03	0.60+0.06	0.66+0.07	0.51+0.09

Values are expressed as means ± SEM.

in cirrhosis, and the lowest concentration was found in the group of
patients with deep encephalopathy (2.77 +0.15 g/dl, $P < 0.001$ vs
controls, $P < 0.005$ vs coma 0, NS vs coma 1-2); b) unconjugated
bilirubin was elevated significantly in cirrhosis compared to normal controls (1.6 ± 0.2 vs 0.5 ± 0.1 mg/dl, $P < 0.05$), and also in
patients with deep coma compared to nonencephalopathic patients
($P < 0.005$, coma 3-4 vs coma 0); c) FFA were increased in all cirrhotic patients without any significant differences among the three
subgroups. However, when linear regression analyses were performed
neither albumin ($r = -0.21$) nor bilirubin ($r = 0.26$) nor FFA
($r = 0.05$) showed any significant correlation with the unbound amino
acid. Table 2 reports the molar ratios of tryptophan on NAA compared
to the ratio between BCAA and the sum phenylalanine + tyrosine. The
ratio free tryptophan/NAA showed a significant rise in patients with
stable cirrhosis ($P < 0.02$ vs controls), but no significant changes
between patients with and without encephalopathy. On the contrary,
the molar ratio total tryptophan/NAA was affected only in patients
with deep encephalopathy ($P < 0.05$ vs controls). Data obtained from
the study of nine encephalopathic patients before and after five
days of parenteral nutrition are reported in Table 3. The results

Table 2. Molar ratios between total or free tryptophan and NAA
         in comparison to the molar ratio NAA/TYR+PHE in normal
         controls and patients with liver cirrhosis

	Controls (32)	Coma 0 (80)	Coma 1-2 (53)	Coma 3-4 (16)
Total try / NAA	0.114+0.009	0.130+0.023	0.130+0.022	0.069+0.018
Free try / NAA	0.006+0.001	0.024+0.004	0.030+0.005	0.033+0.010
BCAA / PHE+TYR	3.32+0.17	1.44+0.13	0.95+0.07	1.28+0.40

Values are expressed as means $\pm$ SEM.

Table 3. Plasma NAA concentrations and molar ratios between
         tryptophan and NAA in encephalopathic patients sub-
         mitted to parenteral nutrition (A) or lactulose and
         oral diet (B)

	A		B	
	Pre	Post	Pre	Post
Free try	22.5+5.5	8.8+1.6 **	13.8+1.5	12.1+1.5
Tyr	132 +15	152 +15	152 +25	133 +20
Phe	108 + 9	128 +11	97 + 7	104 + 6
Val	129 +12	174 +21 *	140 +10	145 + 7
Leu	68 + 2	92 + 5 **	79 + 6	79 + 3
Ile	37 + 1	55 + 4 **	39 + 3	38 + 2
Free try/NAA	0.046	0.014 *	0.027	0.024
BCAA/Phe+Tyr	1.01	1.22	1.00	1.01

Values are expressed as means $\pm$ SEM (nmol/ml)
  * $P < 0.05$ ** $P < 0.005$.

are compared with those observed in eight more patients treated with
oral protein intake restriction and lactulose. Parenteral nutrition
was performed by giving 1000 ml daily (from 0800 to 2200) of a
glucose-amino acid solution rich in BCAA and allowing a caloric
intake of about 1200 Cal per day. Patients submitted to such a treatment recovered from encephalopathy earlier than patients treated
with lactulose and oral diet. Before starting the treatment, the
concentration of free tryptophan was higher in the first group of
patients (22.5+5.5 vs 13.8+1.5 nmol/ml, P < 0.05). After five days
of therapy free tryptophan appeared significantly reduced in patients
under parenteral nutrition (8.87+1.6 nmol/ml, P < 0.05 vs pretreatment level) and unchanged in control patients (12.1+1.5 nmol/ml).

Therefore, the final concentration of plasma free tryptophan
was significantly lower in patients treated with solutions rich in
BCAA (P < 0.05). The molar ratio free tryptophan/NAA improved after
five days of infusions (from 0.046+0.011 to 0.014+0.005, P < 0.05),
but it was unchanged after lactulose and oral diet (from 0.027 +0.008
to 0.024 + 0.007).

Animal Study

Rate submitted to PCA showed changes of plasma NAA concentrations such as those found in patients with advanced cirrhosis
(Table 4). Compared to sham-operated animals, rats with PCA had the
same concentration of total tryptophan and a double level of free
tryptophan (22.5 + 8.3 vs 11.25 + 2.35 nmol/ml, P < 0.02). Also the
ratio between free tryptophan and NAA was significantly higher in
rats with PCA (0.036 + 0.03 vs 0.019 + 0.006, P < 0.01). Accordingly, after PCA tryptophan rose significantly in brain tissue
(15.3 + 5.1 vs 3.7 + 0.7 ug/g, P < 0.001), leading to raised concentrations of 5-HIAA (1.23 + 0.3 vs 0.43 + 0.03 ug/g, P < 0.02)
but not of 5HT (1.05 + 0.16 vs 0.9 + 0.07 ug/g, NS).

The activity of the transport system specific for NAA through
the BBB was considerably enhanced in rats with PCA compared to sham-
operated controls, as shown for tryptophan and leucine (Table 5).
On the contrary, BUI of ornithine, a basic amino acid, was markedly
reduced. When PCA rats were studied four days after the induction
of diabetes with streptozotocin injection, BUI of leucine was not
statistically different from that observed in sham-operated animals
without diabetes.

DISCUSSION

The role of tryptophan in the pathogenesis of hepatic encephalopathy has been supported by several authors.[1,2,3,11,22,23]
However, a relationship between plasma or cerebrospinal (CSF) tryptophan and the stage of encephalopathy is still controversial,[24]
while the mechanism by which tryptophan should exert its toxic

Table 4. Plasma and brain NAA and brain indoleamines in PCA
and sham-operated rats

	Plasma (nmol/ml)		Brain (nmol/g)	
	Controls (8)	PCA (12)	Controls (8)	PCA (12)
Try (free)	11.2+ 1.9	22.5+ 8.3[•]	18.1+0.8	75.2+25.2[•]
Tyr	87.3+ 6.6	108 +21	24.8+2.2	96 + 3.6[•]
Phe	106 + 4.8	158 + 4.8[•]	29.7+3.0	124 + 8.5[•]
Val	205 + 9.4	165 +20.5	47 +1.7	34 + 1.7[*]
Leu	99 + 5.3	110 +22.8	33.6+3.2	39.7+ 1.5
Ile	67 +12.2	70 +10.6	15.3+1.5	13 + 3.0
5-HT			5.1+0.4	6.03+ 0.9
5-HIAA			2.25+0.15	6.4+ 1.58

Values are expressed as means $\pm$ SEM
$*$ P < 0.01 $•$ P < 0.001

effect on CNS remains poorly investigated. Tryptophan circulates in
blood in two forms, bound and unbound.[25] The proportion of tryptophan that is bound could be modified by physiologic or pathologic
events. The present study shows that plasma total tryptophan is
reduced in patients with liver cirrhosis and deep encephalopathy,
while it is normal in the other groups of cirrhotic patients. Such
a result could be explained taking into account that patients with
deep coma are frequently in a catabolic state[26,27] and quite invariably in a fasting state. Fasting and diseases characterized by a
catabolic state are both associated to low tryptophan plasma level.
[23,28] Free tryptophan was increased in all patients investigated
and well correlated with the grade of encephalopathy. The molar
ratio free tryptophan/NAA showed a comparable behavior. These findings are consistent with those previously reported by Cascino.[2] In
the past years, evidence has been accumulated that plasma free
tryptophan and its ratio to NAA play the major role in determining
the entry of tryptophan into the CNS.[5,16,29] Therefore, it is
conceivable, by means of our findings, that brain tryptophan is
progressively increasing in patients with liver cirrhosis up to a
maximum concentration in those with overt encephalopathy. Moreover,
patients who recovered from coma following parenteral infusion of
solutions rich in BCAA showed a significant fall of their free
tryptophan plasma levels as well as of the ratio between free tryptophan and NAA. Although CSF tryptophan concentrations have not
been determined in the present study, it is conceivable that also
brain tryptophan was decreased after recovery from coma. Such
hypothesis is supported by the previous evidence that BCAA injected

Table 5. BUI for amino acids in PCA or sham-operated rats.
          Effects of the streptozotocin-induced diabetes

	Controls	PCA	Controls + diabetes	PCA + diabetes
Try	29.3+1	44.4+1.8	----	----
Leu	12.6+1.25	25.8+3.2	7.5+0.4	14.8+1.06
Orn	19.1+1.40	6.5+0.8	----	6.8+0.9

Values are expressed as means + SEM.

intraperitoneally was able to reduce significantly both tryptophan
and 5-HT in the brain of anhepatic rats.[30] These data, taken all
together, indicate that the control of plasma free tryptophan levels
play a relevant role in patients with chronic liver disease. Unfortunately the mechanism underlying the rise of free tryptophan in
cirrhosis is still to be elucidated. The main hypothesis is that the
binding of tryptophan to albumin is impaired both by reduced serum
albumin[1,2] and by accumulation of factors competing with tryptophan
for albumin binding as FFA[1] and unconjugated bilirubin.[3] In our
experience no correlation was found between free tryptophan levels
and either albumin or FFA or unconjugated bilirubin. These data do
not exclude a real influence of the abovementioned factors on tryptophan binding ability; however, it can be suggested that the
equilibrium between bound and unbound tryptophan in a pathologic
state as liver cirrhosis is regulated by a more complicated process,
probably depending from changed affinity of the amino acid for the
peripheral tissues transport sites.

     One of the most impressive findings in favor of the implication
of peripheral tryptophan in hepatic coma has been recently obtained
by Rossi-Fanelli[12] who induced a coma state in normal dogs by intracarotid infusion of tryptophan and phenylalanine. In that experiment
tryptophan rose markedly in the liquor after injection, suggesting
that also brain tryptophan was consistently increased. Although
other mechanisms were not ruled out, enhanced turnover of 5-HT
appeared to be the easiest way by which high tryptophan concentrations
would produce undesirable effects.[1] However, in our experimental
study, rats with PCA performed four weeks before showed a relatively
small increase of brain 5-HT compared to tryptophan and 5-HIAA. Such
a result, which is consistent with those of Bloxam,[31] would imply
that 5-HT brain turnover is only partly enhanced by tryptophan rise
in PCA animals. In accord with this hypothesis, cirrhotic patients
with encephalopathy were shown to have an unchanged brain 5-HT turnover when CSF 5-HIAA was measured after probenecid administration.[32]

Thus, it is conceivable that the high brain tryptophan levels determined by PCA allowed a reduced activity of tryptophan-hydroxylase, the rate limiting step in 5-HT synthesis. Recently, Neckers[33] showed an inverse relationship between tryptophan and tryptophan-hydroxylase when the amino acid brain concentration was modified by pharmacological manipulations. This finding has been considered a mechanism to shield serotonergic neurons from global changes in blood or brain tryptophan levels. On the basis of these new acknowledgements, one can speculate that the neurological dysfunction induced by giving high tryptophan amounts to both humans and animals[9,10,11,12] were due to unknown mechanisms not involving 5-HT de novo synthesis. Otherwise, it is well known that cerebral changes produced in experimental animals by the administration of L-tryptophan are not limited to indoleamine turnover. This because both the cathecolaminergic system and probably several peptidergic systems are influenced by the entry of tryptophan into the CNS.[7,34]

A further means by which tryptophan accumulates in the CNS of cirrhotic animals is the enhanced activity of the transport system through the BBB specific for NAA. This finding, firstly reported by James,[35] justifies that brain tryptophan rose to a higher extent than plasma free tryptophan did. Change in the brain intake ability for NAA in PCA rats has been attributed hypothetically to the parallel accumulation of glutamine in CNS.[36] In the present study, clear evidence is reported that circulating insulin plays a causing role. Insulin was shown to modulate the brain uptake of tyrosine and tryptophan in normal animals.[37,38] PCA is invariably associated to hyperinsulinemia, and the injection of streptozotocin, a drug destroying b cells of the pancreas, normalized the BUI of leucine in PCA rats.

REFERENCES

1. J. Ono, D. G. Hutson, R. S. Dombro, J. U. Levi, A. Livingstone, and R. Zeppa, Tryptophan and hepatic coma, Gastroenterology 74: 196 (1978).
2. A. Cascino, C. Cangiano, V. Calcaterra, F. Rossi-Fanelli, and L. Capocaccia, Plasma amino acid imbalance in patients with liver disease, Am. J. Dig. Dis. 23: 591 (1978).
3. F. Salerno, F. S. Dioguardi, and R. Abbiati, Tryptophan and hepatic coma, Gastroenterology 75: 769 (1978).
4. W. H. Oldendorf, Brain uptake of radiolabelled amino acids, amines and hexoses after arterial injection, Am. J. Physiol. 221: 1629 (1971).
5. J. Perez-Cruet, T. Chase, and D. L. Murphy, Dietary regulations of brain tryptophan metabolism by plasma ratio of free tryptophan and neutral amino acids in humans, Nature (Lond.) 248: 693 (1974).
6. W. H. Oldendorf and J. Szabo, Amino acid assignment to one of three blood-brain barrier amino acid carriers, Am. J. Physiol.

230: 94 (1976).

7. R. J. Baldessarini and J. E. Fischer, Serotonin metabolism in rat brain after surgical diversion of the portal venous circulation, Nature (New Biol.) 245: 25 (1973).

8. D. W. Woolley, "The Biochemical Bases of Psychoses or the Serotonin Hypothesis about Mental Disease," John Wiley and Sons, New York (1962).

9. B. Smith and D. J. Prockop, Central-nervous-system effects of ingestion of L-tryptophan by normal subjects, N. Eng. J. Med. 267: 1338 (1962).

10. K. Ogihara, T. Mozai,and S. N. Hirai, Tryptophan as cause of hepatic coma, N. Eng. J. Med. 275: 1255 (1966).

11. C. Hirayama, Tryptophan metabolism in liver disease, Clin. Chim. Acta 32: 191 (1971).

12. F. Rossi-Fanelli, H. Freund, R. Krause, A. R. Smith, J. H. James, S. Castorina-Ziparo,and J. E. Fischer, Induction of coma in normal dogs by the infusion of aromatic amino acids and its prevention by the addition of branched-chain amino acids, Gastroenterology 83: 664 (1982).

13. R. D. Adams and J. M. Foley, Neurological disorder associated with liver disease, Res. Publ. Assoc. Res. Nerv. Ment. Dis. 32: 198 (1958).

14. J. E. Fischer, H. M. Rosen, A. M. Ebeid, J. H. James, J. M. Keaney,and P. B. Soeters, The effect of normalization of plasma amino acids in hepatic encephalopathy in man, Surgery 78: 276 (1976).

15. W. D. Denkla and H. K. Dewey, The determination of tryptophan concentration in plasma, liver and urine, J. Lab. Clin. Med. 69: 160 (1967).

16. A. Tagliamonte, G. Biggio, L. Vargiu,and G. L. Gessa, Free tryptophan in serum controls brain tryptophan levels and serotonin synthesis, Life Sci. 12: 277 (1973).

17. E. Stefanini and G. Biggio, A simple method for determination of free tryptophan in serum, Riv. Farmacol. Ter. 6: 49 (1975).

18. S. Laurell and G. Tibbling, Colorimetric microdetermination of free fatty acids in plasma, Clin. Chim. Acta 16: 57 (1967).

19. G. E.Miller and J. D. Rice Jr., Determination of the concentration of blood ammonia by use of cation exchange resin, J. Lab. Clin. Med. 60: 170 (1962).

20. J. M. Funovics, M. G. Cummings, L. Shuman, J. H. James,and J. E. Fischer, An improved nonsuture method for portocaval anastomosis in the rat, Surgery 77: 661 (1975).

21. G. Curzon and A. R. Green, Rapid method for the determination of 5-hydroxytryptamine and 5-hydroxyindolacetic acid in small regions of rat brain, Br. J. Pharmacol. 39: 653 (1970).

22. G. Marchesini, M. Zoli, C. Dondi, L. Cecchini, A. Angiolini, F. B. Bianchi,and E. Pisi, Prevalence of subclinical hepatic encephalopathy in cirrhotics and relationship to plasma amino acid imbalance, Dig. Dis. Sci. 25: 763 (1980).

23. M. L. Zeneroli, C. Cremonini, F. Licari, G. Pinelli, C. Gollini, L. Pranzini, and E. Ventura, Effect of short-term fasting on plasma tryptophan in liver cirrhosis, Ital. J. Gastroenterol. 13: 186 (1981).

24. D. G. Hutson, J. Ono, R. S. Dombro, J. U. Levi, A. Livingstone, and R. Zeppa, A longitudinal study of tryptophan involvement in hepatic coma, Am. J. Surgery 137: 235 (1979).

25. R. H. McMenamy and J. L. Oncley, The specific binding of tryptophan to serum albumin, J. Biol. Chem. 233: 1436 (1958).

26. G. Marchesini, M. Zoli, A. Angiolini, C. Dondi, F. B. Bianchi, and E. Pisi, Muscle protein breakdown in liver cirrhosis and the role of altered carbohydrate metabolism, Hepatology 1: 294 (1981).

27. F. Fiaccadori, F. Ghinelli, G. Pedretti, G. Pelosi, D. Sacchini, and G. Spadini, Negative nitrogen balance in cirrhotics, La Ricerca Clin. Lab. 11: 259 (1981).

28. S. A. Adibi, A. L. Drash, and E. D. Livi, Hormone and amino acid levels in altered nutritional states, J. Lab. Clin. Med. 76: 722 (1970).

29. J. C. Fernando, P. J. Knott, and G. Curzon, The relevance of both plasma free tryptophan and insulin to rat brain tryptophan concentrations, J. Neurochem. 27: 343 (1976).

30. J. H. James, P. M. Herlin, L. Edwards, C. A. Nachbauer, and J. E. Fischer, Effect of infusing the branched-chain amino acids on concentrations of amino acids in plasma and brain and on brain catecholamines after total hepatectomy in the rat, Life Sci. 30: 1361 (1982).

31. D. L. Bloxam and G. Curzon, A study of proposed determinants of brain tryptophan concentration in rats after portocaval anastomosis or sham operation, J. Neurochem. 34: 1255 (1978).

32. S. Lai, A. Aronoff, E. Garelis, T. L. Sourkes, S. Young, and C. E. de la Vega, Cerebrospinal fluid homovanillic acid, 5-hydroxyindolacetic acid, lactic acid and pH before and after probenecid in hepatic coma, Clin. Neurosurg. 22: 142 (1975).

33. L. M. Neckers, G. Biggio, E. Moja, and J. L. Meek, Modulation of brain tryptophan hydroxylase activity by brain tryptophan content, J. Pharmacol. Exp. Ther. 201: 110 (1977).

34. C. B. Lamers, J. E. Morley, P. Poitras, B. Sharp, H. E. Carlson, J. M. Hershman, and J. H. Walsh, Immunological and biological studies on cholecystokinin in rat brain, Am. J. Physiol. 239: E232 (1980).

35. J. H. James, J. Escourrou, and J. E. Fischer, Blood-brain amino acid transport activity is increased after portocaval anastomosis, Science 200: 1395 (1978).

36. J. H. James, B. Jeppsson, V. Ziparo, and J. E. Fischer, Hyperammonemia, plasma amino acid imbalance and blood-brain amino acid transport: a unified theory of portal-systemic encephalopathy, Lancet 2: 772 (1979).

37. M. G. DeMontis, M. C. Olianas, B. Haber, and A. Tagliamonte,

Increase in large neutral amino acid transport into brain
by insulin, J. <u>Neurochem</u>. 30: 121 (1978).

NEW METHODS FOR THE DETERMINATION OF SERUM AND BREATH MERCAPTANS

AND ITS APPLICATION IN LIVER CIRRHOSIS AND HEPATIC ENCEPHALOPATHY

A. Tangerman, M. T. Meuwese-Arends and J. H. M. Van Tongeren

Department of Medicine, Division of Gastroenterology
St. Radboud Hospital, University of Nijmegen
6500 HB Nijmegen, The Netherlands

INTRODUCTION

Mercaptans are extremely toxic compounds that appear to be largely derived from colonic bacterial metabolism of methionine. They have been suggested as being one of the endogenous factors responsible for hepatic coma.[1,2] The reports in literature on breath[3,4] and serum or blood mercaptans[5-7] are highly conflicting. This is probably due to differences in assay and to technical difficulties to measure mercaptans in a reproducible way. The reports on serum and blood mercaptans[4-6] all focus on the use of zinc and acid to release the mercaptans, assuming that the mercaptans are largely covalently bound to proteins in a disulfide linkage. However, this reaction is a very agressive and aspecific one. It gives all kinds of unwanted side reactions, such as degradation of methionine, resulting in falsely elevated levels of methanethiol and dimethylsulfide.

This paper presents new methods for the measurement of volatile sulfur compounds in breath and serum. Very mild and specific methods for the release of sulfur volatiles from serum have been developed. The released volatiles are assayed quantitatively by exhaustive sampling of the headspace gas, concentration of the headspace gas on to Tenax, and gas chromatography of the concentrated sample, using a specific sulfur detector.

METHODS

Breath

The sampling procedure is shown in figure 1B. After 15 s of

108 A. TANGERMAN ET AL.

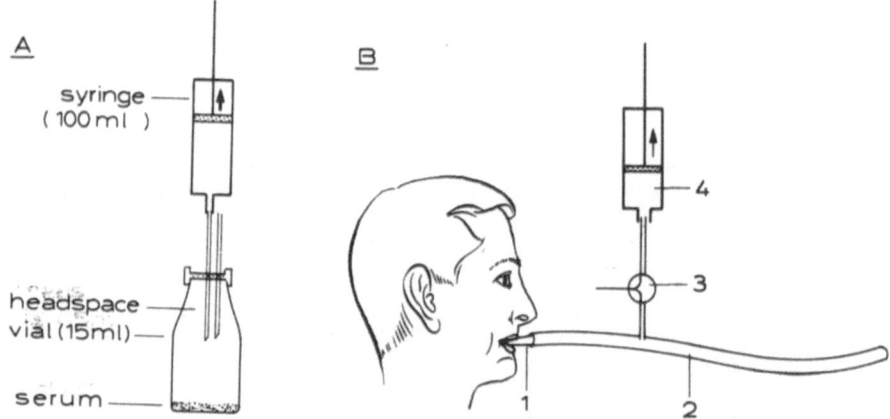

A: Sampling of the serum headspace gas
B: Sampling of breath

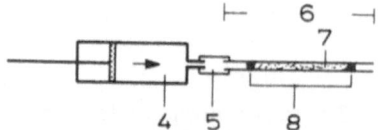

Concentration of mercaptans onto Tenax

Fig. 1. Sampling procedures for serum and breath and concentration of mercaptans onto Tenax. 1, mouthpiece; 2, polypropylene tubing (2 m length, 1 cm i.d.); 3, polypropylene three-way valve; 4, polypropylene gas-tight syringe (100 ml capacity); 5, connecting tubing; 6, glass trap tube (length: 8 cm; i.d. 4 mm), containing 200 mg of Tenax GC; 7, Tenax GC (80-100 mesh); 8, glass wool.

breath-holding, the subject breathes through a polypropylene tubing. Towards the end of a prolonged uninterrupted expiration, 100 ml of breath was collected out of the tube by means of a gas-tight syringe. The breath was then passed through the Tenax glass trap tube (see Figure 1). The glass trap tube could replace the glass liner in the injection port of the gas chromatograph within seconds. The adsorbed sulfur compounds were then thermally liberated directly into the carrier gas stream and transferred to the gas chromatographic column.

Serum

Release of methanethiol (MT) by acid (fraction P). To 250 μl of serum in a 15 ml stoppered septum vial were added 250 μl HCl (5 Mol/1). The mixture was vortexed during 10 s and left at room temperature for 1 minute after which time the release of MT was complete. One sampling of 60 ml of headspace gas (see Fig. 1A), concentration on to Tenax and gas chromatography, gave a yield of 80% of the released MT.

Release of MT by dithiothreitol (fraction Q). To 250 μl of serum in a 15 ml stoppered septum vial were added 100 μl of an aqueous solution of dithiothreitol (10 mg/ml). The mixture was vortexed during 10 s at room temperature after which time the release of MT was complete. One sampling of 60 ml of headspace, concentration onto Tenax and gas chromatography gave a yield of 80% of the released MT.

Release of dimethylsulfide (DMS) from whole blood. DMS is a neutral volatile molecule and is not covalently bound in serum or blood. It escapes in the open air during blood centrifugation. Its determination must therefore be performed in whole blood. Two ml of blood were injected into a 15 ml stoppered vial immediately after withdrawal from the patient. Five consecutive samplings of 60 ml of headspace at room temperature, concentration onto Tenax and gas chromatography gave a 100 per cent recovery of DMS.

Gas Chromatography

A Packard gas chromatograph, type 429, equipped with a flame photometric detector, was used for analysis. Column: 2 m x 4 mm i.d., glass, packed with 20% SE-30 on Chromosorb P 60–80 mesh. Column temperature: 65°C; injector: 200°C; detector; 180°C. N_2 (carrier gas), 30 ml/min; H_2, 140 ml/min; Air 1,80 ml/min; Air 2, 110 ml/min. All glass-ware was coated with dichlorodimethylsilane (5% in toluene). Calibration was performed by injecting standard amounts of the sulfur volatiles into the large sampling syringe, containing 60–100 ml of air. This gas mixture was then treated in the same way as described for breath and serum headspace. The lines produced by plotting the logarithm of dose vs the logarithm of peak height were used for calibration. A gas chromatogram of a standard mixture of sulfur volatiles is shown in Figure 2.

RESULTS

Metabolites of Methanethiol in Serum

MT released by acid (fraction P). To study the origin of the acid-hydrolysable MT fraction, diaflo filtration experiments were carried out. The concentration of fraction P in the filtrate, using the Amicon diaflo filter UM 05 > 500 MW, was the same as that in whole serum. This means that this MT fraction is covalently bound in serum to a compound with a molecular mass <500. A thiolester is proposed (Figure 3).

MT released by dithiothreitol (fraction Q). Dithiothreitol has been reported[8] to be a specific reagent for the quantitative reduction of disulfides. Diaflo filtration experiments, using the filter

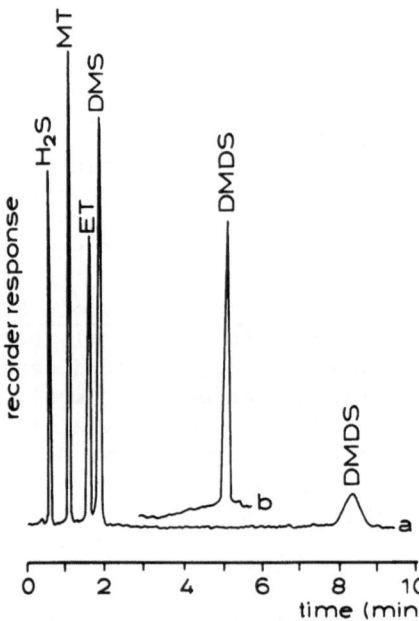

Fig. 2. Gas chromatogram of a standard mixture of H$_2$S (1 ng), MT
(1.5 ng), ET (3.0 ng), DMS (3.0 ng), and DMDS (6.0 ng).
(a) Isothermal run, 65°C; (b) programmed run; initial
temperature of 65°C for 2.2 min, then programming to a
final temperature of 105°C at a rate of 35°C per minute.
Detector attenuation: 10x32.

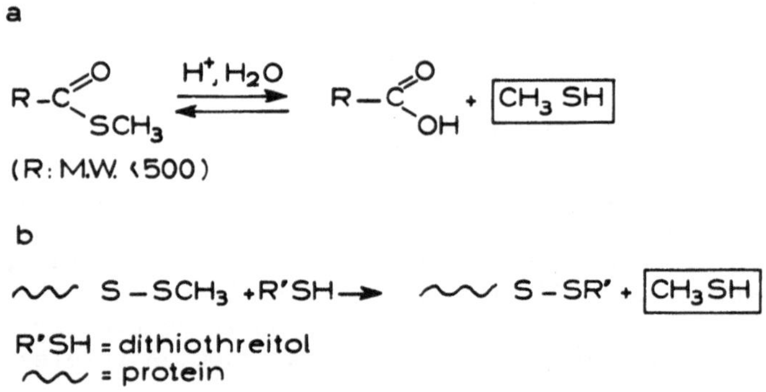

a

$$R-C \overset{O}{\underset{SCH_3}{\big<}} \quad \overset{H^+, H_2O}{\rightleftarrows} \quad R-C \overset{O}{\underset{OH}{\big<}} + \boxed{CH_3\,SH}$$

(R: M.W. ‹500)

b

$$\sim\!\!\sim S-SCH_3 +R'SH \longrightarrow \sim\!\!\sim S-SR' + \boxed{CH_3SH}$$

R'SH = dithiothreitol
$\sim\!\!\sim$ = protein

Fig. 3. Release of MT from serum by addition of acid (fraction P)
(a) and by addition of dithiothreitol (fraction Q) (b).

Table 1. Volatile sulfur compounds in breath and serum of normals, cirrhotics and patients in hepatic coma

BREATH

		DMS (Means ± SEM, ng/1)
Normals	(N = 20)	21.1 ± 1.7 (8 - 40)•
Liver Cirrhosis	(N = 35)	113.4 ± 189.3 (5 - 823)

SERUM

		MT (Means ± SEM, µmol/1)	
		P	Q
Normals	(N = 20)	0.19+0.01 (0.12-0.28)	0.15+0.01 (0.05-0.30)
Liver Cirrhosis	(N = 60)	0.30+0.02 (0.11-0.90)	0.15+0.01 (0.05-0.30)
Hepacic Coma	(N = 5)	2.44+1.08 (0.86-6.56)	0.17+0.04 (0.04-0.29)

• Values in parentheses represent the observed range.

PM30 > 30,000 MW, showed that this MT fraction Q is completely bound
to serum proteins. It is therefore concluded that this MT fraction
is covalently bound to serum proteins in a disulfide linkage (Figure 3).

Serum and Breath Mercaptans

The results are compiled in Table 1.

The DMS concentration in the breath of cirrhotics is significantly elevated compared to controls. MT was not present in
detectable amounts in the breath of normals. Of the 35 cirrhotic
patients only 5 had small amounts of MT in the breath (0.0 - 11.0
ng/l). Ethanethiol (ET) and dimethyldisulfide (DMDS) were absent in
the breath of both normals and cirrhotics.

As concerning serum, there is no significant difference in the
concentration of the disulfide bound MT fraction (Q) between
normals, cirrhotics and patients in hepatic coma. In contrast, the
acid-hydrolysable MT fraction (P) differs for all three groups.
Fraction P in the group of cirrhotics is significantly elevated
compared to controls, although there is much overlap between these
two groups. Fraction P in patients with hepatic coma is highly
elevated compared to both normals and cirrhotics. ET and DMDS were
absent in the serum of all three groups.

The concentration of DMS in the blood of normals was very low
and could hardly be detected. Patients with elevated DMS breath
levels also had elevated DMS levels in their blood.

DISCUSSION

DMS, disulfide bound MT fraction (Q) and acid-hydrolysable MT
fraction (P) have been positively identified as metabolites of MT
in serum. ET and DMDS were absent in both serum and breath.

Fraction Q seems to be of minor importance in the field of
hepatoencephalopathy because no differences were observed in
fraction Q between normals, cirrhotics and patients in hepatic
coma. In contrast, fraction P was highly elevated for patients in
hepatic coma. A thiolester is proposed for fraction P. Such esters
are easily hydrolyzed by acid resulting in the formation of a
carboxylic acid and a thiol.[9] Thiolesters may be formed by carboxy-
lation of MT.[10]

REFERENCES

1. L. Zieve, W. M. Doizaki, and F. J. Zieve, Synergism between
    mercaptans and ammonia or fatty acids in the production of

coma: a possible role for mercaptans in the pathogenesis of
hepatic coma, J. Lab.Clin. Med. 83: 16 (1974).

2. C. J. McClain, L. Zieve, W. M. Doizaki, S. Gilberstadt, and G.
   R. Onstad, Blood methanethiol in alcoholic liver disease with
   and without hepatic encephalopathy, Gut 21: 318 (1980).

3. S. Schen L. Zieve, and V. Mahadevan, Mercaptans and dimethyl
   sulfide in the breath of patients with cirrhosis of the liver,
   J. Lab. Clin. Med. 75: 628 (1970).

4. H. Kaji, M. Hisamura, N. Saito, and M. Murao, Evaluation of
   volatile sulfur compounds in the expired alveolar gas in
   patients with liver cirrhosis, Clin. Chim. Acta 85: 279 (1978).

5. W. M. Doizaki and L. Zieve, An improved method for measuring
   blood mercaptans, J. Lab. Clin. Med. 90: 849 (1977).

6. G. Brunner and P. Scharff, Untersuchungen über den diagnostische
   Wert der Bestimmung von Mercaptanen im Serum bei Leberer-
   krankungen, Dtsch. Med. Wochenschr. 103: 1796 (1978).

7. H. A. Mardini, K. Bartlett, and C. O. Record, An improved gas
   chromatographic method for the detection and quantitation of
   mercaptans in blood, Clin. Chim. Acta 113: 35 (1981).

8. W. W. Cleland, Dithiothreitol, a new protective reagent for SH
   groups, Biochemistry 3: 480 (1964).

9. M. J. Janssen, Thiolo, thiono and dithio acids and esters, in:
   "The Chemistry of Carboxylic Acids and Esters", S. Patai, ed.
   Interscience Publishers, London (1969).

10. J. M. Westendorf and D. B. McCormick, Isolation of volatile
    sulfur-containing microbial catabolites of biotin, Intern. J.
    Vit. Nutr. Res. 50: 150 (1980).

PLASMA INFLUENCE ON THE ALTERED BLOOD-BRAIN BARRIER TO AMINO ACIDS

AFTER PORTACAVAL SHUNT: PRELIMINARY RESULTS

G. Zanchin, P. Rigotti, P. Vassanelli, D. Salassa, and
L. Battistin

Clinica Neurologica and Clinica Chirurgica III, University
of Padova, Italy

INTRODUCTION

The increased cerebral levels of aromatic amino acids are likely
to play an important role on the pathogenesis of hepatic encephalopathy.[5] Liver impairment is accompanied with changes in the levels
of neurotransmitters,[6] possibly consequent to the high brain concentrations of their precursors amino acids: brain serotonin is elevated, due to high cerebral levels of tryptophan;[4,14] the false neurotransmitters phenylethanolamine and octopamine are increased,
probably because the raised cerebral levels of tyrosine and phenylalanine partially divert the cathecolamine synthesis pathway.[7,15]

It was thought that the cerebral elevation of the aromatics
cound be secondary to their increase in the plasma, along with the
decrease of branched chain amino acids; all these compounds are
neutral amino acids sharing a common carrier and therefore they
compete at the blood-brain barrier (BBB) transport sites[5]: indeed,
the possibility of modifying the cerebral amino acid profile mani-
pulating the plasmatic concentration of these compounds has been
well established.[2,5]

However, recent studies have demonstrated a specific alteration
of the BBB in rats after portacaval shunt (PCS), consisting in an
increased permeability for the neutrals and a decreased one for the
basics.[3,8,11,16]

Both the altered amino acid profile in plasma and the modified BBB permeability could contribute to the increased passage of
the neutral amino acids into the brain and therefore to the cerebral
increase of the aromatics.

Our investigation was designed to study the relevance of these two mechanisms in the rat after experimental PCS.

MATERIALS AND METHODS

Male Sprague-Dawley rats, weighing 270-320 g, were used. Animals were either sham operated or submitted to end-to-side PCS.[10] BBB permeability was studied four weeks later, using the well-known Oldendorf's technique, that is a short term intracarotid injection of a bolus containing ^{14}C-labeled amino acids and tritiated water, used as a free-diffusible internal reference.[12] [13]. Blood samples from 5-6 controls or from 5-6 shunted animals were separately collected in heparinized test tubes and centrifuged for 10 minutes at 3000 g. Portions of the plasma from each animal were pooled separately for the two groups and aliquots of 0.2 ml were used as injection bolus, adding the ^{14}C-labeled amino acid and tritiated water.

To study the transport, four groups of 6-8 rats were used for each amino acid. A first group of control rats was injected with the tested amino acid and plasma of control rats. A second group of controls was injected with the same amino acid but with plasma of shunted rats. Likewise, a third group consisting of shunted rats was injected with control plasma, and a fourth group, of shunted animals, was injected with plasma of shunted rats. The cerebral extraction of the amino acid was expressed as "brain uptake index" (BUI) and calculated as ($^{14}C/^{3}H$ ratio in the tissue): ($^{14}C/^{3}H$ ratio in the injected solution) x100.[12]

Tritiated water and ^{14}C-labeled amino acids (injected in tracer amounts) were purchased from Amersham-Searle.

RESULTS AND DISCUSSION

Figure 1 and Figure 2 report the BUI of two neutral amino acids, phenylalanine and tyrosine respectively, in the four experimental conditions described. Control rats injected with control plasma (C+CP1) have a BUI significantly lower than shunted rats injected with shunted plasma (S+SP1).

An increased neutral amino acid permeability after PCS has been well established[8,11 16] with injection of the tested compound in an artifical bolus, and therefore in a relatively unphysiological condition, that is in absence of the competing amino acids in the plasma: Oldendorf's technique indeed allows minimal mixing with plasma of the injected solution, and therefore the passage of the studied amino acid takes place at the bolus-cerebral endothelium contact surfaces, without competition by substances contained in

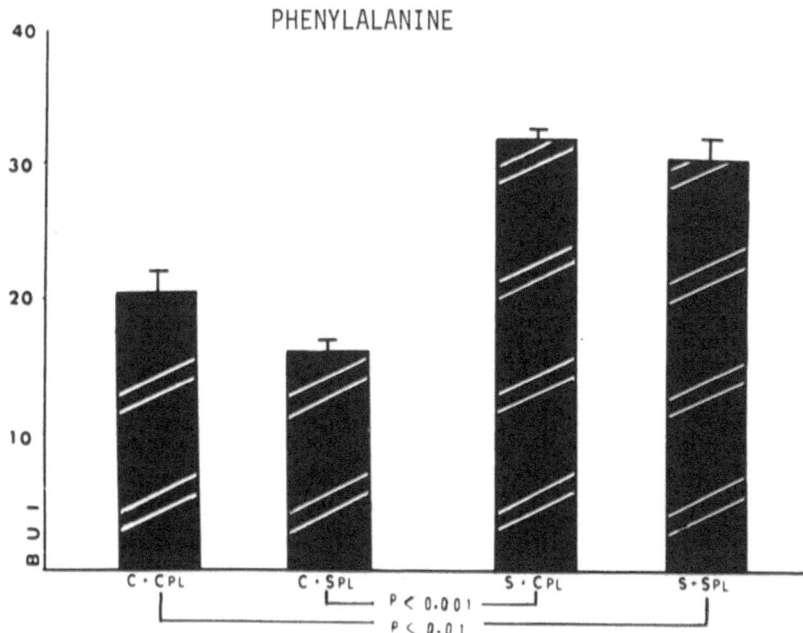

Fig. 1. C + CP1 = control rats injected with plasma from controls;
         C + SP1 = control rats injected with plasma from shunted
         animals; S + CP1 = shunted rats injected with plasma from
         controls; S + SP1 = shunted rats injected with plasma from
         shunted animals. Results expressed as BUI $\pm$ SEM. N = 6-8.
         Significance at the Student's t test is reported.

the blood.[13]

     Our results demonstrate that the already described higher up-
take occurs also when the tested amino acid is competing with the
other plasma compounds sharing the BBB transport sites.

     If we now consider, in the same figures, what happens when we
inject control animals with shunted plasma (C+SP1), we observe a
slight, not significant inhibition of the uptake in comparison with
control rats injected with control plasma (C+CP1): we would expect
the opposite, that is an uptake enhancement, should amino acid
permeability depend on plasmatic amino acid levels.

     Moreover, the injection of shunted animals with plasma from
controls (S+CP1) causes no differences to the BUI in comparison
with shunted rats injected with plasma from shunted animals (S+SP1):
whereas, should be the amino acid profile in the plasma influencing
amino acid permeability, in the latter condition we would expect a

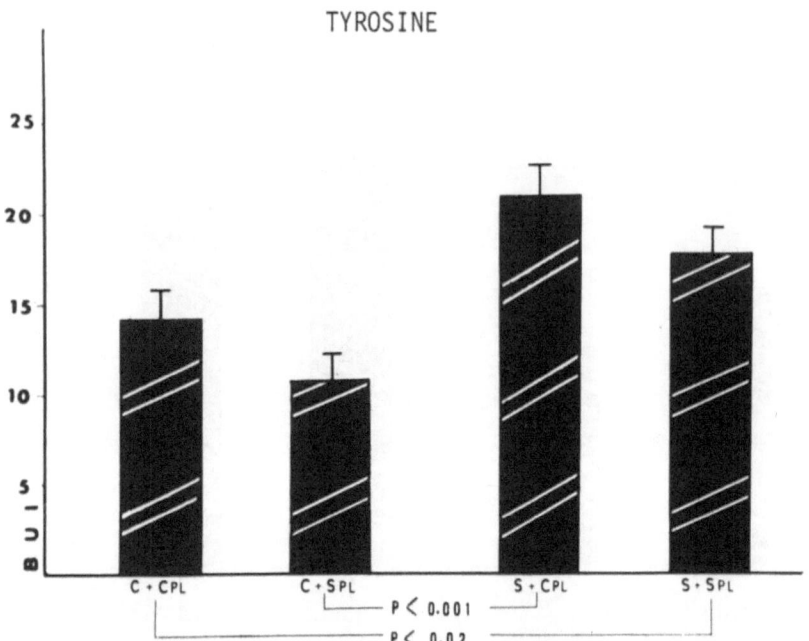

Fig. 2.   Legend as in Fig. 1.

decrease of the BUI.

We are obtaining preliminary data, not reported here, that seem to confirm similar observations also for the basic amino acids: the decreased BBB permeability reported for these compounds[16] is confirmed also in our experimental conditions and seems to be unchanged when plasma from shunted animals is injected in control rats and vice-versa.[17]

Therefore, we conclude that the altered amino acid levels observed in the plasma seem not to be a determining factor in the changes of BBB permeability that have been well-established after PCS.

These observations, stressing the importance of a "barrier factor" instead of plasma, would indirectly support a recent hypothesis, explaining the altered permeability for the neutral amino acids after PCS as an enhanced exchange, through the cerebral capillary cells, between these compounds in the plasma and the brain glutamine.[9]

Experiments are in progress in our laborarory to confirm and complete these results.

REFERENCES

1. R. J. Baldessarini and J. E. Fischer, Substitute and alternative
    neurotransmitters in neuropsychiatric illness, Arch. Gen.
    Psychiat. 34: 958 (1977).
2. L. Battistin, A. Grynbaum, and A. Lajtha, The uptake of various
    amino acids by the mouse brain in vivo, Brain Res. 29: 85
    (1971).
3. P. Cardelli-Cangiano, C. Cangiano, J. H. James, B. Jeppsson, W.
    Brenner, and J. E. Fischer, Uptake of aminoacids by brain mi-
    crovessels isolated from rats after portacaval anastomosis,
    J. Neurochem. 36: 627 (1981).
4. G. Curzon, B. G. Kantamaneni, J. C. Fernando, M.S.Woods, and J.B.
    Cavanagh, Effects of chronic portocaval anastomosis on brain
    tryptophan, tyrosine and 5-hydroxytryptamine, J. Neurochem.
    24: 1065 (1975).
5. J. F. Fischer, J. M. Funovics, A. Aguirre, J. H. James, J. M.
    Keane, R. I. C. Wesdorp, N. Yoshimura,and T. Westman, The role
    of plasma amino acids in hepatic encephalopathy, Surgery 78:
    276 (1975).
6. A. M. Hoyumpa and S. Schenker, Perspectives in hepatic encephalo-
    pathy, J. Lab. Clin. Med. 100: 477 (1982).
7. J. H. James, J. M. Hodeman, J. M. Funovics, and J. E. Fischer,
    Alterations in brain octopamine and brain tyrosine following
    portacaval anastomosis in rats, J. Neurochem. 27: 223 (1976).
8. J. H. James, J. Escourrou, and J. E. Fischer, Blood-brain neutral
    amino acid transport activity is increased after portacaval
    anastomosis, Science 200: 1395 (1978).
9. J. H. James, V. Ziparo, B. Jeppsson, and J.E. Fischer, Hyperammo-
    naemia, plasma aminoacid imbalance, and blood-brain amino-
    acid transport: a unified theory of portal-systemic encepha-
    lopathy, Lancet 2: 772 (1979).
10. S. H. Lee and B. Fisher, Porto-caval shunt in the rat, Surgery
    50: 668 (1961).
11. A. M. Mans, J. F. Biebuyck, K. Shelly, and R. A. Hawkins, Regional
    blood-brain barrier permeability to amino acids after porta-
    caval anastomosis, J. Neorochem.38: 705 (1982).
12. W. H. Oldendorf, Measurement of brain uptake of radiolabeled
    substances using a tritiated water internal standard, Brain
    Res. 24: 372 (1970).
13. W. H. Oldendorf, Brain uptake of radiolabeled amino acids,
    amines and hexoses after arterial injection, Am. J. Physiol.
    221: 1629 (1971).
14. G. Simert, A. Nolin, E. Rosengren, and J.Vang, Neurotransmitter
    changes in the rat brain after portocaval anastomosis, Eur.
    Surg. Res. 10: 73 (1978).
15. A. R. Smith, F. Rossi-Fanelli, V. Ziparo, H. J. James, B. A.
    Perelle, and J. E. Fischer, Alterations in plasma and CSF ami-
    noacids, amines and metabolites in hepatic coma, Ann. Surg.

187: 343 (1978).

16. G. Zanchin, P. Rigotti, N. Dussini, P. Vassanelli, and L. Battistin, Cerebral amino acid levels and uptake in rats after portocaval anastomosis: II. Regional studies in vivo, J. Neurosci. Res. 4: 301 (1979).

17. G. Zanchin, P. Rigotti, P. Vassanelli, and L. Battistin, Blood-brain barrier after portocaval shunt (PCS) in the rat: plasma influence on the altered amino acid transport. 9th International Congress of Neuropathology (abstracts). Vienna (1982).

HEPATIC ENCEPHALOPATHY IS ASSOCIATED WITH DECREASED NUMBERS OF RECEPTORS FOR EXCITATORY AMINOACID NEUROTRANSMITTERS *

P. Ferenci,* C. S. Pappas,** E. A. Jones**

I. Universitätsklinik für Gastroenterologie und
Hepatologie, Vienna, Austria; Liver Diseases Section
Niaddk, NIH, Bethesda Md, USA**

The pathogenesis of hepatic encephalopathy (HE) is still poorly understood. In a recent editorial Zieve[1] mentioned 20 different metabolic abnormalities which are associated with liver failure and which could conceivably contribute to the mediation of this syndrome. Several observations have suggested that in liver failure impairment of cerebral neurotransmission may occur. In the "false neurotransmitter hypothesis" of the pathogenesis of HE proposed by Fisher and Baldessarini[2] it was assumed that a decrease in the cerebral content of dopamine and the presence of competitive inhibitors of dopamine impaired the function of the dopaminergic neurotransmitter system and thereby induce neural inhibition. However an increasing body of evidence at variance with the hypothesis has been generated.[3] Numerically dopaminergic neurons constitute only a small fraction of the total number of neurons in the central nervous system (CNS). In contrast, the number of neurons which mediate aminoacid-induced neurotransmission constitute a very large proportion of the total neurons in the CNS.[4]

Several recent observations in an animal model of fulminant hepatic failure suggest that the development of HE may be associated with changes in the gamma aminobutyric acid (GABA) neurotransmitter system.[5] GABA is the principal inhibitory neurotransmitter of the mammalian brain. In this model HE was associated with a more than tenfold increase in the serum concentration of GABA, a decrease in the activity of GABA-transaminase - the enzyme responsible for GABA

---

* Paper selected for publication.

catabolism - in the brain and an increase in the number of receptors
for GABA on postsynaptic neurons.

There is a paucity of data relating to the status of excitatory
aminoacid neurotransmitter systems in HE. Glutamate is believed to
be the principal excitatory neurotransmitter in the brain. About
90% of neurons will be depolarized when exposed to glutamate by
iontophoresis.[6] The role of glutamate as an excitatory neurotransmitter in the hippocampus, entorhinal cortex, cerebellum and some
cortical projections has been firmly established.[7] A second
excitatory aminoacid neurotransmitter, aspartate, has been less
well characterized. Its potency to induce membrane depolarization
appears to be similar to that of glutamate but its regional distribution in the brain differs from that of glutamate.[7]

Besides their function as neurotransmitters both glutamate and
aspartate serve important metabolic functions in the brain. As the
brain lacks the enzymes of the urea cycle, ammonia fixation by
glutamate and aspartate appears to be important in the detoxification
of ammonia within the brain. Hyperammonemia, which is believed to
play a role in the pathogenesis of HE, has been shown to decrease
the cerebral concentration of glutamate and aspartate in vivo.[8]
Furthermore ammonia inhibits glutaminase, the enzyme that catalizes
the formation of glutamate in the synaptic endings, and the evoked
release of glutamate from neurons in hippocampal slices in vitro.[9,10]
Thus, changes in the glutamatergic neurotransmitter system could be
present in HE. Most valuable information relating to this possibility would be the demonstration of a change in the concentration of
glutamate or aspartate at the site where they influence neurotransmission, namely the synaptic cleft. Direct measurements of neurotransmitters at this site are currently not feasible. However changes
in receptors for a neurotransmitter on neural membranes may constitute "foot prints" of synaptic events and may provide indirect
information relating to the concentration of that neurotransmitter
in the synaptic region. Accordingly measurements were made of receptors for excitatory neurotransmitter aminoacids on synaptic membranes prepared from the brains of normal rabbits and rabbits with
liver failure. The model of HE used in this study was galactosamine-
induced fulminant hepatic failure, a highly reproducible model which
resembles human fulminant hepatic failure in all important res-
pects.[11]

Specific receptors for excitatory aminoacid neurotransmitters
have been characterized on synaptic membranes. There are at least
three different receptor sites, which recognize glutamate, aspartate
and kainic acid respectively. Kainic acid is a potent neuroexcita-
tory aminoacid found in marinae algae. It has not been detected in
the mammalian brain and the endogenous ligand for the kainic acid
binding site is unknown.[7]

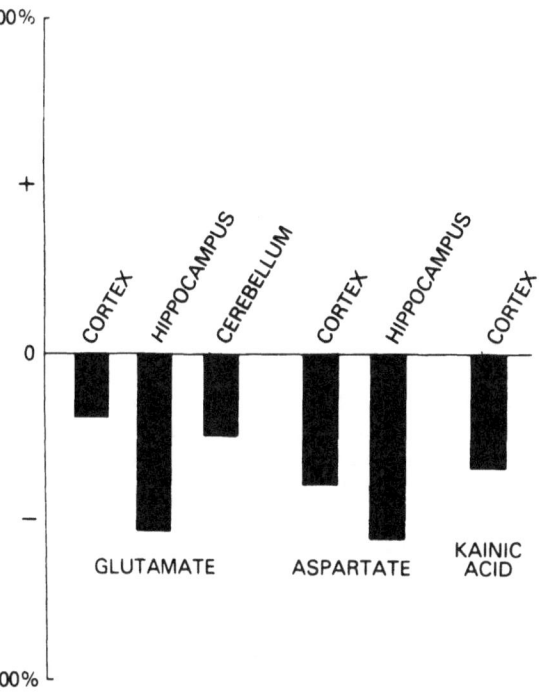

Fig. 1. Percentage changes in the density (B_{max}) of receptors for excitatory aminoacid neurotransmitters on synaptic membranes of rabbits with hepatic encephalopathy.

Data on the specific binding of ^{3}H-glutamate, ^{3}H-aspartate and of ^{3}H-kainic acid were determined using established assay procedures.[12,13,14] Specific binding of all three ligands was found to be decreased in rabbits with HE as compared to control animals. Scatchard plot analysis of the binding data revealed that the decrease in the specific binding of each of these ligands could be attributed to a decrease in the number of binding sites (B_{max}). The affinity of each of these receptors remained unchanged in HE. It was shown for the glutamate and aspartate receptors that the extent of the observed changes in HE varied in different brain areas. The decrease in glutamate binding sites was greatest in the hippocampus (-39%) but was also present in the cerebellum and the cerebral cortex (-23% and -20% respectively). The decrease in aspartate receptors was also more marked in the hippocampus (-50%) than in the cerebral cortex (-29%) (Fig. 1). To determine whether the changes observed in HE are specific for this syndrome or merely reflect a phenomenon common to metabolic encephalopathies in general, glutamate binding to synaptic membranes prepared from the brains of rabbits in uremic encephalopathy was also studied. Uremia was induced by bilateral ureteral ligation. In contrast to the observations in HE, the number of glutamate receptors in uremic encephalopathy was similar to that in sham operated controls.

Together with the previously described increase in the number of receptors for inhibitory aminoacid neurotransmitters in HE[5,15] suggest that liver failure is associated with a distinctive pattern of changes in receptors for neurotransmitters. The regulation of the expression of neurotransmitter receptors in the brain under physiologic conditions is poorly understood. However extrapolations of well substantiated concepts relating to other receptor systems such as the insulin receptor[16] to neurotransmitter receptors in the brain may facilitate interpretation of the new findings. Accordingly a decrease in the number of binding sites for excitatory aminoacid neurotransmitters in HE could reflect an increase in the synaptic concentration of these aminoacids and/or a decrease in the sensitivity of postsynaptic neurons to glutamate and aspartate mediated excitation. Whether such extrapolations are shown to be justified or not, the observed changes in neurotransmitter receptors in the brains of rabbits with HE probably imply that liver failure is associated with fundamental disturbances of neurotransmission which may be responsible for the development of the syndrome of neural inhibition which characterizes HE.

REFERENCES

1. L. Zieve, The mechanism of hepatic coma, Hepatology 1: 360 (1981).
2. J. E. Fischer and R. J. Baldessarini, False neurotransmitters and hepatic failure, Lancet II: 75 (1971).
3. False neurotransmitters and hepatic failure (editorial), Lancet I: 86 (1982).
4. P. L. McGeer, J. C. Eccles, and E. G. McGeer,"Molecular Neurobiology of the Mammalian Brain,"Plenum Press, New York (1978).
5. D. F. Schafer and E. A. Jones, Hepatic encephalopathy and the gamma-aminobutyric acid neurotransmitter system, Lancet I: 18 (1982).
6. D. R. Curtis and G. A. R. Johnston, Aminoacid transmitters in the mammalian central nervous system, Ergebn. Physiol. 69: 97 (1974).
7. G. P. Chiara and G. L. Gessa, Glutamate as a neurotransmitter, Raven Press, New York (1981).
8. B. Hindfelt, F. Plum, and Th. E. Dubby, Effect of acute ammonia intoxication on cerebral metabolism in rats with portacaval shunts, J. Clin. Invest. 59: 386 (1977).
9. H. F. Bradford and H. K. Ward, On glutaminase activity in mammalian synaptosomes, Brain Res. 110: 115 (1976).
10. A. Hamberger, B. Hedquist, and B. Nystroem, Ammonium ion inhi-

bition of evoked release of endogenous glutamate from
hippocampal slices, J. Neurochem. 33: 1295 (1979).

11. B. J. Blitzer, J. G. Waggoner, E. A. Jones, H. R. Gralnick, D.
Towne, J. Butler, V. Weise, I. J. Kopin, I. Walters, P. F.
Teychenne, D. C. Goodmann, and P. D. Berk, A model of fulminant hepatic failure in the rabbit, Gastroenterology 74: 664
(1978).

12. T. Honore, J. Lauridsen, and P. Krogsgaard-Larsen, Ibotemic acid
analogues as inhibitors of ^{3}H-glutamic acid binding to cerebellar membranes, J. Neurochem. 36: 1302 (1981).

13. N. A. Sharif and P. Roberts, L-aspartate binding sites in rat
cerebellum: a comparison of the binding of L-^{3}H-aspartate
and L-^{3}H-glutamate to synaptic membranes, Brain Res. 211:
293 (1981).

14. J. R. Simon, J. F. Contrera, and M. J. Kuhar, Binding of ^{3}H-
kainic acid, an analogue of L-glutamate, to brain membranes,
J. Neurochem. 26: 141 (1976).

15. P. Ferenci, S. C. Pappas, and E. A. Jones, Changes in receptors
for neurotransmitter aminoacids may promote neural inhibition in hepatic encephalopathy, Hepatology 2: 708 (1982).

16. R. G. Kahn, Membrane receptors for hormones and neurotransmitters, J. Cell. Biol. 70: 261 (1974).

BRAIN GAMMA AMINO-BUTYRIC ACID IN ACUTE HEPATIC ENCEPHALOPATHY

IN DOGS FOLLOWING HEPATECTOMY WITH OR WITHOUT ABDOMINAL EVISCERATION*

G. Pomier-Layrargues[*], P. Bories[*], D. Mirouze[*], J. Giordan[**],
B. Feneyrou[*], H. Bellet-Hermann[***], G. Marchal[**], and H.
Michel[*]

[*]Clinique des Maladies de l'Appareil Digestif, Hôpital
Saint-Eloi, Montpellier, France; [**]Clinique Chirurgicale
C, Hôpital Saint-Eloi, Montpellier, France; [***]Laboratoire
de Biochimie B, Faculté de Médicine, Montpellier, France

INTRODUCTION

The mechanism of acute hepatic encephalopathy (H.E.) is still
unknown. Several hypotheses have been proposed but none of them can
explain the entire clinical and biochemical picture.[1] The present
study was designed to evaluate the gamma aminobutyric acid (GABA)
neuroinhibitory system in acute HE following hepatectomy in dogs;
indeed, several features of HE are quite similar to coma produced
by substances like barbiturates and benzodiazepines which enhance
the GABA ergic system. Since the enteric flora is supposed to
synthesize GABA, we also examined the effect of abdominal evisceration on acute HE induced by hepatectomy.

MATERIALS AND METHODS

Animals

18 mongrel dogs were studied. They were all anesthesized with
a bolus IV injection of thiopental (15 mg/kg) followed by an infusion
of alphaxalone (30 µg/kg/mn). Six dogs underwent a side-to-side
portacaval shunt followed by a one time total hepatectomy. Six dogs
underwent an abdominal evisceration together with the hepatectomy.
Six dogs were sham-operated: the portal vein was clamped during 20
minutes and the abdomen was left open during 3 hours; the dogs were
allowed to recover from anesthesia until they became fully alert;
they were then sacrificed with a potassium chloride injection.

* Paper selected for publication.

All dogs were monitored with continuous EEG recordings; serum glucose was maintained between 1 and 2 g/l by an appropriate infusion of 10% dextrose solution. Serial biochemical determinations including blood glucose, hematocrit, prothrombin time, BUN, creatinine and electrolytes were done at each four-hour intervals until death or sacrifice; arterial ammonia was measured according to Dropsy et al.,[2] plasma amino acids were determined using an autoanalyser 121 M Beckman[3] and plasma thiopental levels were measured as previously described.[4]

Brain samples

Immediately after death, dogs were exsanguinated and brain samples were taken in the following brain areas: frontal cortex, caudate nucleus, thalamus, hypothalamus and putamen. The specimens were weighed, wrapped into aluminium foil, then quickly frozen in liquid nitrogen. The entire procedure lasted between 20 and 30 minutes.

Brain aminoacids assay

Brain GABA, glutamate and glutamine were measured in the five brain areas using an autoanalyser 121 M Beckman, as previously described for plasma amino acids.[3]

Statistical calculations

The data in the 3 groups of animals were compared using the non parametric Mann and Withney's test for unpaired values.

RESULTS

The survival was 20 ± 3 hours (mean $\pm$ SEM) in the hepatectomized dogs and 15 ± 1 hours in the eviscerated dogs. This difference was not statistically significant. In these 2 groups, the clinical evolution followed the same pattern; they aroused from anaesthesia approximately 2 hours after the end of surgery, fell into stupor and progressive coma until death supervened. Electroencephalographic changes began to appear 2-3 hours after hepatectomy or evisceration with a predominance of "slow" sleep pattern followed by increasing changes which consisted of alteration, then disappearance of spindles of high voltage waves, predominance of slow waves, depression of voltage and finally flat tracing.

Gross abnormalities of coagulation tests were observed in both groups as soon as 4 hours after surgery. Plasma thiopental levels were undetectable 8-10 hours before death in these two groups. In control dogs, thiopental had disappeared from plasma at the time of sacrifice.

Plasma samples (Table 1)

In the plasma samples obtained just before death, arterial
ammonia was highly significantly elevated in hepatectomized and
eviscerated dogs when compared to controls, and this elevation was
more important in hepatectomized dogs. Plasma glutamate levels
increased to the same extent in the two liverless groups. Glutamine
was higher in these 2 groups when compared to controls, and was more
elevated in eviscerated dogs.

Brain samples

The values of brain GABA, glutamate and glutamine are shown
in the figures 1, 2 and 3. Brain GABA and glutamate levels were not
significantly different in five brain areas in the 3 groups; brain
glutamine levels were significantly higher in these five brain areas
in the two liverless groups of dogs when compared to controls and
this elevation was more striking in hepatectomized dogs than in
eviscerated dogs.

DISCUSSION

GABA is the main neuroinhibitory neurotransmitter of the
mammalian brain and may play a role in the pathogenesis of hepatic
coma. The metabolism of GABA is intimately related to that of
ammonium. The former substance is produced by the decarboxylation
of glutamate. This represents an alternative to the glutamine
synthetase reaction which is the main route for ammonium disposal
by extrahepatic tissue. But GABA and glutamate may also contribute
to the brain energy metabolism in the citric acid cycle.

As previously shown in rats,[5] abdominal evisceration did not
modify the clinical and electroencephalographic pattern of acute
HE following total hepatectomy and this argues against the role of
putative gut toxic substances in the pathogenesis of HE. Arterial
ammonia was elevated in hepatectomized dogs. As expected this
increase in arterial ammonia was less striking in eviscerated dogs
than in hepatectomized dogs because ammonia is partly synthetized
by gut bacteria and is also produced from glutamine which is used
by the gut as an energetic substrate.[6,7] This is probably why plasma
glutamine levels were more increased in eviscerated dogs.

In the brain, the ammonia should have been more elevated in
hepatectomized dogs when compared to eviscerated dogs. Glutamine
does not cross easily the blood brain barrier[8] so brain glutamine
mostly results from local synthesis from brain glutamate and brain
ammonia. Consequently brain glutamine was lower in eviscerated dogs
than in hepatectomized dogs.

GABA is synthetized by gut bacteria.[9] It has been postulated

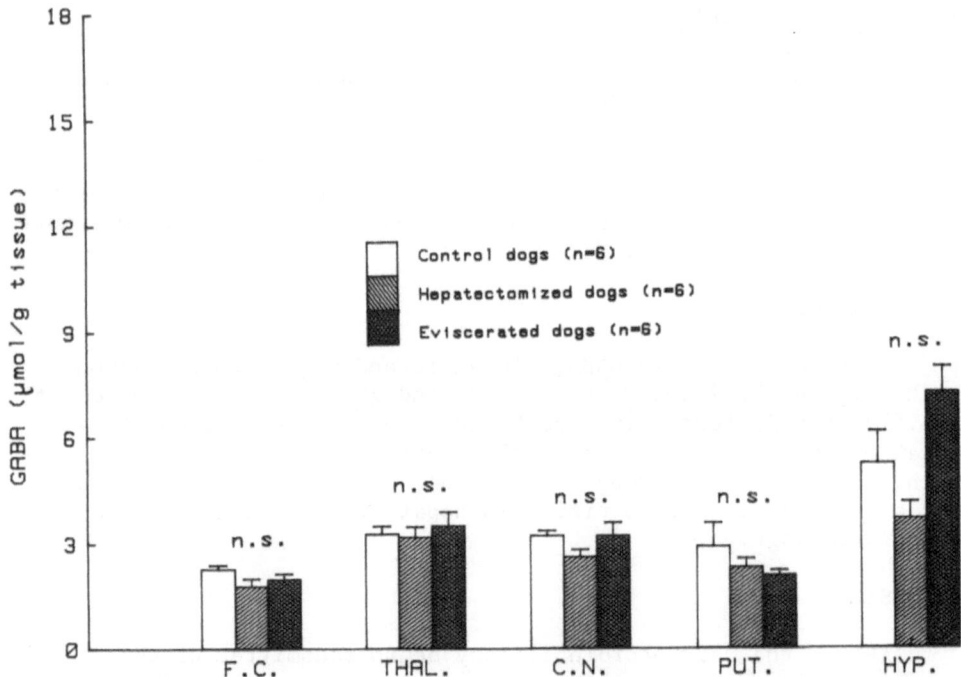

Fig. 1. Brain GABA levels (FC, frontal cortex; THAL, thalamus;
CN, caudate nucleus; PUT, putamen; HYP, hypothalamus).
Values are expressed as mean $\pm$ SEM.

that hepatic coma is associated with increased levels of GABA in
plasma, and increased permeability of the blood brain barrier; thus
the activity of the brain GABA neuroinhibitory system would be
enhanced.[10] In this study, plasma GABA levels were not measured
because plasma GABA concentrations can only be accurately determined
by measuring the ability of plasma to displace ^3H GABA from normal
post synaptic membranes and, unfortunately this technique was not
available in our laboratory. However, brain GABA levels were not
increased in hepatectomized dogs. Similar findings have been reported
in rats with acute hepatic coma[11] or with chronic liver disease.[12]
One explanation could be that the blood brain barrier permeability
for plasma GABA is not enhanced in hepatic coma.

Moreover, abdominal evisceration should have abolished the
elevation in the plasma GABA levels induced by the hepatectomy. But
this did not result in any change in the brain GABA of the eviscerated dogs.

Brain GABA could have been disturbed by anaesthetics but serial
plasma samples showed that thiopental had disappeared in the plasma

Table 1. Plasma levels of arterial ammonia, glutamate and glutamine after death

	Sham-operated (n = 6)	Hepatectomized (n = 6)	Eviscerated (n = 6)
Arterial ammonia (μmoles/l)	1158 ± 115	3950 ± 433 *♦	1795 ± 207°
Glutamate (μ moles/l)	34 ± 10	87 ± 6 *	86 ± 16°
Glutamine (μ moles/l)	702 ± 74	1582 ± 76 *♦	3058 ± 299°

Values are expressed as mean ± SEM.

P < 0.001 * hepatectomized versus sham-operated
° eviscerated versus sham-operated
♦ hepatectomized versus eviscerated

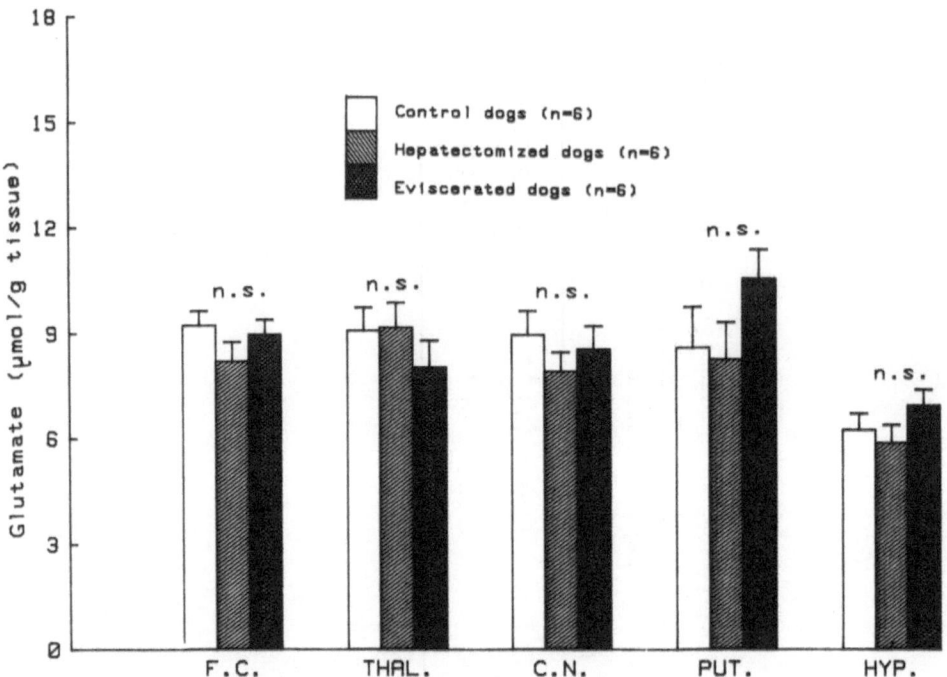

Fig. 2.   Brain glutamate levels (FC, frontal cortex; THAL, thalamus;
          CN, caudate nucleus; PUT, putamen; HYP, hypothalamus).
          Values are expressed as mean ± SEM.

a long time before death. We also maintained serum glucose higher
than 1g/l to avoid the effect of hypoglycemia on the brain
neurotransmitter metabolism.

One might argue against the sampling methods. Indeed the brain
GABA level rises very soon after death but remains quite stable from
one to eight hours after death.[13] To avoid this post-mortem elevation, the brain specimens should be taken within 30 seconds after
death. Obviously, this was not possible in studies using dogs.
However, the brain sampling technique was identical in the 3 groups
of animals such that post-mortem rise in brain GABA should be the
same in all dogs.

In conclusion, hepatectomy did not change the brain levels of
GABA in dogs. When an abdominal evisceration was performed together
with the hepatectomy, the brain GABA content was not modified.
However, despite unchanged brain GABA levels, the GABA neuroinhibitory system might be enhanced because it has been recently
suggested that there is an increase in the brain GABA receptors in
rats with hepatic coma.[14]

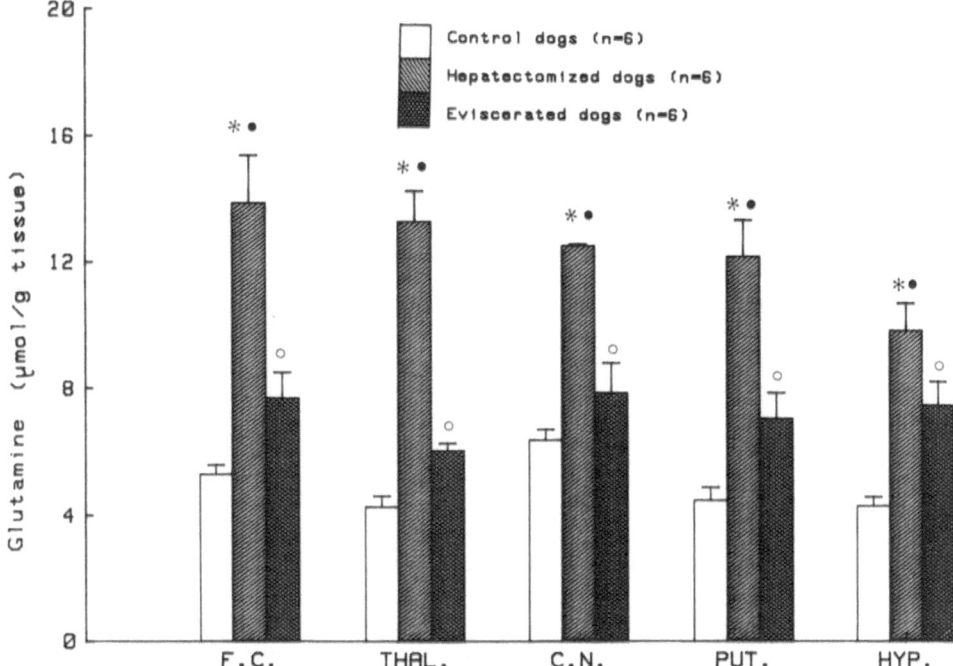

Fig. 3.   Brain glutamine levels (FC, frontal cortex; THAL, thalamus;
          CN, caudate nucleus; PUT, putamen; HYP, hypothalamus).
          Values are expressed as mean ± SEM. P < 0.05. Hepatectomized
          versus sham-operated; ° eviscerated versus sham-operated;
          ⁎hepatectomized versus eviscerated.

REFERENCES

1. L. Zieve, The mechanism of hepatic coma, Hepatology 4: 360
    (1981).
2. G. Dropsy and J. Boy, Determination de l'ammionémie (Méthode
    automatique par dialyse), Ann. Biol. Clin. 19: 313 (1961).
3. S. Moore and W. H. Stein, Chromatography of amino acids on
    sulfonated polystirene resins, J. Biol. Chem. 92: 663 (1951).
4. M. M. Ghoneim and M. S. Van Hamme, Pharmacokinetics and thio-
    pentone: effects of enflurane and nitrous oxide anaesthesia
    and surgery, Brit. J. Anaesth. 50: 1237 (1978).
5. F. Degos, J. D. Degos, D. Boudriau, M. Peignoux, D. Pranzi,
    J. Roche-Sicot, C. Sicot, B. Rueff, and J. P. Benhamou,
    Experimental acute hepatic encephalopathy: comparison of
    the electroencephalographic changes in the liverless and
    in the eviscerated rat, Clin. Sci. Mol. Med. 47: 599 (1974).
6. F. L. Weber and G. L. Veach, The importance of the small
    intestine in gut ammonium production in the fasting dog,
    Gastroenterology 77: 235 (1979).

7. H. G. Windmueller and A. E. Spaeth, Uptake and metabolism of plasma glutamine by the small intestine, J. Biol. Chem. 249: 5070 (1974).

8. W. H. Oldendorf and J. Szabo, Amino acid assignment to one of the three blood-brain barrier amino acid carrier, Am. J. Physiol. 230: 94 (1976).

9. D. F. Shafer, J. M. Fowler, L. E. Brody, and A. E. Jones, Hepatic coma and inhibitory neurotransmission: the enteric bacterial flora as a source of γ-amino-butyric-acid, Gastro-enterology 79: 1052A (1980).

10. D. F. Shafer and E. A. Jones, Hepatic encephalopathy and the amino-butyric-acid neurotransmitter system, Lancet 8262: 18 (1982).

11. J. M. Funovics and J. E. Fisher, Brain energy metabolism and alterations of transmitter profiles in acute hepatic coma, J. Neural Transmission Suppl. 14: 61 (1978).

12. J. S. Goetcheus and L. T. Webster, γ-amino-butyrate and hepatic coma, J. Lab. Clin. Med. 64: 257 (1965).

13. T. L. Perry, S. Hansen, and S. S. Gandham, Post-mortem changes in amino compounds in human and rat brain, J. Neurochem. 46: 406 (1981).

14. M. Baraldi and M. L. Zeneroli, Experimental hepatic encephalo-pathy: changes in the binding of γ-amino-butyric acid, Science 216: 427 (1982).

SECTION   2

METABOLIC AND PROPHYLACTIC ASPECTS OF HEPATIC ENCEPHALOPATHY

CARBOHYDRATE METABOLISM IN LIVER DISEASE

P. B. Soeters, J. E. G. de Boer, R. J. Oostenbroek, and M. A. Janssen

Departments of Surgery and Biochemistry, St. Annadal Hospital, University of Limburg, Maastricht The Netherlands

INTRODUCTION

The purpose of this chapter is not to give a comprehensive overview of all aspects of fat and carbohydrate metabolism but to focus on glucose intolerance, its possible causes and the possible relationship with changes in fat metabolism. Facts with regard to metabolic disorders in liver disease are accumulating rapidly but the mechanisms involved are far from understood.

CAUSES OF GLUCOSE INTOLERANCE

Glucose intolerance in several forms of hepatic disease has been well established in the fifties and earlier,[1-3] so that the term "hepatogenic diabetes" resulted. In the late sixties, papers appeared reporting hyperinsulinism in cirrhotic patients, first from a Swiss group,[4] later from American groups[5] and many others. The presence of both glucose intolerance and hyperinsulinism in liver disease includes that some form of insulin resistance is present.

Finally, in the early seventies it was demonstrated by Marco and coworkers[6] and by Sherwin and coworkers in 1974[7,8] that glucagon levels were elevated in cirrhotic patients, both in the basal state and after stimulation with arginine or alanine respectively.

All this results in the typical picture presented by Marco and his group, demonstrating increased basal levels of insulin and glucagon in cirrhotics and augmented increases after stimulation with arginine. After a glucose tolerance test, cirrhotics exhibited increased glucose and insulin levels, and diminished glucagon suppressibility by glucose. In the meantime, initially as a byproduct of these studies it became apparent that many cirrhotics but also patients with other types of liver disease exhibited increased free fatty acid levels.[9]

Many other metabolic changes and derangements occur in hepatic disease and several of these changes may interfere with carbohydrate metabolism.[10]

Recently with the advent of a sensitive assay for plasma catecholamines, it is appreciated that plasma catecholamines are equally increased in hepatic cirrhosis.[11]

It is highly likely that atrophy or damage of hepatic parenchymal cells in some way interfere with metabolism but the question remains what the mechanism is. A diminished capacity to store glycogen may indeed explain an exaggerated rise in plasma glucose levels after an oral or intravenous glucose load. It does not explain increased plasma glucose- and insulin-levels after overnight- or longer fasting. Increased glucagon levels or decreased sensitivity to insulin might also explain diminished glycogen synthesis and glucose intolerance. It is not known however if insensitivity to insulin applies to the liver, to the peripheral tissues or both. Undernutrition, albeit often present is not solely responsible for glucose intolerance. Likewise, a degree of glucose intolerance persists when potassium depleted liver patients are repleted. The counterregulatory hormones may have important effects on glucose intolerance and insulin resistance, and recently it is appreciated that all 3 counterregulatory hormones are increased in liver disease.[9,11,12]

COUNTERREGULATORY HORMONES

Simultaneous elevation of all three hormones exerts important influences on hepatic glucose production, hepatic glucose disposal and peripheral glucose disposal.[13] Severe illness or trauma is associated with glucose intolerance and insulin resistance. Severe stress may even cause a diabetic state with fasting hyperglycemia which persists as long as stress persists.[14] These metabolic derangements are generally ascribed to the release of epinephrine, glucagon, cortisol and growth hormone.

The relative contribution of these hormones have recently been elucidated in more detail by the work of Sherwin,[13] Deibert and others. Their work suggests that epinephrine interferes especially with glucose utilization in splanchnic and peripheral tissues, not with glucose production in the liver. Glucagon has little effect on glucose tolerance. None of the counterregulatory hormones alone elicit a persistent glucose intolerance. In humans, simultaneous elevations of cortisol, epinephrine and glucagon are necessary to

produce hyperglycemia in the postabsorptive state. In insulin dependent diabetics, epinephrine alone suffices to cause severe hyperglycemia.

These counterregulatory hormones if anything are elevated in
hepatic disease.[9,11,12] Individual hormonal levels do not always
correlate with the degree of glucose intolerance but it transpires
from the work of Sherwin[13] that simultaneous increases are necessary
to produce intolerance. Simultaneous increases are also present in
many forms of liver disease which suggests that identical mechanisms
may underlie the glucose intolerance of hepatic disease and severe
stress or illness. At this point, it is unknown what stimulus
elicits hypersecretion of these hormones in hepatic disease. In some
way, diminished liver function, diminished hepatic metabolic capacity elicits directly or indirectly secretion of catecholamines and
cortisol, although many of these patients have (for instance) stable
cirrhosis with portal hypertension and portal systemic shunting
without seeming to be chronically in stress or severely ill. Nor
is it known how exactly these hormones integrate at the tissue
level.

Much work has been done on the third counterregulatory hormone:
glucagon and concomitantly on insulin in hepatic disease. The
infusion of glucagon in human volunteers produces only a transient
elevation in plasma glucose level and in glucose production and
therefore does not seem to contribute to glucagon intolerance.[13,15]
It is however unclear how legitimate conclusions from such experiments are.

Does glucagon or any other counterregulatory cause stress or
is it caused by stress? In other words: Is any conclusion drawn from
the results of glucagon infusions legitimate as long as in these
experiments the stimulus for glucagon secretion is absent? This
is less theoretical than it seems, with regard to glucagon, epinephrine and insulin. A world of literature exists depicting insulin
and glucagon as hepatotrophic substances, promoting hepatic regeneration and therefore being useful to the organism. On the other hand,
glucagon (and epinephrine) are considered to cause glucose intolerance justifying measures to block the secretion of glucagon (and
epinephrine) to improve glucose intolerance.[16] Also hyperinsulinemia has been named detrimental in hepatic disease because it
might provoke hepatic encephalopathy.[17]

Until this point, we have indiscriminately discussed glucose
intolerance, increases in diabetogenic hormones, hyperinsulinemia
etc. without specifying hepatic disease. Hyperinsulinemia does not
occur in all forms of liver disease. Normal fasting insulin levels
are encountered for instance in patients with liver damage due to
paracetamol.[18] Hypoinsulinemia occurs in patients with chronic
active hepatitis.[19] It has been suggested that this is due to

autoimmune pancreatic damage. There is no question however that in most other forms of liver disease, clear hyperglucagonism and hyperinsulinism are present.[6-8] Many workers have tried to define the relative roles of liver cell damage and portal systemic shunting in the genesis of hyperinsulinism and hyperglucagonism, and have tried to distinguish between hypersecretion and diminished degradation if these hormones. In an endeavour to define the role of portal systemic shunting, insulin and glucagon were measured in dogs before 1 week and 4 weeks after performing a portal systemic shunt and when these dogs became encephalopathic.[20]

Postabsorptive insulin and glucagon levels rose slightly after portal systemic shunting. Glucagon however rose precipitously when portal systemic encephalopathy supervened. These findings suggest that hepatic insufficiency and not portal systemic shunting induced hypersecretion of glucagon. It should be realized that hepatic architecture demonstrates atrophy[21] but only discrete signs of cellular damage and no clear necrosis after portal systemic shunting.[22] Contrasting data were reported by Sherwin.[8] Patients with surgical porta-caval shunts exhibited highest plasma glucagon levels. Cirrhotics with demonstrated portal hypertension and signs of portal systemic shunting had moderate rises in glucagon. Patients with cirrhosis without portal hypertension did not differ from normal controls. These data from humans do seem to be contradictory with the data in dogs. They can be reconciled however. Portal systemic shunting apart from correlating with glucagon levels in humans correlates relatively well with ammonia tolerance and the capacity to produce urea.[23] This is unlikely to be caused by the absence of a first pass effect in portal systemic shunting, rather is it due to diminished total hepatic blood flow due to portal systemic shunting. Indirect support may be derived from Burchell[24-25] who demonstrated that prognosis after portal systemic shunting in cirrhotics with variceal bleeding was determined by the ability of the hepatic artery to increase its flow.

So, although hepatic architecture may not dramatically change after portal systemic shunting, total metabolic capacity may be decreased due to diminished total hepatic flow of blood and diminished total hepatic exposure to hepatotrophic substances.

On the other hand, total metabolic capacity may change by cellular damage like in severe acute viral hepatitis. In conclusion, both residual hepatic cell mass after severe cell damage and total hepatic flow determine total metabolic capacity. There is no question that elevated glucagon levels in liver disease result from hypersecretion. Normal hepatic degradation of glucagon is low, and glucagon degradation occurs at other sites.[25] In addition, glucagon levels are increased severalfold, so that this cannot be explained on the basis of diminished degradation. Sherwin[8] demonstrated that the biologically active form of glucagon, which is the 3500 dalton component was increased in cirrhotics with portal hypertension and that the clearance rate of this component was normal, indicating that indeed hypersecretion takes place.

What signal elicits glucagon hypersecretion? The pancreatic alpha cell is under direct nervous control,[26,27] autonomous nerve fibers ending in its direct neighbourhood. Nervous outflow from the brain is no prerequisite for glucagon secretion however because adequate glucagon secretion occurs in glucopenia in sympathectomized man.[28] Similarly catecholamines are reported to enhance glucagon secretion[29-32] but bilateral adrenalectomy does not abolish adequate glucagon secretion in response to glucopenia.[33] Other reports also question the physiologic significance of the sympathoadrenal system in controlling glucagon secretion.[34]

Hypoglycemia can directly stimulate the pancreatic alpha cell to produce glucagon. Aminoacids are well known to stimulate glucagon secretion. Especially glucogenic aminoacids have a large secretory capacity. A fall in the level of free fatty acids results in a rise of glucagon. A rise in plasma free fatty acids causes a fall of glucagon and an inhibition of the stimulatory effect of aminoacids. This hypothetical feedback mechanism involving free fatty acids and glucagon appears to be of minor importance compared to the other major energy fuels.[35,36] Pancreozymin and glucocorticoids potentiate glucagon secretion[37] but the relevance hereof in liver disease is questionable.

Finally, it has been suggested[8] that changes in hepatic responsiveness to the effects of pancreatic glucagon may be important in regulating the secretion of this hormone. That still raises the question what the signal is. In the liver, glucagon raises the intracellular concentrations of cyclic AMP and this stimulates glycogenolysis and gluconeogenesis at the same time assimilating tricarbon fragments, stimulating ureagenesis, stimulating ketogenesis and assimilating NH_3 and other aminoacid derived nitrogen. Glucagon also stimulates entry of aminoacids into the liver.

The glycemic response to glucagon has been shown to be diminished[8] in cirrhotic patients with portal systemic shunting and it has been suggested that this diminished metabolic capacity to produce glucose is the feed back signal to the alpha cell to secrete more glucagon. Likewise, the diminished hepatic capacity to assimilate small nitrogen-containing molecules[38] or to produce ketone bodies may provide the feed back signal to secrete glucagon.

In this way, a new set point may be reached with relatively normal metabolic hepatic capacity at the expense of increased glucagon levels enhancing the function described. Free fatty acids do not seem to play a role because their role in glucagon secretion is

minor and if anything increased free fatty acid levels in hepatic
disease would favor decreased glucagon secretion. The role of the
nervous system and of the catecholamines remains to be established.
Especially the catecholamines are interesting as they appear to be
elevated.[11] In fact, many metabolically stable cirrhotics with signs
of portal systemic shunting exhibit all signs of a stress response
including elevated plasma levels of glucagon, catecholamines, growth
hormone and cortisol, and exhibiting glucose intolerance and insulin
resistance, without clinically exhibiting clear signs of stress.
The sensitivity of the tissues to catecholamines is not yet fully
established,[39] but preliminary reports demonstrate normal tissue
sensitivity.[11]

In conclusion, hyperglucagonism may be the result of a diminished
capacity of the liver to produce glucose, ketones and urea and to
assimilate tricarbon fragments and nitrogen containing molecules.
Hyperglucagonism sustains these functions.

INSULIN

Hyperinsulinism is well established in many forms of liver
disease.[40] No agreement exists on the role of portal systemic shunting. In dogs[20] walking happily around 1 and 4 weeks after surgical
porta-caval shunt increased postabsorptive insulin levels are encount-
ered.So porta-caval shunt appears to induce hyperinsulinism by itself.
Discrete cellular damage cannot be ruled out however.[22] Johnston,
Alberti and Coworkers[41-43] find normal insulin levels in patients
with longstanding portal vein thrombosis, spontaneous portal systemic
shunting and relatively normal hepatic architecture. Hyperinsulinism,
found in cirrhotics, hepatitis etc., is therefore ascribed to hepatic
cellular damage rather than portal systemic shunting.

Another question is if hyperinsulinism results from hypersecretion or from diminished degradation.[40] The liver is the primary organ
of insulin clearance. Hyperinsulinism in peripheral blood of liver
patients may therefore result from diminished insulin degradation
rather than hypersecretion.[42] Proinsulin, the precursor of insulin,
is cleaved in the pancreatic beta cell to insulin and C-peptide
which are released into the circulation in equimolar quantities.
Unlike insulin, C-peptide is claimed not to be degraded by the
liver[44,45] and peripheral C-peptide concentration might therefore
be a better index of insulin secretion than peripheral insulin
resistance. On the basis of this assumption, C-peptide and insulin
were measured in patients with cirrhosis and patients with portal
venous block with and without cellular damage.[41,42] Fasting C-peptide
and insulin levels from patients with portal vein block without apparent hepatic damage did not differ from normals. Most cirrhotic
patients had fasting hyperinsulinemia with a reduced C-peptide/
insulin ratio. After glucose administration, the C-peptide/insulin

ratio in portal vein block patients without cellular damage did not differ from controls. When cellular damage was superimposed the C-peptide/insulin ratio was significantly reduced like in the cirrhotics. From these studies and others, it was suggested that portal systemic shunting in the presence of a normal liver does not influence hepatic insulin metabolism and that the hyperinsulinism of cirrhosis is therefore a feature of liver damage. Unfortunately, recent doubt has risen with regard to the validity of the assumption that C-peptide is a good measure for insulin secretion in liver disease. It has been shown by Kühl and coworkers [46] that C-peptide is significantly removed from the circulation by the liver. In addition, other groups have demonstrated increased basal levels of C-peptide compared to normal controls suggesting that hypersecretion of C-peptide and insulin occurs. Data from another group raise also doubt with regard to the assumption that C-peptide is cleared normally in liver disease.[12]

In conclusion, hyperinsulinism in liver disease results in part from diminished degradation, chiefly caused by hepatic parenchymal damage, but some degree of hypersecretion may occur. Portal systemic shunting in experimental animals increases insulin levels, but that this is equally due to discrete cellular damage cannot be ruled out.

If hypersecretion occurs, many factors may be responsible. Hyperglucagonism itself may be responsible for hypersecretion of insulin. It should not be forgotten that simultaneous infusions of epinephrine, glucagon and corticosteroids[13] induce glucose intolerance and elevated insulin levels. That this is due to increased secretion of insulin instead of diminished degradation is likely but remains to be established. All the counterregulatory hormones are generally elevated in liver disease, so that this may directly or indirectly via glucose intolerance be responsible for hypersecretion of insulin.

GLUCOSE INTOLERANCE

Glucose intolerance is recently well established in liver disease. Creutzfeldt's group and recently Vannini and others[47,48] have clearly established diminished tissue sensitivity to insulin in cirrhotic patients maintaining euglycaemic hyperinsulinism employing a glucose clamp technique. Diminished sensitivity to insulin and glucose intolerance was demonstrated. Creutzfeldt however ascribes hyperinsulinism in cirrhotics to diminished degradation, leading to downregulation of insulin receptors leading to insulin resistance of peripheral tissues and liver leading to reduced utilization of glucose. This hypothesis totally relies on decreased insulin binding to its receptors. Taylor and coworkers[49] confirmed glucose intolerance in cirrhotics maintaining euglycemia with a constant insulin infusion.

Monocytes and adipocytes from these patients were isolated. Normal insulin binding was demonstrated to monocytes and slightly decreased binding to adipocytes demonstrating slightly decreased insulin receptors in adipocytes. Also this study does not give the final answer leaving room for additional explanations for glucose intolerance and insulin resistance.

Many possible causes have been mentioned in the introduction of this chapter, most of which are unlikely or individually do not explain the whole process.

The work of Sherwin[13] demonstrates that simultaneous infusions of all three counterregulatory hormones are necessary to produce glucose intolerance. The likelihood that elevation of these hormones during injury are responsible for the same phenomena, and the fact that plasma levels of all three counterregulatory hormones are elevated in cirrhotic patients, suggest that glucose intolerance and insulin resistance after severe injury and during severe liver disease result from similar mechanisms. Black and others recently[14] demonstrated that after injury the maximal rate of glucose disposal is diminished and that insulin resistance results from a post-receptor defect.

Glucose intolerance in liver disease has been linked to NEFA but until recently, no good correlation was established.

Riggio and associates[12] demonstrated via stepwise linear regression analysis that basal free fatty acids correlated significantly with the degree of glucose intolerance in cirrhotic patients. Free fatty acids may play a role in carbohydrate intolerance after fasting, stress and other disorders by directly interfering with peripheral glucose utilization according to the glucose-fatty acid-ketone body cycle as formulated by Randle and Newsholme. [50,51] The cycle postulates the following mechanisms: adipose tissue releases fatty acids, which are oxidized by muscle. This reduces glucose utilization in muscle. In the liver, fatty acids are converted to ketone bodies. Ketone bodies are oxidized in brain and muscle, reducing glucose utilization in these tissues. In addition, high levels of ketone bodies can restrict lipolysis directly via an unknown mechanism or indirectly by stimulating insulin release. Randle and Newsholme already in 1963 [50] postulated a crude version of the cycle and stated that control of the cycle was modified by growth hormone, corticosteroids and adrenaline by accelerating release of fatty acids from adipose tissue and muscle triglycerides. Through this action, glucose uptake by muscle is inhibited and insulin sensitivity at the post-receptor level is reduced.

How the cycle is disrupted in liver disease is unknown, but the primary effect obviously resides in the liver. It might be that ketone body production in the liver is inappropriate so that lipo-

lysis is not restricted. The counterregulatory hormones may at the
same time enhance fatty acid release which is not inhibited by
adequate ketone body production in a compromised liver. Nor does
hyperinsulinism inhibit lipolysis like it would after feeding when
no stress or liver disease is present. Many parallels can be distinguished between liver disease and other stress states, suggesting
that identical mechanisms are operative despite the fact that not
all glucose intolerant cirrhotics appear to be stressed clinically.

REFERENCES

1. C. M. Leevy, C. M. Ryan, and J. C. Fineberg, Diabetes mellitus
    and liver dysfunction: etiologic and therapeutic considera-
    tions, Am. J. Med. 8: 290 (1950).
2. P. K. Bondy, Some metabolic anormalities in liver disease, Am.
    J. Med. 24: 428 (1958).
3. R. Hed, Clinical studies in chronic alcoholism. I. Incidence
    of diabetes mellitus in portal cirrhosis, Acta Med. Scand.
    162: 189 (1958).
4. J. P. Felber, P. Magnenat, and A. Vannotti, Tolérance au glucose
    diminuée et réponse insulinique élevée dans la cirrhose,
    Schweiz. Med. Wschr 97: 1537 (1967).
5. J. R. Collins and O. B. Crofford, Glucose intolerance and
    insulin resistance in patients with liver disease, Arch.
    Int. Med. 124: 142 (1969).
6. J. Marco, J. Diego, M. L. Villanueva, M. Diaz-Fierros, I. Val-
    verde, and J. M. Segovia, Elevated plasma glucagon levels
    in cirrhosis of the liver, New Engl. J. Med. 89: 1107 (1973).
7. R. Sherwin, P. Joshi, R. Hendler, Hyperglucagonemia in Laennec's
    cirrhosis. The role of portal-systemic shunting, New Engl.
    J. Med. 290: 239 (1974).
8. R. S. Sherwin, M. Fisher, J. Bessoff, N. Snyder, R. Hendler,
    H. O. Conn,and P. Felig, Hyperglucagonemia in cirrhosis:
    altered secretion and sensitivity to glucagon, Gastroente-
    rology 74: 1224 (1978).
9. A. Mortiaux and A. M. Dawson, Plasma free fatty acid in liver
    disease, Gut 2: 304 (1961).
10. K. G. M. M. Alberti and D. G. Johnston, Carbohydrate Metabolism
    in Liver Disease in :"Liver and Biliary Disease, Pathophy-
    siology, Diagnosis, Management" R. Wright, ed., W. B.
    Saunders Company Ltd., London, Philadelphia, Toronto (1979).
11. H. Ring-Larsen, B. Hesse, J. H. Henriksen,and N. J. Christensen,
    Sympathetic nervous activity and renal and systemic hemo-
    dynamics in cirrhosis: Plasma norepinephrine concentration,
    hepatic extraction and renal release Hepatology 2: 304
    (1982).
12. O. Riggio, M. Merli, C. Cangiano, R. Capocaccia, A. Cascino,
    A. Lala, F. Leonetti, M. Mauceri, M. Pepe, F. Rossi-Fanelli,
    M. Savioli, G. Tamburrano,and L. Capocaccia, Glucose into-
    lerance in liver cirrhosis, Metabolism 31: 627 (1982).

13. R. S. Sherwin, Effect of epinephrine on fuel metabolism in man:
    Role in the response to stress. Proceedings of the 4th Espen
    Congress, Vienna. In press (1982).
14. P. R. Black, D. C. Brooks, P. Q. Bessey, R. R. Wolfe, and D. W.
    Wilmore, Mechanisms of insulin resistance following injury,
    Ann. Surg. 196: 420 (1982).
15. D. C. Deibert and R. A. DeFronzo, Epinephrine-induced insulin
    resistance in man, J. Clin. Invest. 65: 717 (1980).
16. J. E. Liljenquist and D. Rabin, Lack of a role for glucagon
    in the disposal of an oral glucose load in normal man, J.
    Clin. Endocrinol. Metab. 49: 937 (1979).
17. R. H. Unger and L. Orci, Role of glucagon in diabetes, Arch.
    Int. Med. 137: 482 (1977).
18. H. N. Munro, D. Fernstrom,and R. J. Wurtman, Insulin, plasma
    amino acid imbalance and hepatic coma, Lancet 1: 722 (1975).

19. C. O. Record, R. A. Chase, K. G. M. M. Alberti,and R. Williams,
    Disturbances in glucose metabolism in patients with liver
    damage due to paracetamol overdose, Clin. Sci. Mol. Med.
    49: 473 (1975).
20. K. G. M. M. Alberti, C. O. Record, D. H. Williamson, and R.
    Wright, Metabolic changes in active chronic hepatitis, Clin.
    Sci. Mol. Med. 42: 591 (1972).
21. P. B. Soeters, G. Weir, A. M. Ebeid, and J. E. Fischer, Insulin,
    glucagon, portal systemic shunting and hepatic failure in
    the dog, J. Surg. Res. 23: 183 (1977).
22. P. Rous and L. D. Larimore, Relation of the portal blood to
    liver maintenance: A demonstration of liver atrophy condi-
    tion on compensation, J. Exp. Med. 31: 600 (1920).
23. T. E. Starzi, K. Watanabe, and K. A. Porter, Effect of insulin,
    glucagon and insulin/glucagon infusions on liver morphology
    and cell division after complete portacaval shunt in dogs,
    Lancet 1: 821 (1976).
24. H. O. Conn, Ammonia tolerance as an index of portal-systemic
    collateral circulation in cirrhosis, Gastroenterology 41:
    97 (1961).
25. A. R. Burchell, A. H. Moreno, W. F. Panke, and T. F. Nealon,
    Hepatic artery flow improvement after portacaval shunt: a
    single haemodynamic clinical correlate, Ann. Surg. 184:
    289 (1976).
26. P. J. Lefebvre and A. S. Luyckx, Effect of acute kidney exclu-
    sion by ligation of renal arteries on peripheral plasma
    glucagon levels and pancreatic glucagon production in the
    anesthetized dog, Metabolism 24: 1169 (1975).
27. S. C. Woods and D. Porte, Jr., Neural control of the endocrine
    pancreas, Physiol. Rev. 54: 596 (1974).
28. L. Orci, A portrait of the pancreatic beta cell, Diabetologia
    10: 163 (1974).
29. J. P. Palmer, D. P. Henry, J. W. Benson, D. G. Johnson, and
    J. W. Ensinck, Glucagon response to hypoglycemia in sympa-

tectomized man, J. Clin. Invest. 57: 522 (1976).

30. J. Iversen, Adrenergic receptors and the secretion of glucagon and insulin from the isolated perfused canine pancreas, J. Clin. Invest. 52: 2102 (1973).

31. J. E. Gerich, J. H. Karam, and P. H. Forsham, Stimulation of glucagon secretion by epinephrine in man, J. Clin. Endocrin. Metab. 37: 479 (1973).

32. J. E. Gerich, M. Langlois, C. Noacco, V. Schneider, and P. H. Forsham, Adrenergic modulation of pancreatic glucagon secretion in man, J. Clin. Invest. 53: 1441 (1974).

33. E. J. Rayfield, D. T. George, H. L. Eichner, and T. H. Tsu, L-Dopa stimulation of glucagon secretion in man, New Engl. J. Med. 293: 589 (1975).

34. J. W. Ensinck, R. M. Walter, J. P. Palmer, R. G. Brodows, and R. G. Campbell, Glucagon responses to hypoglycemia in Adrenalectomized Man, Metabolism 25: 227 (1976).

35. J. P. Palmer, J. Halter, and P. L. Werner, Differential effect of isoproterenol on acute glucagon and insulin release in man, Metabolism 28: 237 (1979).

36. A. S. Luyckx and P. J. Lefebvre, Arguments for a regulation of pancreatic glucagon secretion by circulating plasma free fatty acids, Proc. Soc. Exp. Biol. Med. 133: 524 (1970).

37. S. S. Andrews, S. A. Lopez, and W. G. Blackard, Effect of lipids on glucagon secretion in man, Metabolism 24: 35 (1975).

38. J. K. Wise, R. Hendler, and P. Felig, Influence of glucocorticoids on glucagon secretion and plasma amino acid concentrations in man, J. Clin. Invest. 52: 2774 (1973).

39. E. Holm, Personal communication.

40. M. R. Lunzer, S. P. Newman, A. G. Bernard, K. K. Manghani, S. P. V. Sherlock, and J. Ginsburg, Impaired cardiovascular responsiveness in liver disease, Lancet 2: 382 (1975).

41. D. G. Johnston, K. G. M. M. Alberti, O. K. Faber, and C. Binder, Hyperinsulinism of hepatic cirrhosis: diminished degradation or hypersecretion? Lancet, January 1: 10 (1977).

42. D. G. Johnston, K. G. M. M. Alberti, R. Wright, G. Smith-Laing, A. M. Stewart, S. Sherlock, O. Faber, and C. Binder, C-peptide and insulin in liver disease, Diabetes 27 (Suppl. 1): 201 (1978).

43. G. Smith-Laing, S. Sherlock, and O. K. Faber, Effects of spontaneous portal-systemic shunting on insulin metabolism, Gastroenterology 76: 685 (1979).

44. A. I. Katz and A. H. Rubenstein, Metabolism of pro-insulin, insulin and C-peptide in the rat, J. Clin. Invest. 52: 1113 (1973).

45. R. W. Stoll, J. L. Touber, L. A. Menahan, and R. H. Williams, Clearance of porcine, insulin, pro-insulin and connecting peptides by the isolated rat liver, Proc. Soc. Exp. Biol. Med. 133: 894 (1970).

46. C. Kühl, O. K. Faber, P. Hornnes, and S. Jensen Lindkaer, C-

peptide metabolism and the liver, Diabetes 27 (Suppl. 1): 197 (1978).

47. G. Oehler, H. Bleyl, and K. J. Matthes, Glucose tolerance and serum insulin in different chronic liver diseases. VI International Congress of Liver Diseases, Basel, October 15-17, Abstract no. 145 (1982).

48. P. Vannini, G. Forlani, G. Marchesini, and E. Pisi, Evaluation of insulin resistance in liver cirrhosis by means of the glucose clamp technique, Ital. J. Gastroenterol. 13: 255 (1981).

49. R. Taylor, R. Heine, J. Collins, K. G. M. Alberti, and O. F. W. James, No marked impairment of insulin binding to adipocytes in insulin resistant cirrhotics. VI International Congress of Liver Diseases. Basel, October 15-17, 1982. Abstract no. 193 (1982).

50. P. J. Randle, C. N. Hales, P. B. Garland, and E. A. Newsholme, The glucose fatty-acid cycle, its role in insulin sensitivity and the metabolic disturbances of diabetes mellitus, Lancet 1: 7285 (1963).

51. E. A. Newsholme and C. Start, Regulation of fat metabolism in liver. Introduction. in:"Regulation in Metabolism," Chapter 7. John Wiley, London, New York, Toronto (1974).

PROTEINS AND AMINO ACIDS IN LIVER FAILURE [°]

G. Marchesini, M. Zoli, C. Dondi, and G. P. Bianchi

Istituto di Patologia Medica 1, Università di Bologna
Policlinico S. Orsola, Via Massarenti 9 - 40138 Bologna
Italy

INTRODUCTION

Patients with liver cirrhosis scarcely tolerate protein thus large nitrogen loads are likely to induce hepatic coma. A protein load, either as a protein rich meal or a gastrointestinal bleeding, which increase nitrogen reabsorption, or an intravenous administration of protein hydrolisates, may produce stupor and drowsiness up to deep coma, at the same time increasing blood ammonia. This clinical observation forms the basis of the 'ammonia' theory of hepatic encephalopathy.

In recent years, however, this theory was questioned and considerable attention was turned from protein to the single amino acids. Again, the first suggestions came from the clinical observation that not all protein foods were equally harmful. Bessman et al.[1] in 1958 first reported that whole blood was more toxic to patients with advanced liver disease than an equivalent amount of casein protein. In 1966 Fenton et al.[2] proved an apparent beneficial effect of a milk-and-cheese diet in patients with liver cirrhosis and porta-caval anastomosis as compared to a diet comprising an equivalent amount of protein of different sources. The Authors were unable to explain the reasons of improvement.

A reasonable answer came several years later, when Fischer and Baldessarini[3] proposed the 'false neurotransmitters' theory. The basis of this theory lies in the imbalance of the plasma amino acid profile of patients with cirrhosis, characterized by increased levels of aromatic amino acids (phenylalanine and tyrosine) and free tryptophan, and decreased levels of branched-chain amino acids (valine,

---

(°) Supported by Research Contract N°800038504 from the National Research Council (CNR), Rome.

isoleucine, and leucine = BCAAs). The entry into the brain of
different amino acids, and hence the synthesis of putative neurotransmitters is regulated by their plasma concentration and mainly
by the balance between the single neutral amino acids. Because of
the disturbed plasma profile, the passage of aromatic amino acids
is increased, the synthesis of putative neurotransmitters is decreased
and large amounts of 'false' neurotransmitters (tyramine, octopamine,
B-phenylethanolamine)are produced, leading to considerable disturbances in neurotransmission. The role of decreased BCAAs in the
pathogenesis of hepatic coma has grown after the demonstration that
large amounts of i.v. BCAAs may ameliorate che neuropsychiatric
symptoms,[4,5] possibly preventing and reversing the influx of aromatic
amines and the synthesis of false neurotransmitters. These data may
explain the beneficial effects of a milk-and-cheese diet, since
casein is rich in BCAAs and poor in aromatic amino acids.

Pathogenesis of Amino Acid Imbalance

     The above mentioned study, and the clinical implications which
are derived, raised an impressive series of experiments and hypotheses trying to define the pathogenesis of the altered plasma amino
acid imbalance of cirrhotics. Because of its position between portal
and systemic circulation, the liver exercises a regulatory and homeo-
static function on the levels of substrates which are derived from
gastrointestinal absorption. Several factors may contribute to the
changes in plasma amino acid profile. The liver is the sole site of
degradation of most essential amino acids.[6] This may explain the
peculiar increase in phenylalanine and tyrosine. To support this
hypothesis, Zoli et al.[7] studied a large series of patients with
cirrhosis without overt encephalopathy and correlated plasma levels
of amino acids with different tests of liver function and portal-
systemic shunting. A significant correlation was observed between
the sum of phenylalanine and tyrosine and galactose elimination
capacity r = -0.657) or the ammonia tolerance test (r = 0.758). A
direct role of shunting is however questioned by the data of Iwasaki
et al.[8] who found that in patients with idiopathic portal hypertension and normal liver histology, aromatic amino acids are in the
normal range. In cirrhotics both the shunting of blood around the
liver and reduced liver cell mass may contribute to decrease the
handling of these substrates. A third pathogenic factor in the increased levels of aromatic amines may be the endogenous breakdown
of lean body mass,[9] partly due to the reduced intake of nutrients
(mainly by the alcoholics), or to the hormonal imbalance associated
with cirrhosis.[10] Most patients with cirrhosis show a negative
nitrogen balance[11] and increased muscle protein breakdown rates.[12]
In rats with end-to-side porta-caval shunt, whose plasma amino acid
profile is similar to the one of patients with cirrhosis, the achieve-
ment of a positive nitrogen balance significantly reduced plasma and
brain levels of phenylalanine and tyrosine in a dose-related relationship.[13] A role of increased-myofibrillar breakdown is also

supported by the recent finding that patients with increased protein
catabolic rates have higher levels of phenylalanine and tyrosine than
patients whose protein turnover, as assessed by 3-methylhistidine
and creatinine excretion, is in the normal range.[14]

Similar considerations possibly apply to plasma tryptophan. In
this case, also albumin levels may play an additional role, regulating
the amount of the free amino acid in plasma, and consequently its
removal and metabolism by liver cells.

The most puzzling abnormality of plasma amino acid profile in
patients with cirrhosis is the decrease in BCAAs. Valine, isoleucine,
and leucine are always reduced, also in well-nourished and compensated patients, indipendently from the presence of hepatic encephalopathy.[15] In 1975 Munro et al.[16] suggested a role of hyperinsulinaemia,
which is almost always present in advanced cirrhotics, in decreasing
BCAA levels. The primary site of BCAA metabolism is skeletal muscle,
into which amino acid entry is regulated by insulin levels.[17] By
contrast, in the basal postabsorptive state no changes in BCAA levels
occur after the passage of blood through the liver.[18] Several data
in patients with various diseases seem to support this hypothesis.
In Type 1 (insulin-dependent) diabetes mellitus after insulin with-
drawl, BCAAs are very high,[19] and this alteration is corrected by
insulin treatment.[20,21] In patients with insulinomas, BCAAs are low,
possibly as effect of hyperinsulinaemia.[22] In both groups of patients,
and mainly in diabetics, strict correlations were found between BCAAs
and the blood levels of several insulin-dependent substrates: glucose,
free fatty acids, glycerol, and ketone bodies.[22]

In patients with liver cirrhosis, however, only few data were
available to support this hypothesis. No correlation could be found
between decreased BCAAs and insulin levels.[23] Similarly in dogs with
end-to-side porta-caval shunt no relationship is present between
insulin and BCAAs.[24] Although a few studies claimed that BCAA metabolism is accelerated in the muscle of cirrhotics,[25,26] this was
related to hyperammonaemia and not to hyperinsulinaemia,[26] Soeters
et al.[27] did not show any increased uptake of labelled ^{14}C-leucine
in the muscle of shunted rats, whose BCAAs are greatly reduced. Most
importantly, increased uptake of BCAA in muscle should lead to increased muscle mass and decreased myofibrillar catabolism,[28] which
does not occur. From a clinical point of view the cirrhotics show a
striking loss of muscle mass.

The relationship between insulin levels and BCAAs may change
according to peripheral insulin resistance (Table 1). In uncontrolled
Type 2 (non-insulin dependent) diabetes, BCAAs, as well as different
insulin-dependent substrates, increase, in spite of high insulin
levels.[29] In patients with cirrhosis the presence of high normal
blood glucose levels and intolerance to oral glucose,[30] associated
to hyperinsulinaemia and an exaggerated insulin response to oral

Table 1. Insulin and insulin-dependent substrates in various diseases and in states of insulin resistance.

Disease	Insulin	Blood glucose	Branched-chain amino acids	Free fatty acids	Insulin resistance
Type 1 (insulin-dependent) diabetes mellitus					
uncontrolled	absent	high	high	high	absent
under therapy	present	normal	normal	normal	absent
Insulinoma	high	low	low	low	sometimes present
Type 2 (non-insulin-dependent) diabetes mellitus	high	high	high	high	strongly present
Liver cirrhosis	high	high	low	high	strongly present

glucose,[31] is in keeping with a strong insulin resistance.

The Protein Meal Test in Cirrhotics

A more accurate assessment of the influence of liver physiology and disease, peripheral tissue metabolism, and hormonal balance on plasma levels of different amino acids may be obtained after stimulus.

Following a protein meal, muscle nitrogen repletion is due to the uptake of the amino acids which enter the systemic circulation from the splanchnic bed.[32] BCAAs show the greatest and more prolonged increments in plasma levels, due to their selective escape of hepatic metabolism,[33],[34] The rise in plasma insulin[35] favours BCAA oxidation in muscle,[17] where BCAA balance turns from a net output to a net uptake.[34] In insulin-deficient states (Type 1 diabetes mellitus after insulin withdrawal), peripheral BCAAs are unusually largely increased after a protein meal, and only a transient leg uptake was observed.[34]

We evaluated the metabolic effects of a protein meal in 20 patients with cirrhosis without encephalopathy and 10 age- and sex-matched controls.[35] The test meal consisted of 200 g of lean boiled beef (protein content about 22%), to be eaten after an overnight fast in 10 to 15 minutes. As it appears from Figure 1, a greater and more prolonged insulin response was observed in cirrhotics, whose basal insulin levels were higher than in controls (19 $\pm$ 2 μU/ml versus 11 $\pm$ 1; p < 0.05). BCAA levels, which were reduced in cirrhotics in the basal state (365 $\pm$ 15 nmol/ml versus 498 $\pm$ 18; p < 0.001), increased in controls and, more largely, in cirrhotics. At 180 min plasma BCAA levels were higher in cirrhotics (795 $\pm$ 56 versus 719 $\pm$ 35). The total BCAA response to protein ingestion was markedly higher in cirrhotics (259 $\pm$ 27 nmol/ml·min versus 153 $\pm$ 14; p < 0.02). The levels of most amino acids increased as well, in both cirrhotics and controls, but an exaggerated increase comparable to that of BCAAs was only observed in aromatic amino acids and tryptophan, which are exclusively metabolized by the liver (Figure 2). The sum of phenylalanine and tyrosine increased by 37 $\pm$ 2 nmol/ml·min in controls and 64 $\pm$ 7 in cirrhotics (p < 0.02), while tryptophan increased by 12 $\pm$ 2 nmol/ml·min and 17 $\pm$ 1 respectively (p < 0.02). In summary, the exaggerated BCAA response was one of the most striking abnormalities we could observe, in spite of increased insulin and lack of importance of liver damage.

To prove a role of insulin resistance, the metabolic effects of the protein meal were compared to those of an oral glucose load (75 g). Glucose response to oral glucose was abnormal in the presence of hyperinsulinaemia, and significantly correlated to the BCAA response to protein ingestion (r = 0.714). For a better assessment of insulin sensitivity, in 8 subjects with cirrhosis an euglycaemic glucose clamp was also performed, according to De Fronzo et al.,[36] with minor modifications. The measure of insulin activity on glucose metabolism,

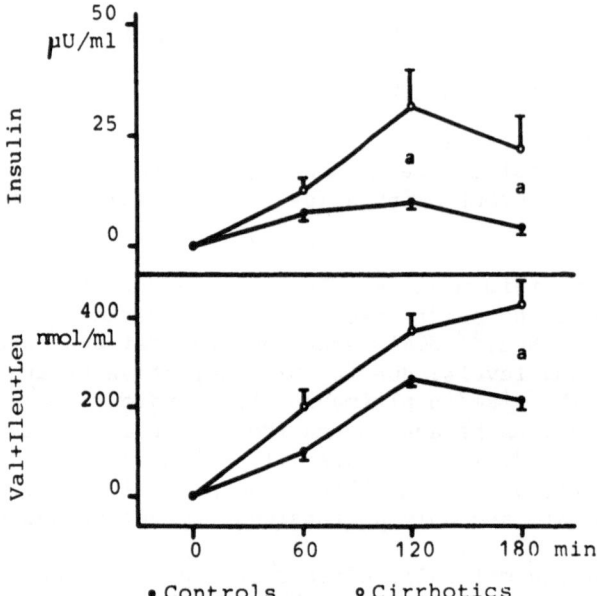

Fig. 1.   Increase in plasma insulin and branched-chain amino acid
          levels following a protein meal in 10 controls and in 20
          cirrhotics (means ± SEM). (a) Significance of difference:
          p < 0.05 or less.

which was obtained, significantly correlated with the insulinogenic
index following oral glucose (r = -0.777), or the ratio of insulin
response to BCAA response after protein, a tentative index of insulin
activity on BCAA metabolism (r = -0.847).

    These data are in keeping with the hypothesis that insulin
resistance remarkably affects BCAA metabolism. This conclusion is
also supported by amino acid levels during the euglycaemic clamp.[38]
In the second hour of insulin infusion, at similar steady-state
levels of 72 ± 5 µU/ml in controls and 82 ± 5 in cirrhotics, BCAAs
fell from 366 ± 32 nmol/ml to 300 ± 21 in controls and from 350 ± 11
to 316 ± 19 in cirrhotics. In agreement with previous data,[39] BCAA
decrease per µU of circulating insulin was reduced in cirrhotics
(0.21 ± 0.06 nmol/µU versus 0.46 ± 0.09; p < 0.01). A significant
correlation was present between the index of insulin resistance,
during insulin infusion, and the fall in BCAA levels (r = -0.868).

Conclusions

    These studies suggest three important considerations. First,
they question the hypothesis that decreased BCAA levels in patients

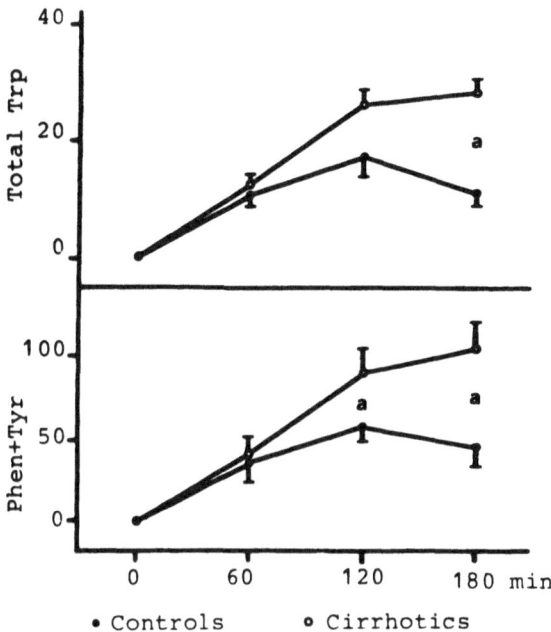

Fig. 2.   Increase in peripheral plasma amino acid levels following
          a protein meal in 10 control and in 20 cirrhotic subjects
          (means $\pm$ SEM in nmol/ml). (a) Significance of difference:
          $p < 0.05$ or less.

with cirrhosis are merely due to hyperinsulinaemia. Insulin resistance is likely to vanish the metabolic effect of hyperinsulinaemia
on protein metabolism, as well as on glucose metabolism, where it
does not induce hypoglycaemia. Soeters et al.[27] suggested a possible degradation of BCAAs in tissues other than muscle, and proved
an increased uptake of ^{14}C-leucine in adipose tissue, where these
substrates might be utilized more rapidly because of altered meta-
bolizing capacity.[40] However, also in adipocytes, leucine utilization is under insulin control. Beside the liver, the kidney is an
organ where a marked gluconeogenesis takes place. The activity or
concentration of the BCAA transaminases is high in kidneys of
animals following portacaval shunt.[41] The renal medulla glucose
uptake is not under insulin control. Non-insulin-dependent metabolic
pathways of BCAA degradation in organs other than skeletal muscle,
and especially in the kidney, may be suggested, and require further
consideration.

    The second point regards the site of insulin resistance in
cirrhosis. We showed that BCAA and insulin responses to protein
ingestion look like glucose and insulin curves after the oral glucose load. More than 50% of ingested glucose, absorbed from the
splanchnic bed, is retained within the liver. In patients with liver
cirrhosis, the diabetic-like blood glucose response to glucose

ingestion may therefore be due to the shunting of blood around the
liver, which prevents hepatic glucose uptake, or to the unresponsi-
veness of peripheral tissues to insulin. The evaluation of a substrate which is not metabolized by the liver may provide clues on this
problem. The altered BCAA response to protein is consistent with
the hypothesis that peripheral insulin activity is decreased as well.
Greco et al.[42] proved that insulin binding to monocytes is reduced
in cirrhotics. Record et al.[43] confirmed a reduction of peripheral
insulin receptors in cirrhotics, with and without glucose intolerance. They conclude that peripheral insulin resistance is not an
important determinant of glucose intolerance, as compared to reduced
hepatic retention of the glucose load. Functional or anatomic shunting possibly prevents hepatic glucose uptake. The peripheral hyper-
glycaemia which ensues massively stimulates insulin secretion; hyperinsulinaemia is enhanced by reduced hepatic removal of insulin, and
leads to changes in peripheral insulin activity. Insulin resistance
further impairs glucose metabolism, and reduces muscular BCAA uptake
as well. Whether the decreased peripheral insulin activity is due to
defects in either receptor concentration or affinity, or to a post-
receptor defect,[44] remains to be determined, although recent data
favour the second hypothesis.[45]

     Finally, the decreased BCAA removal after protein load may have
important therapeutic implications in the treatment of hepatic encephalopathy. They might balance the effects of decresed aromatic amino
acid clearance, and prevent the entry of tryptophan across the blood-
brain barrier. The effects of insulin resistance on BCAA metabolism
should also be considered in the therapeutic trials of hepatic encephalopathy using oral BCAA.

REFERENCES

1. A. N. Bessman, G. S. Mirik, and R. Hawkins, Blood ammonia levels
    following the ingestion of casein and whole blood, J. Clin.
    Invest. 37: 990 (1958).
2. J. C. Fenton, E. J. Knight, and P. L. Humpherson, Milk-and-
    cheese diet in portal-systemic encephalopathy, Lancet 1:
    164 (1966).
3. J. E. Fischer and R. Baldessarini, False neurotransmitters
    and hepatic failure, Lancet 2: 74 (1971).
4. J. E. Fischer, J. M. Funovics, A. Aguirre, J. H. James, J. M.
    Keane, R. I. C. Wesdorp, N. Yoshimura, and T. Westman, The
    role of plasma amino acids in hepatic encephalopathy,
    Surgery 78: 276 (1975).
5. J. E. Fischer, H. M. Rosen, A. M. Ebeid, J. H. James, J. M.
    Keane, and P. B. Soeters, The effects of normalization of
    plasma amino acids in hepatic encephalopathy in man, Surgery
    80: 77 (1976).
6. L. L. Miller, The role of the liver and the non-hepatic tissues
    in the regulation of free amino acid levels in the blood, in:

   "Amino Acid Pools," J. T. Holden, ed., Elsevier Publishing
   Co., Amsterdam, 708-721 (1962).

 7. M. Zoli, G. Marchesini, A. Angiolini, C. Dondi, F. B. Bianchi,
     and E. Pisi, Plasma amino acids as markers of liver dysfunc-
     tion in cirrhotics, Scand. J. Gastroenterol. 16: 689 (1981).

 8. Y. Iwasaki, H. Sato, A. Ohkubo, T. Sanjo, S. Futagawa, M. Sugiu-
     ra, and S. Tsuji, Effect of spontaneous portal-systemic shun-
     ting on plasma insulin and amino acid concentrations, Gastro-
     enterology 78: 677 (1980).

 9. H. M. Rosen, N. Yoshimura, J. M. Hodgman, and J. E. Fischer,
     Plasma amino acid patterns in hepatic encephalopathy of dif-
     fering etiology, Gastroenterology 72: 483 (1977).

10. G. Marchesini, M. Zoli, A. Angiolini, C. Dondi, F. B. Bianchi,
     and E. Pisi, Muscle breakdown in liver cirrhosis and the
     role of altered carbohydrate metabolism, Hepatology 1: 294
     (1981).

11. F. Fiaccadori, F. Ghinelli, G. Pedretti, G. Pelosi, D. Sacchini,
     and G. Spadini, Negative nitrogen balance in cirrhotics, Ric.
     Clin. Lab. 11: 259 (1981).

12. M. Zoli, G. Marchesini, C. Dondi, G. P. Bianchi, and E. Pisi,
     Myofibrillar protein catabolic rates in cirrhotic patients
     with and without muscle wasting, Clin. Sci. 62: 683 (1982).

13. H. M. Rosen, P. B. Soeters, J. H. James, J. Hodgman, and J. E.
     Fischer, Influences of exogenous intake and nitrogen balance
     on plasma and brain aromatic amino acid concentrations, Meta-
     bolism 27: 393 (1978).

14. M. Zoli, G. Marchesini, G. P. Bianchi, C. Dondi, A. Melli, S.
     Cassarani, and V. Bua, The role of muscle protein catabolism
     in the plasma amino acid profile of cirrhotics, Ital. J.
     Gastroenterol. 15: in press (1983).

15. G. Marchesini, M. Zoli, C. Dondi, L. Cecchini, A. Angiolini,
     F. B. Bianchi, and E. Pisi, Prevalence of subclinical hepatic
     encephalopathy in cirrhotics and relationship to plasma amino
     acid imbalance, Dig. Dis. Sci. 25: 763 (1980).

16. H. N. Munro, J. D. Fernstrom, and R. J. Wurtman, Insulin, plasma
     amino acid imbalance, and hepatic coma, Lancet 1: 722
     (1975).

17. T. Pozefsky, P. Felig, J. D. Tobin, S. Soeldner, and G. F.
     Cahill, Amino acid balance across tissues of the forearm
     in postabsorptive man. Effects of insulin at two dose levels,
     J. Clin. Invest. 48: 2273 (1969).

18. J. Wahren, P. Felig, E. Cerasi, and R. Luft, Splanchnic and
     peripheral glucose and amino acid metabolism in diabetes
     mellitus, J. Clin. Invest. 51: 1870 (1972).

19. P. Felig, E. B. Marliss, J. L. Ohman, and J. F. Cahill, Plasma
     amino acid levels in diabetes ketoacidosis, Diabetes 19:
     727 (1970).

20. A. Carlsten, B. Hallgren, R. Jagenburg, A. Svanborg, and L.
     Werko, Amino Acids and free fatty acids in plasma in diabe-
     tes, Acta Med. Scand. 179: 361 (1966).

21. A. K. Hanna, B. Zinman, A. F. Nakhoda, H. L. Minuk, E. F. Stokes,
     M. Albisser, B. S. Leibel, and E. B. Marliss, Insulin, glu-
     cagon, and amino acids during glycaemic control by the arti-
     ficial pancreas in diabetic man, Metabolism 29: 321 (1980).
22. M. Berger, H. Zimmerman-Telschow, P. Berchtold, M. Drost, W. A.
     Muller, F. A. Gries, and H. Zimmerman, Blood amino acid
     levels in patients with insulin excess (functioning insu-
     linoma) and insulin deficiency (diabetic ketosis), Metabolism
     27: 793 (1978).
23. G. Marchesini, G. Forlani, M. Zoli, A. Angiolini, M. P. Scolari,
     F. B. Bianchi, and E. Pisi, Insulin and glucagon levels in
     liver cirrhosis: relationship with the plasma amino acid im-
     balance of chronic hepatic encephalopathy, Dig. Dis. Sci.
     24: 594 (1979).
24. P. B. Soeters, G. Weir, A. M. Ebeid, and J. E. Fischer, Insulin,
     glucagon, portal-systemic shunting, and hepatic failure in
     the dog, J. Surg. Res. 23: 183 (1977).
25. V. Job, W. W. Coon, and M. Sloan, Free amino acids in liver,
     plasma, and muscle of patients with cirrhosis of the liver,
     J. Surg. Res. 7: 41 (1967).
26. M. Hayashi, H. Ohnishi, Y. Kawade, Y. Muto, and Y. Takahashi,
     Augmented utilization of branched-chain amino acids by
     skeletal muscle in decompensated liver cirrhosis in special
     relation to ammonia detoxication, Gastroenterol. Jpn. 16:
     64 (1981).
27. P. B. Soeters and J. E. Fischer, Insulin, glucagon, amino
     acid imbalance, and hepatic encephalopathy, Lancet 2: 880
     (1976).
28. G. Marchesini, M. Zoli, C. Dondi, G. P. Bianchi, M. Cirulli,
     and E. Pisi, Anticatabolic effects of branched-chain amino
     acid-enriched solutions in patients with liver cirrhosis,
     Hepatology 2: 420 (1982).
29. P. Vannini, G. Marchesini, G. Forlani, A. Angiolini, A. Ciava-
     rella, M. Zoli, and E. Pisi, Branched-chain amino acids and
     alanine as indices of the metabolic control in type 1 (insu-
     lin-dependent) and type 2 (non-insulin-dependent) diabetes,
     Diabetologia 22: 217 (1982).
30. C. Megyesi, E. Samols, and V. Marks, Glucose tolerance and
     diabetes in chronic liver disease, Lancet 2: 1051 (1967).
31. J. R. Collins and O. B. Crofford, Glucose intolerance and
     insulin resistance in patients with liver disease, Arch.
     Intern. Med. 124: 142 (1969).
32. D. D. Van Slyke and G. M. Meyer, The fate of protein decompo-
     sition products in the body. III. The absorption of amino
     acids from the blood by the tissues, J. Biol. Chem. 16: 197
     (1913).
33. E. G. Frame, The levels of individual free amino acids in the
     plasma of normal man at various intervals after a high
     protein meal, J. Clin. Invest. 37: 1710 (1958).
34. J. Wahren, P. Felig, and L. Hagenfeldt, Effect of protein in-

gestion on splanchnic and leg metabolism in normal man and in patients with diabetes mellitus, J. Clin. Invest. 57: 987 (1976).

35. J. C. Flyod, S. S. Fajans, J. W. Conn, R. F. Knopf, and J. Rull, Insulin secretion in response to protein ingestion, J. Clin. Invest. 45: 1479 (1966).

36. R. A. Fronzo, J. D. Tobin, and R. Andres, Glucose clamp technique: a method for quantifying insulin secretion and resistance, Am. J. Physiol. 237: E214 (1979).

37. P. Vannini, G. Forlani, G. Marchesini, and E. Pisi, Evaluation of insulin resistance in liver cirrhosis by means of the glucose clamp technique, Ital. J. Gastroenterol. 13: 225 (1981).

38. G. Marchesini, G. Forlani, M. Zoli, C. Dondi, G. P. Bianchi, V. Bua, P. Vannini, and E. Pisi, Effect of euglycaemic insulin infusion on plasma levels of branched-chain amino acids in patients with liver cirrhosis, Hepatology 3: in press (1983).

39. P. Ferenci, P. Bratusch-Marrain, W. Waldhausl, A. Korn, and P. Novotny, Insulin resistance in patients with cirrhosis-associated defects of plasma clearance of amino acids, Gastroenterology 80: 1332 (1981).

40. J. E. G. De Boer, R. J. Costenbroek, M. A. Janssen, J. J. van Dongen, and P. B. Soeters, Influence of porta-caval shunting on the fate of leucine in rat muscle and adipose tissue, Proceedings of the 17th Meeting of the European Association for the Study of the Liver (EASL), Göteborg: 21 (1982).

41. J. E. Fischer, and R. J. Baldessarini, Pathogenesis and therapy of hepatic coma, in: "Progress in Liver disease," H. Popper, F. Schaffner, eds., Grune and Stratton, New York and London, 5: 363 (1976).

42. A. V. Greco, A. Bertoli, G. Ghirlanda, R. Manna, L. Altomonte, and A. G. Rebuzz, Insulin resistance in liver cirrhosis: decreased insulin binding to circulating monocytes, Horm. Metab. Res. 12: 577 (1980).

43. C. O. Record, M. C. Bramble, J. Whittaker, M. Piniewska, and K. G. M. M. Alberti, Impaired monocyte insulin binding in cirrhosis, Gut 22: 869 (abs.) (1981).

44. A. Biel, D. Robbins, E. Drodny, G. Baumann, and A. Rubenstein, Insulin resistance in cirrhosis: a receptor study, Gastroenterol. 80: 1331 (abs.) (1981).

45. J. Iversen and N. Tygstrup, Carbohydrate metabolism in relation to liver physiology and disease, in: "The Liver," I. M. Arias, M. Frenkel, J. A. P. Wilson, eds., Excerpta Medica, Amsterdam, Oxford, Princeton, 2: 1 (1982).

THE METABOLIC FATE OF BRANCHED-CHAIN AMINO ACIDS

E. Holm, H. Leweling, U. Staedt, J.-P. Striebel, and
St. Jacob

Dept. of Pathophysiology, 1st Med. Clinic Mannheim
University of Heidelberg, FRG

INTRODUCTION

This contribution is, at first, concerned with data which indicate that portal-systemic shunting (PSS) of blood and hepatic
failure exert differential effects on the plasma levels of branched-
chain amino acids (BCAA). Following this, recent findings pertaining
to amino acid clearance rates in cirrhotic patients are presented.
Special interest is given to metabolic mechanisms underlying the
reduction in the plasma levels of BCAA in patients with liver cirrhosis and in animals with portocaval anastomosis (PCA). From the
metabolic alterations outlined, provisional therapeutic principles
can be derived. Finally, the concentrations of BCAA produced in
plasma and muscle by therapeutic administration of these substances
require a brief discussion.

1. DIFFERENTIAL EFFECTS OF PORTAL-SYSTEMIC SHUNTING AND LIVER CELL DAMAGE ON THE PLASMA LEVELS OF BCAA

In patients with liver cirrhosis, it is perhaps impossible, or
at least very difficult, to identify and to separate from one another,
the effects of PSS and of an impairment of hepatic function on the
plasma levels of BCAA. Therefore, we want to refer to a series of
experiments carried out on a total of 82 cats (Fig. 1). 29 animals
served as healthy controls. 46 animals were given a PCA; 13 of them
were additionally injected with thioacetamide. The remaining 7 cats
had microspheres injected into the portal vein; they developed portal
hypertension. In the cats which had undergone only the shunt operation as well as in those treated with microspheres, neither structural alterations of the hepatocytes nor liver insufficiency could be
assessed by histological examinations and conventional blood chemi-

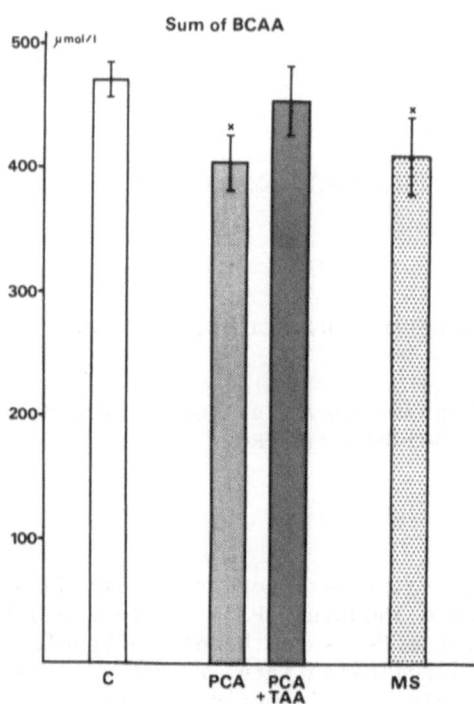

Fig. 1.   Plasma BCAA concentrations in experiments on cats (means
          + S.E.M.). C: healthy controls (n=29); PCA: animals given
          a portacaval anastomosis (n=33); PCA + TAA: animals with
          portacaval anastomosis and additional liver cell damage
          induced by thioacetamide (5 times 20 mg/kg i.p., with 48-hr
          intervals between the single injections; n = 13); MS: ani-
          mals which had microspheres injected into the portal vein
          (n=7).   p ≤ 0.05, compared to the healthy controls (U-test).

stry. There was a fall in the plasma levels of BCAA in these cats.
The combination of PCA with moderate liver cell damage induced by
thioacetamide resulted in a less marked decrease or even in normal
values of BCAA concentrations. In patients, a condition of extensive
portal-systemic shunting without significant deficits of hepatic
function occurs in the form of idiopathic portal hypertension which
is also characterized by lowered BCAA levels in plasma.[1] Thus, only
PSS insufficiency can exert the opposite effect.[2,3]

     Whenever the plasma levels of a particular group of amino acids
are regulated by a common mechanism, these amino acids are likely to
show co-varying values from individual to individual. A good overall
view of the correlations between many variables can be provided by
factor analysis. This method was applied to the plasma concentra-

tions of amino acids measured in 76 cirrhotic patients.[4] Five factors
resulted (Table 1). Each factor represents co-variations of the
levels of several substances in plasma. For the purposes of this
contribution, three of the five factors are relevant. As can be seen
from factor 3, there were strong correlations between valine, leucine
and isoleucine, probably because the BCAA concentrations are mainly
determined by the degree of PSS. According to factor 1, methionine,
phenylalanine, tyrosine, and two other amino acids, the values of
which depend primarily on overall hepatic function,[5] form an extra
group. Factor 2 comprises amino acids which play an important role
in gluconeogenesis. Since the factors are independent of one another,
one can conclude that, in plasma, no constant relationship exists
between the concentrations of branched-chain, aromatic, and glycogenic amino acids. The lack of a co-variation of branched-chain and
glycogenic amino acids is reported in section 3.2.

A second factor pattern was calculated from data which had been
obtained in 33 cats with PCA.[6] This pattern confirms the first one,
in that it also fails to reveal any correlation between the plasma
levels of the aforementioned three groups of amino acids (Table 2).

2. PLASMA CLEARANCE OF BCAA IN PATIENTS WITH LIVER CIRRHOSIS

The reduction in the plasma levels of BCAA has often been considered to be related to an increased clearance rate of these amino
acids. Leweling and Holm determined amino acid clearances in 8
healthy volunteers used as controls and in 24 cirrhotic patients
during continuous infusion of a BCAA-enriched amino acid solution
under steady state conditions.[7] For the cirrhotics, the mean values
resulting from 62 infusion periods are available, because each
patient was repeatedly investigated. The clearance rate of the total
of the amino acids was 110.3 ml/kg.min in the controls but reached
only 68.6 ml/kg.min in the cirrhotics (Fig. 2). The clearance rate
of the BCAA proved to be almost equal in the two groups in terms
of the absolute values. However, while in the controls the clearance
of BCAA accounted for only 22.9% of the total amino acid clearance,
it accounted for 32.7% in the cirrhotics (Fig. 2). At least two
conclusions can be drawn from these findings. First, the absolute
clearance of BCAA does not help to explain the lowered plasma concentrations in cirrhotics, probably because the metabolism during
an amino acid infusion is, to some extent, determined by factors
other than those present in the postabsorptive state. Second, nutritional regimens which include a relatively large quantity of BCAA
are likely to be adequate for cirrhotic patients.

3. MECHANISMS OF THE REDUCTION IN THE PLASMA LEVELS OF BCAA - META-
BOLISM OF BCAA IN MUSCLE AND FATTY TISSUE

The metabolic routes of BCAA chiefly reside in peripheral tissues,[8] the degradation taking place independently of hepatic function.

Table 1. Factor pattern of amino acid and ammonia concentrations in the venous plasma of 76 patients with liver cirrhosis[a]

Variables	Factors				
	1	2	3	4	5
Methionine	+.86				
Phenylalanine	+.81				
Thyrosine	+.68				
Lysine	+.62				
Histidine	+.63	+.53			
Valine			+.83		
Leucine			+.82		
Isoleucine			+.69		
Alanine		+.68			
Threonine		+.63			
Serine		+.70			
Glycine		+.90			
Ammonia					+.75
Glutamic acid					+.71
Ornithine				+.90	
Arginine				+.58	

[a]Principal component method. Since the correlation matrix had five eigenvalues above 1, five factors were extracted and then varimax-rotated. The five factors account for 74.4 per cent of the total variance. Only loadings exceeding $\pm$ 0.50 are indicated.

Reversible transamination is the first step of degradation. It is followed by oxidative decarboxylation of the ketoanalogues and then by beta-oxidation of their metabolites. Because the uptake of BCAA by the liver is not significant, these amino acids pass through the liver for use in other organs.[9] Transamination can be carried out especially by muscle, brain, and fatty tissue.[9,10,11] Active in the oxidation of the carbon skeleton are liver and kidney, fatty tissue and heart.[9,10,11,12] Muscle, although showing only minor activities of the oxidizing enzymes, also plays an important role in the latter process,[9,10] since muscle comprises up to 40% of body mass.

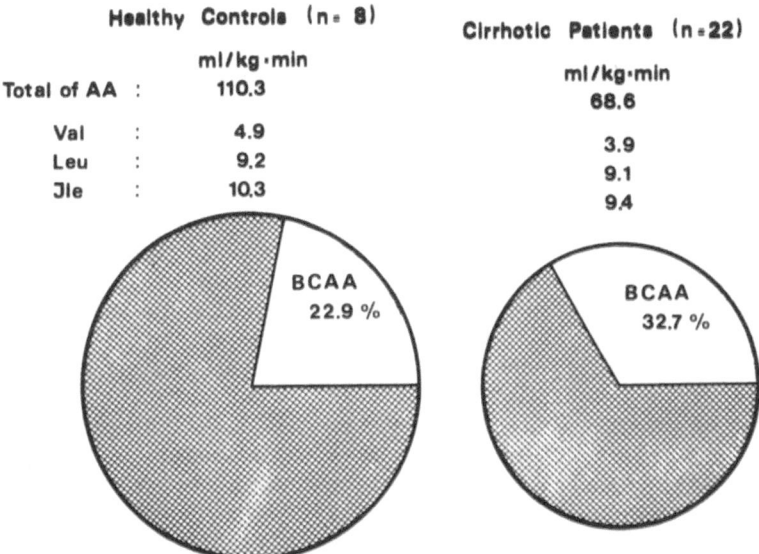

Fig. 2. Absolute and percentage plasma clearance rates (means) of
amino acids (AA) in two groups of subjects. Results obtained
by Leweling and Holm.[7] Further comments are given in the
text.

Several attempts have been made to explain the decrease in the
plasma concentrations of BCAA in patients with liver cirrhosis and
in animals with PCA.

3.1 The "Insulin Hypothesis"

Above all, the "insulin hypothesis" needs to be discussed.
Hyperinsulinemia is very common in cirrhotic patients[13,14] and is
also typical of shunted animals.[15] Insulin has been thought to remove
BCAA from plasma into muscle, thereby reducing their plasma levels.
[16,17] In addition, insulin is known to stimulate branched-chain
keto acid (BCKA) dehydrogenase, i.e. the rate-limiting enzyme
complex in the degradation of BCAA.[18]

The well-known negative correlations between the levels of
insulin and BCAA in patients with insulinomas and diabetic ketosis[19,20] as well as in brief starvation[21,22,23] and after infusion
of somatostatin[24] are compatible with the assumption that in liver
cirrhosis insulin is mainly responsible for the decreased concentrations of BCAA, although in the case of brief starvation the
combination of low insulin with high BCAA levels was explained by
an increased muscular release of BCAA.[22] Additional support for
the "insulin hypothesis" comes from the observation of an inverse
relationship between plasma insulin and plasma BCAA in shunted and

diabetic rats.[25] Furthermore, it has been demonstrated that the peripheral uptake of labelled leucine - especially by muscle - is
increased in PCA animals,[26] and that the administration of insulin
causes a decline in the muscular release of BCAA in the human forearm.[27]

The cited findings, however, do not provide a proof that there
is a decisive role of insulin in cirrhotics or in shunted animals.
The above-mentioned reduction in the levels of BCAA in patients
with idiopathic portal hypertension[1] occurred despite a normal
plasma insulin concentration. Furthermore, in patients with liver
cirrhosis a correlation between the insulin and BCAA levels was
lacking;[1,28] according to the results of a factor analysis, a co-
variation of glucose and BCAA in plasma does not exist, either.[29]
The infusion of ammonium salts in dogs caused a fall in the levels
of BCAA; since this effect of exogenous hyperammonemia was also
observed after pancreatectomy, it could not have been mediated by
insulin.[30] In addition, it must not be overlooked that muscle
degrades more BCAA in starvation which is characterized by a low
plasma insulin concentration than it does in the fed state associated with an increase of insulin.[10,18,31,32,33,34] Finally, there
are proven effects of insulin resistance on BCAA metabolism in
cirrhotic patients;[35] the latter aspect does not invalidate, but
only restricts the "insulin hypothesis". In view of the arguments
against this hypothesis, mechanisms other than hyperinsulinemia
have to be looked for, in order to explain the subnormal values
of BCAA.

3.2 The "Glucagon Hypothesis"

Regarding the fact that pronounced hyperglucagonemia is brought
about by PSS in patients[13] and in animals,[15] one could consider
the following sequence of metabolic processes: Hepatic gluconeogenesis, intensified by PSS, diminishes the plasma level of alanine;
as a consequence of this, muscle forms and releases more alanine
than under physiological conditions; since the nitrogen of alanine
is provided by BCAA, these substances are released to a smaller
extent than normal.

Several observations are in favor of the "glucagon hypothesis".
The administration of glucagon[36,37] as well as hyperglucagonemia
induced by starvation[37,38] result in a marked decrease of the glycogenic amino acids alanine, glycine, and serine in plasma. The same
is true for PSS in patients with idiopathic portal hypertension,[1]
in shunted animals,[6,39] and in cats treated with microspheres.[40]
Skeletal muscle has been shown to react to the reduction in the
plasma levels of glycogenic amino acids by releasing these amino
acids into the circulation, a process which at least limits the
extent of their fall in the blood.[37,38] Now the question arises
whether alanine is synthetized de novo or whether it is provided by

protein breakdown. If the former process took place, the muscular
alanine production could account for a deficiency of BCAA, because
it may be coupled to their degradation. It has, in fact, been
demonstrated that the synthesis of alanine in muscle can utilize
amino groups which are generated in the degradation of BCAA and
then transferred to alpha-ketoglutarate and pyruvate by repeated
transamination.[18,34] BCAA oxidation and alanine production are both
accelerated in starvation,[18,27] although only prolonged starvation
is associated with a simultaneous reduction in the plasma levels of
BCAA and alanine.[21,22] The finding that, in dogs with PCA, alanine
feeding partly reversed the lowering of plasma BCAA levels[39] is also
in keeping with the outlined theory.

   In spite of the aforementioned evidence for the "glucagon
hypothesis", this hypothesis does not seem to be valid in the cases
of liver cirrhosis and experimental PSS. Substantial objections can
be raised. Cirrhotic patients can simultaneously display diminished
plasma concentrations of BCAA and a normal concentration of alanine.
[41] According to the results of our two factor analyses (see section
1), a correlation between the plasma levels of BCAA and alanine
exists neither in cirrhotics nor in shunted cats. Especially infor-
mative in this context is the finding that, in patients with liver
cirrhosis, the postabsorptive peripheral alanine release is reduced.
[42] An indication that the amino group of BCAA is carried predominantly to alpha-ketoglutarate and glutamate rather than being
further transferred to pyruvate comes from observations which were
made after the administration of BCAA. In healthy individuals the
infusion of leucine was followed by an increased muscular release
of glutamine, but not of alanine.[43] PCA cats which were infused with
a BCAA-enriched amino acid solution showed a marked rise in the
intracellular BCAA and glutamate concentrations of muscle, whereas
the intracellular quantity of alanine was not influenced (see
section 3.4); the plasma levels of alanine also remained unchanged.
All in all, a lot of data is at variance with the suggestion that
glucagon-induced alanine consumption is responsible for the
lowering of the plasma levels of BCAA.

3.3 The hypothesis of decreased hepatic BCKA reamination

   Occasionally, the possibility has been put forward that a decreased reamination of BCKA by the liver - due to hepatic failure
or PSS - could be a mechanism of the reduction in the plasma concentrations of BCAA. However, there is hardly any evidence for this
hypothesis. In plasma, the quantity of BCKA is 5-7 times less than
that of BCAA.[44,45] Although the liver can release BCAA in vitro,[46]
it does not do so in vivo; studies of amino acid balances across
the liver of human subjects showed that the liver is not a source
of plasma BCAA, neither in the postabsorptive state nor in starvation, the levels of these amino acids always being lower in hepatic
venous blood than in arterial blood.[22] One might argue that liver

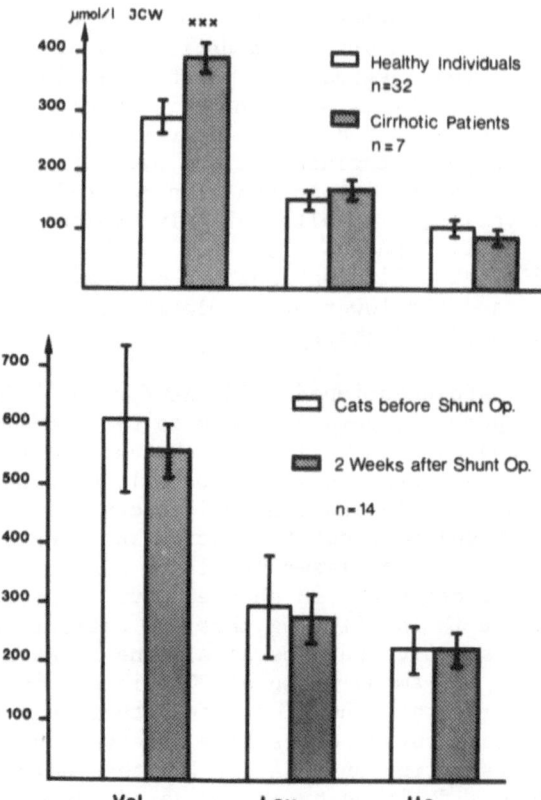

Fig. 3.   BCAA concentrations (means + S.E.M.) in intracellular water
          (ICW) of muscle[48] measured in two groups of human subjects
          (Fürst[49]) as well as in cats before and two weeks after
          construction of a portacaval anastomosis (Staedt et al.[50]).
          ***$p \leq 0.005$.

disease could change this situation. A failure to reaminate orally
administered BCKA has, in fact, been demonstrated in cirrhotic
patients.[47] However, only an impairment of hepatic function would
explain a decreased reamination capacity, while PSS could not. Nevertheless, PSS - and not hepatic failure - is associated with a
reduction in the concentrations of BCAA. A convincing correlation
between the level of overall hepatic function and the total amount
of valine, leucine, and isoleucine in plasma could not be established.[5]

3.4 Conclusions based on recent results

      The reduction in the plasma levels of BCAA in liver cirrhosis
and experimental PSS is likely to be caused, for the most part, by
increased uptake of these amino acids by muscle and fatty tissue,

with increased utilization as metabolic fuel as well as with increased incorporation into muscle protein and fat.

In cirrhotic patients and in PCA cats, the intracellular BCAA concentrations of muscle were found to be largely unchanged, with the exception of valine in the patients (Fig. 3). In experimental PSS, labelled leucine has been shown to enter muscle tissue to a greater extent than normal.[26] De Boer et al. and Soeters et al. reported in vitro results pertaining to the question of what happens to the carbon skeleton of leucine, isoleucine, and valine.[25,51] An intensified oxidation of the BCAA and an augmented incorporation of leucine as well as isoleucine into muscle protein were observed. Leucin-derived carbon metabolized to CO_2 was found to be raised by about 25%, while leucine incorporation into protein was raised by 50-100%.[25,51] Thus, the normal intracellular concentrations of BCAA depicted in Figure 3 appear to reflect an equilibrium between amino acid uptake, oxidation, incorporation, and release as well as protein breakdown, most of these processes being increased.

A considerable muscular uptake of valine, leucine, and isoleucine was noted during the infusion of a BCAA-enriched amino acid solution in cats with PCA (Fig. 4). There was, in addition, an increase of intracellular glutamate, but not of alanine, although the amino acid mixture used did not contain glutamate, but contained alanine (Fig. 4). This finding indicates that, in muscle of shunted animals, the BCAA-derived amino groups are carried predominantly to alpha-ketoglutarate rather than being transferred to pyruvate.

PCA cats display a rise in the intracellular glutamine concentration of muscle (Fig. 5). Most probably, the accumulation of ammonia accounts for the increase of glutamine; it is known that high quantities of ammonia in muscle promote glutamine production and diminish alanine synthesis.[18] The ammonia-induced excessive formation of glutamine is likely to result in a deficit of intracellular alpha-ketoglutarate and glutamate.[52] We are tempted to speculate that an intensified BCAA degradation contributes to at least a partial normalization of the alpha-ketoglutarate and glutamate pools by yielding alpha-ketoglutarate (via succinate from valine and isoleucine) as well as amino groups.[a]

Liver cirrhosis probably resembles diabetes and starvation, in that glucose is oxidized to a lower degree than normal,[53] while BCAA serve as a compensatory source of energy.[10,18,35,54] Expecially leucine can contribute a considerable amount of the energy needs of muscle.[18] Leucine simultaneously inhibits the oxidation of glucose and pyruvate,[18] thus enhancing the demand for BCAA as metabolic fuel.

(a) Suggestion made by J.H. James during discussions.

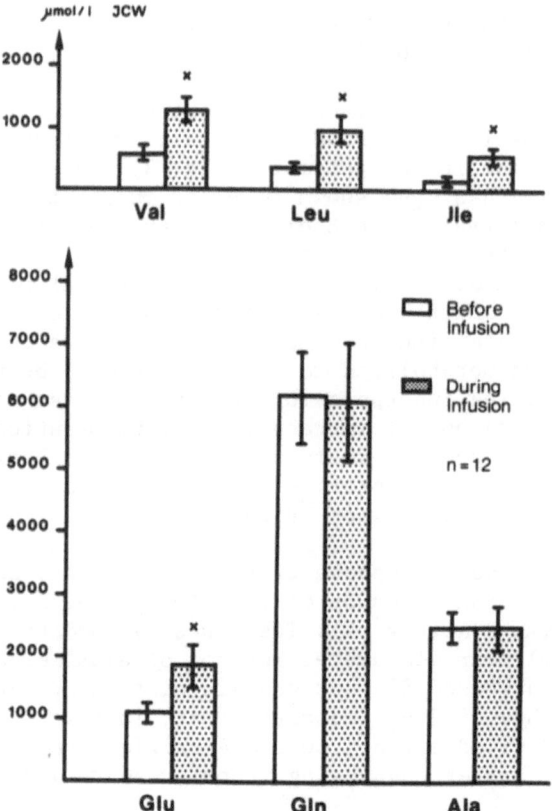

Fig. 4.   Amino acid concentrations (means ± S.E.M.) in intracellular
          water (ICW) of muscle measured in cats with portacaval ana-
          stomosis before and towards the end of a 7-hr parenteral
          nutrition which included a BCAA-enriched amino acid solution.
          *P ≤ 0.05 (Wilcoxon test). Results obtained by Staedt et
          al.[50]

        In addition to muscle, fatty tissue may play an important role
in lowering the plasma levels of BCAA.[25,55] De Boer et al. found
that the oxidation of leucine was increased 1.2 - 1.7 times in the
fatty tissue of PCA rats. An increased incorporation of leucine-
derived carbon into fat was even more pronounced, the incorporation
being raised by a factor of 4.1 - 4.7.[51] As to isoleucine-derived
carbon, parallel changes in CO_2 production and incorporation into
fat were assessed.[25]

4. "THERAPEUTIC" CONCENTRATIONS OF BCAA IN PLASMA AND MUSCLE

        Finally, it seems appropriate to outline data and problems

Table 2. Factor pattern of amino acid and ammonia concentrations in the venous plasma of 33 cats with portacaval anastomosis[a]

Variables	Factors			
	1	2	3	4
Methionine		+.63		
Phenylalanine		+.85		
Tyrosine		+.77		
Threonine		+.64		
Arginine		+.65		
Valine	+.89			
Leucine	+.93			
Isoleucine	+.95			
Alanine			+.64	
Glycine			+.76	
Serine			+.64	
Ammonia			+.63	
Glutamate			+.60	
Glutamine				-.86
Citrulline				+.95

[a]Principal component method. Since the correlation matrix had four eigenvalues above 1, four factors were extracted and then varimac-rotated. The four factors account for 74.5 per cent of the total variance. Only loadings exceeding $\pm$ 0.60 are indicated.

concerning therapeutically induced BCAA concentrations in plasma and muscle. Figure 6 shows median values and quartils of plasma BCAA levels in cirrhotic patients who received 12-hour infusions of glucose and an amino acid mixture similar to F080,[56,57] over a period of two weeks.[58] The dosage of the amino acids was either 50 or 80 g. Blood samples were taken 12 hours after the infusion. In order to examine the extent of normalization of the BCAA levels at that time, we considered only those patients who had exhibited decreased values before treatment. 80 g of amino acids raised the BCAA concentrations into the normal range, whereas 50 g proved to be an insufficient dose in this respect. What is not demonstrated in the Figure 6 diagrams is that during the infusion of 80g

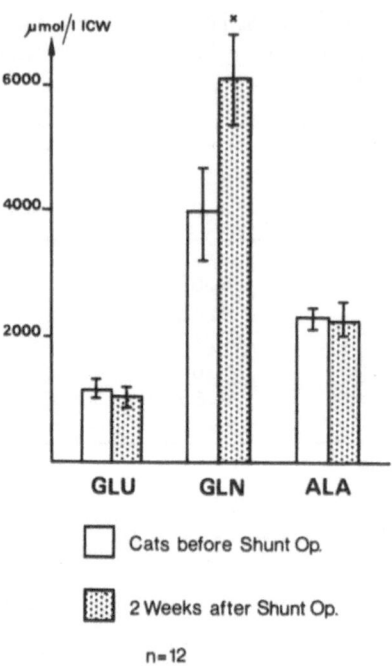

Fig. 5.   Amino acid concentrations (means ± S.E.M.) in intracellular
          water (ICW) of muscle measured in cats before and two weeks
          after construction of a portacaval anastomosis. P ≤ 0.05
          (Wilcoxon test). Results obtained by Staedt et al.[50]

of amino acids the BCAA levels were more than twice as high as normal
values. An excess of BCAA in plasma apperas to be a desirable effect
regarding treatment of encephalopathy.[41,56,57,59] On the other hand,
if such an imbalance results, the nutritional efficacy of the amino
acid administration is perhaps lessened. We would expect that plasma
amino acid levels within or near the physiological range (as depicted in Figure 6) more adequately meet nutritional requirements.

     Considering figure 7, one is confronted with an additional
problem. In shunted cats given a 1-day parenteral nutrition which
included a BCAA-enriched solution, the intracellular BCAA concentrations of muscle were found to be increased up to 16 hours after cessation of treatment. The highly increased intracellular concentrations were associated with normal plasma levels.[50] It must, however,
be added that continuous parenteral nutrition conducted over 6 days
in shunted rats[60] resulted in a steady state of the BCAA levels in
plasma and intracellular water (Fig. 8).

     Plasma amino acid levels were also measured in cirrhotic

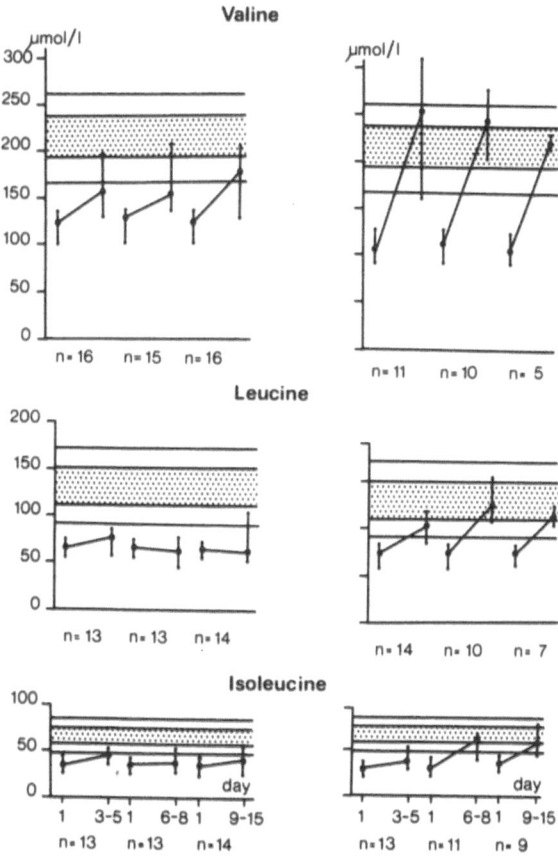

Fig. 6. Plasma BCAA concentrations (median values and quartils) in
cirrhotic patients receiving parenteral nutrition which
included a BCAA-enriched amino acid solution. The dosage
of the amino acids was either 50 g/12 hrs (diagram left)
or 80 g/12 hrs (diagram right). The physiological ranges
are signified by the +1 and +2 standard deviations.

patients undergoing different oral dietary regimens.[61] The patients
first received a standard diet and then a BCAA-supplemented diet.
Representative findings are shown in Figure 9. As a result of the
supplementation, the concentrations of valine, leucine, and isoleucine were raised by about 100%. BCAA given orally are known to
increase protein tolerance;[62] however, anabolic effects of high
levels of these amino acids have, in patients with liver cirrhosis,
until now not sufficiently been established.[40]

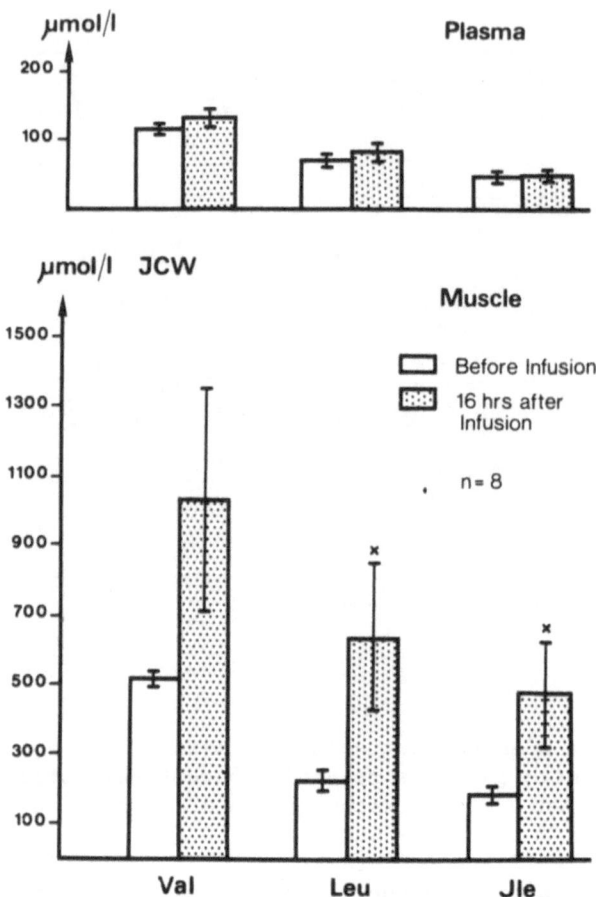

Fig. 7.   BCAA concentrations (means ± S.E.M.) in plasma and intracellular water (ICW) of muscle measured in cats with portacaval anastomosis before and 16 hours after cessation of
parenteral nutrition which included a BCAA-enriched amino
acid solution. * P ≤ 0.05 (Wilcoxon test). Results obtained
by Staedt et al.[50]

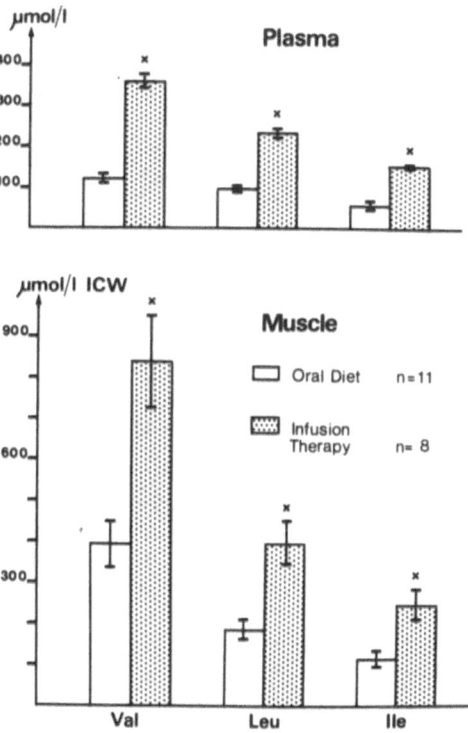

Fig. 8.   BCAA concentrations (means + S.E.M.) in plasma and intra-
          cellular water (ICW) of muscle measured in two groups of
          cats with portacaval anastomosis. One group had an oral
          diet and the other received continuous parenteral nutrition
          which included a BCAA-enriched amino acid solution. All
          measurements were made on the 6th day of the experiments,
          P ≤ 0.005 (U-test). Results obtained by Leweling et al.[60]

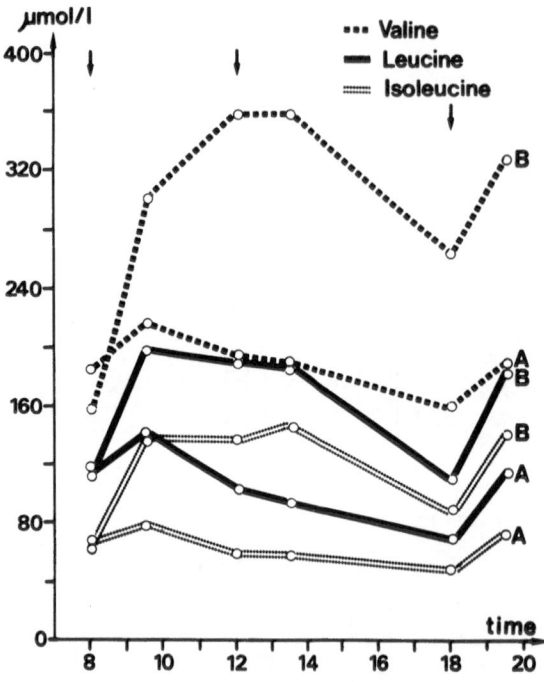

Fig. 9.   Plasma BCAA concentrations in a cirrhotic patient with
          portacaval anastomosis on two consecutive days. On the
          first day (A) the patient received a standard diet contai-
          ning 40 g of natural protein; on the second day (B) this
          diet was supplemented by BCAA (3x5 g).

REFERENCES

1. Y. Iwasaki, H. Sato, A. Ohkubo, T. Sanjo, S. Futagawa, M. Su-
    giura, and S. Tsuji, Effect of spontaneous portal-systemic
    shunting on plasma insulin and amino acid concentrations,
    Gastroenterology 78: 677 (1980).
2. A. Aguirre, N. Yoshimura, T. Westman, and J. E. Fischer, Plasma
    amino acids in dogs with two experimental forms of liver
    damage, J. Surg. Res. 16: 339 (1974).
3. E. Holm, J.-P. Striebel, R. Münzenmaier, and R. Kattermann,
    Pathogenese der hepatischen Enzephalopathie, Leber Magen
    Darm 7: 241 (1977).
4. E. Holm, J.-P. Striebel, W. Langhans, R. Kattermann, and B.
    Werner, Beziehunger zwischen Plasmaammoniak, Plasmaamino-
    säuren und weiteren Parametern bei Leberzirrhose. Zwei
    Hauptkomponentenanalysen, Verh. dt. Ges. inn. Med. 86: 775
    (1980).

5. R. Herz, M. Rössle, U. Schulte, and W. Gerok, Periphere Amino-säuren-Konzentrationen bei eingeschränkter quantitativer Leberfunktion infolge Leberzirrhose, Z. Gastroenterol. 17: 586 (1979).

6. E. Holm, J.-P. Striebel, R. Kattermann, E. Schick, and U. Staedt, Encephalopathy resulting from portacaval anastomosis in cats. Ammonia, amino acids, and cerebral electrical activity, in: "Amino Acid and Ammonia Metabolism in Hepatic Failure", E. Holm, ed., Witzstrock, Baden-Baden - Köln - New York (1982), pp. 58-94.

7. H. Leweling, and E. Holm, in preparation.

8. L. L. Miller, The role of the liver and the non-hepatic tissues in the regulation of free amino acid levels in the blood, in: "Amino Acid Pools", J. T. Holden, ed., Elsevier, Amsterdam - London - New York (1962), pp. 708-721.

9. A. E. Harper and C. Zapalowski, Interorgan relationships in the metabolism of the branched-chain amino and alpha-keto-acids, in: "Metabolism and Clinical Implications of Branched Chain Amino and Ketoacids," M. Walser and J. R. Williamson, eds., Elsevier/North-Holland, New York - Amsterdam - Oxford pp. 195-203 (1981).

10. S. A. Adibi, Metabolism of branched-chain amino acids in altered nutrition, Metabolism 25: 1287 (1976).

11. H. M. Goodman and G. P. Frick, Metabolism of branched chain amino acids in adipose tissue, in: "Metabolism and Clinical Implications of Branched Chain Amino and Ketoacids," M. Walser and J. R. Williamson, eds., Elsevier/North-Holland, New York-Amsterdam - Oxford, pp. 169-180 (1981).

12. K. Brand, Metabolism of alpha-keto acid analogues of leucine, valine and phenylalanine in extrahepatic and hepatic tissues, in: "Metabolism and Clinical Implications of Branched Chain Amino and Ketoacids," M. Walser and J. R. Williamson, eds., Elsevier/North-Holland, New York - Amsterdam - Oxford, pp. 135-142 (1981).

13. R. Sherwin, P. Joshi, R. Hendler, Ph. Felig, and H. O. Conn, Hyperglucagonemia in Laennec's cirrhosis, New Engl. J. Med. 290: 239 (1974).

14. G. Smith-Laing, The glucoregulatory hormones in cirrhosis of the liver, Z. Gastroenterol. 7: 462 (1979).

15. P. B. Soeters, G. Weir, A. M. Ebeid, and J. E. Fischer, Insulin, glucagon, portal systemic shunting and hepatic failure in the dog, J. Surg. Res. 23: 183 (1977).

16. J. H. James, V. Ziparo, B. Jeppson, and J. E. Fischer, Hyper-ammonaemia, plasma aminoacid imbalance, and blood-brain aminoacid transport: a unified theory of portal-systemic encephalopathy, Lancet II: 772 (1979).

17. H. N. Munroe, J. D. Fernstrom, and R. J. Wurtman, Plasma amino acid imbalance and hepatic coma, in: "Klin. Anästhesiol. Intensivther."Bd. 13, F. W. Ahnefeld, H. Bergmann, C. Burri,

W. Dick, M. Halmagyi, and E. Rügheimer, eds., Springer, Berlin-Heidelberg-New York, pp. 103-112 (1977).

18. A. L. Goldberg and T. W. Chang, Regulation and significance of amino acid metabolism in skeletal muscle, Fed. Proc. 37: 2301 (1978).

19. M. Berger, H. Zimmernann-Telschow, P. Berchtold, H. Drost, W. A. Müller, F. A. Gries, and H. Zimmermann, Blood amino acid levels in patients with insulin excess (functioning insulinoma) and insulin deficiency (diabetic ketosis), Metabolism 27: 793 (1978).

20. G. Kleinberger, P. Ferenci, A. Gassner, M. Pichler, and H. Lochs, Unterschiede im Plasmaaminogramm bei Coma hepaticum und Coma diabeticum, Z. Gastroenterol. 16: 752 (1978).

21. Ph. Felig, Amino acid metabolism in man, Ann. Rev. Biochem. 44: 933 (1975).

22. Ph. Felig, O. E. Owen, J. Wahren, and G. F. Cahill, Amino acid metabolism during prolonged starvation, J. Clin. Invest. 48: 584 (1969).

23. T. Pozefsky, R. G. Tancredi, R. T. Moxley, J. Dupre, and J. D. Tobin, Effects of brief starvation on muscle amino acid metabolism in nonobese man, J. Clin. Invest. 57: 444 (1976).

24. B. Limberg and B. Kommerell, Why decreased serum branched-chain amino acids in cirrhosis, Gastroenterology 80: 211 (1981).

25. P. B. Soeters, J. E. G. de Boer, R. J. Oostenbroek, and M. A. Janssen, Fate of branched chain amino acids, in:"New Aspects of Clinical Nutrition," G. Kleinberger, and E. Deutsch, eds., Karger, Basel, pp. 337-345 (1983).

26. P. B. Soeters, J. Hodgman, J. H. James, and J. E. Fischer, Increased catabolism of branched chain amino acids following portacaval shunt, Gastroenterology 69: 867 (1975).

27. T. Pozefsky, Ph. Felig, J. D. Tobin, J. S. Soeldner, and G. F. Cahill, Amino acid balance across tissues of the forearm in postabsorptive man. Effects of insulin at two dose levels, J. Clin. Invest. 48: 2273 (1969).

28. G. Marchesini, G. Forlani, M. Zoli, A. Angiolini, M. P. Scolari, F. B. Bianchi, and E. Pisi, Insulin and Glucagon levels in liver cirrhosis. Relationship with plasma amino acid imbalance of chronic hepatic encephalopathy, Digest. Dis. Sci. 24: 594 (1979).

29. E. Holm, unpublished data.

30. D. R. Strombeck, Q. Rogers, and J. S. Stern, Effects of intravenous ammonia infusion on plasma levels of amino acids, glucagon and insulin in dogs, Gastroenterology 74: 1165 (1978).

31. S. A. Adibi, Roles of branched-chain amino acids in metabolic regulation, J. Lab. Clin. Med. 95: 475 (1980).

32. S. A. Adibi, R. T. Stanko, and E. L. Morse, Modulation of leucine oxidation and turnover by graded amounts of carbohydrate intake in obese subjects, Metabolism 31: 578 (1982).

33. S. M.Hutson, C. Zapalowski, Th. C. Cree, and A. E. Harper,
    Regulation of leucine and alpha-ketoisocaproic acid meta-
    bolism in skeletal muscle, J. Biol. Chem. 255: 3418 (1980).
34. R. Odessey, E. A. Khairallah, and A. L. Goldberg, Origin and
    possible significance of alanine production by skeletal
    muscle, J. Biol. Chem. 249: 7623 (1974).
35. G. Marchesini, G. Forlani, and M. Zoli, Iperinsulinismo e ca-
    duta degli aminoacidi a catena ramificata nel cirrotico:
    causa ed effetto? Il fegato 27: 197 (1981).
36. V. Brodan, M. Brodanova, M. Andel, and E. Kuhn, The effect of
    glucagon on free plasma amino acids in cirrhotics and healthy
    controls, Acta Hepato-Gastroenterol. 25: 23 (1978).
37. P. M. Daniel, O. E. Pratt, and E. Spargo, The mechanisms by
    which glucagon induces the release of amino acids from muscle
    and its relevance to fasting, Proc. R. Soc. London B 196:
    347 (1977).
38. E. Spargo, O. E. Pratt, and P. M. Daniel, Metabolic functions
    of skeletal muscles of man, mammals, birds and fishes: a
    review, J. Roy. Soc. Med. 72: 921 (1979).
39. M. C. Schaeffer, Q. R. Rogers, B. M. Wolfe, and R. A. LeCouteur,
    Effects of glutamine feeding on plasma and cerebrospinal
    fluid ammonia and amino acids in portacaval shunt dogs. 12th
    Int. Congr. Nutr., San Diego, Abstract Book, No. 840 (1981).
40. E. Holm, H. Leweling, and U. Staedt, Metabolism and nutritional
    supply of amino acids in hepatic failure, in :"New Aspects
    of Clinical Nutrition," G. Kleinberger and E. Deutsch., eds.,
    Karger, Basel, pp. 377-399 (1983).
41. E. Holm, J.-P. Striebel, E. Meisinger, P. Haux, W. Langhans,
    and H. D. Becker, Aminosäurengemische zur parenteralen
    Ernährung bei Leberinsuffizienz, Infusionstherapie 5: 274
    (1978).
42. M. Imler, J. L. Schlienger, A. Frick, A. Stahl, and G. Chabrier,
    Study of muscular glutamine and alanine release in cirrhotics
    with hyperammonemia and in ammonium infused rats, in :"Amino-
    säuren- und Ammoniakstoffwechsel bei Leberinsuffizienz," E.
    Holm, ed., Witzstrock, Baden-Baden-Köln-New York, pp. 33-39
    (1982).
43. M. Elia and G. Livesey, Branched chain amino acid and oxo acid
    metabolism in human and rat muscle, in :"Metabolism and
    Clinical Implications of Branched Chain Amino and Ketoacids,"
    M. Walser and J. R. Williamson, eds., Elsevier/North-Holland,
    New York-Amsterdam-Oxford, pp. 257-262 (1981).
44. D. E. Matthews, H. P. Schwarz, R. D. Yang, K. J. Motil, V. R.
    Young, and D. M. Bier, Relationship of plasma leucine and
    alpha-ketoisocaproate during a L-(1-^{13}C)leucine infusion in
    man: A method for measuring human intracellular leucine tracer
    enrichment, Metabolism 31: 1105 (1982).
45. P. Schauder, K. Schröder, H. V. Henning, and U. Langenbeck,
    Some aspects on the role of branched chain keto acids in the

pathophysiology and treatment of uremia. Convegno interna-
zionale su "Problemi metabolici e nutrizionali nell'insuffi-
cienza renale e epatica", Parma 1982, in press.

46. D. L. Bloxam, Nutritional aspects of amino acid metabolism. 2.
     The effects of starvation on hepatic portal-venous differen-
     ces in plasma amino acid concentration and on liver amino
     acid concentrations in the rat, Br. J. Nutr. 27: 233 (1972).

47. P. Ferenci, B. Dragosics, and F. Wewalka, Oral administration
     of branched chain amino acids (BCAA) and keto acids (BCKA)
     in patients with liver cirrhosis (LC), in: "Metabolism and
     Clinical Implications of Branched Chain Amino and Ketoacids,"
     M. Walser and J. R. Williamson, eds., Elsevier/North-Holland,
     New York-Amsterdam-Oxford, pp. 507-512 (1981).

48. J. Bergström, P. Fürst, L.-O. Norée, and E. Vinnars, Intracel-
     lular free amino acid concentration in human muscle tissue,
     J. Appl. Physiol. 36: 693 (1974).

49. P. Fürst, personal communication, (1982).

50. U. Staedt, E. Holm, J.-P. Striebel, and P. Gasteiger, Amino acid
     concentrations in plasma and intracellular water of muscle
     in cats given a portacaval anastomosis. Effects of brief
     intravenous nutrition including a BCAA-enriched solution,
     Clin. Nutr. 1: F 52 (1982).

51. J. E. G. de Boer, R. J. Oostenbroek, M. A. Janssen, R. I. C.
     Wesdorp, and P. B. Soeters, Fate of leucine in muscle and
     adipose tissue in male Sprague-Dawley rats with portacaval
     shunts (PCS), Clin. Nutr. 1: F 51 (1982).

52. E. Roth, personal communication, (1982).

53. E. Mezey, Liver disease and nutrition, Gastroenterology 74:
     770 (1978).

54. P. J. Randle, P. B. Garland, C. N. Hales, and E. A. Newsholme,
     The glucose fatty-acid cycle. Its role in insulin sensitivity
     and the metabolic disturbances of diabetes mellitus, Lancet
     I: 785 (1963).

55. P. B. Soeters and J. E. Fischer, Insulin, glucagon, amino-acid
     imbalance, and hepatic encephalopathy, Lancet II: 880
     (1976).

56. J. E. Fischer, J. M. Funovics, A. Aguirre, J. H. James, J. M.
     Keane, R. I. C. Wesdorp, N. Yoshimura, and Th. Westman, The
     role of plasma amino acids in hepatic encephalopathy, Surgery
     78: 276 (1975).

57. J. E. Fischer, H. M. Rosen, A. M. Ebeid, J. H. James, J. M.
     Keane, and P. B. Soeters, The effect of normalization of
     plasma amino acids on hepatic encephalopathy in man, Surgery
     80: 77 (1976).

58. E. Holm, Parenteral nutrition in patients with hepatic failure,
     J. Drug. Res.6: 41 (1981).

59. E. Holm, Behandlungen mit Aminosäuren bei hepatischer Enzephalo-
     pathie, Fischer, Stuttgart-New York (1976).

60. H. Leweling, E. Holm, U. Staedt, H. Feussner, O. Zelder, and
     J.-P. Striebel, Totale parenterale Ernährung bei Ratten mit

portokavaler Anastomose, Infusionsther. Klin. Ern. 9: 234 (1982).

61. E. Holm, BCAA-enriched diets for oral treatment of patients with liver cirrhosis: A controlled study of biochemical variables, psychometric performance, and the EEG. Ajinomoto Symp., Abstract Book, Raleigh (1982).

62. D. Horst, N. Grace, H. O. Conn, E. Schiff, S. Schenker, A. Viteri, D. Law, and C. E. Atterbury, A double-blind randomized comparison of dietary protein and an oral branched-chain amino acid (BCAA) solution in cirrhotic patients with chronic portal-systemic encephalopathy, Congr. IASL, Abstract Book, No. 157, Hong Kong (1982).

LONG TERM DIETARY SUPPLEMENT WITH BRANCHED CHAIN AMINO ACIDS: A NEW

APPROACH IN THE PREVENTION OF HEPATIC ENCEPHALOPATHY: RESULTS OF A

CONTROLLED STUDY IN CIRRHOTICS WITH PORTO-CAVAL ANASTOMOSIS

O. Riggio, C. Cangiano, A. Cascino, M. Merli, M. Stortoni,
F. Rossi Fanelli, °°V. Ziparo, °°M. Anzà, and °°R. Lupino
III Clinica Medica, University of Rome, °° IV Patologia
Chirurgica, University of Rome

INTRODUCTION

Recurrent episodes of hepatic encephalopathy (HE) frequently
occur in patients with cirrhosis of the liver especially after surgical portal systemic anastomosis.[1] The prevention of these recurrent
episodes of HE is based on neomycin, purging of the gastrointestinal
tract, lactulose and restriction of protein intake.[2]

Protein restriction is particularly objectable. In fact a
protein intake less than 30-40 gr/day contributes to the negative
nitrogen balance, to the protein catabolism and finally to the malnutrition present in cirrhotic patients.[3]

Fischer and subsequently other authors have demonstrated the
relationship between protein catabolism, altered plasma amino acids
profile and HE,[4,5] as well as the possibility of treating HE by nor-
malizing the amino acid pattern through the intravenous infusion of
solutions enriched[6] or containing exclusively branched chain amino
acids (BCAA): valine, leucine and isoleucine.[7,8] Using these solutions a cirrhotic patient may be given his daily protein requirement
without precipitating HE.[6]

As in parenteral administration it is conceivable that, oral
supplementation of BCAA to the diet may allow cirrhotic patients
to tolerate an adequate protein intake and permit an effective pro-
phylaxis of HE at the same time.

In this prospective randomized controlled study we investigated
such possibilities in a group of cirrhotic patients at high risk of
HE.

Patients and Protocol

     Twenty-eight patients were selected from a large group of cir-
rhotics with surgical portal-systemic anastomosis (PSA). All were
followed as outpatients in the 5th Department of Surgery of the
University of Rome. The selected patients suffered from chronic
recurrent hepatic encephalopathy, as most of them had experienced
more than one episode of HE in the past. All of them were on a
restricted protein diet and lactulose to prevent recurrent episodes.
23 of the 28 patients were males. They varied in age from 47 to 74 yrs
(mean 54). Fourteen had alcoholic, nine cryptogenic and five post-
necrotic cirrhosis. All patients had had at least one episode of
gastrointestinal bleeding. As for the type of PSA, 12 had side-to-
side porto-caval shunts and 16 had meso-caval anastomosis with
autologous jugular vein interposition.

     All patients had been maintained on a protein restricted diet
(0.5 g/Kg/day) and oral lactulose since their operation. After randomization the 28 patients were divided into two groups of 14
patients each. As shown in Table 1 the two groups were comparable
in age, sex, type of cirrhosis, type of PSA, time since operation,
number of previous episodes of HE and also (Table 2) in routine
blood chemistry values.

     The two groups were subjected to 2 different treatments:

Group A - Pts. included in this Group were given a restricted protein
          diet of 0.5 g/Kg/day for 60 days and of 0.8 g/Kg/day for
          the following 30 days. In addition they took 0.3 g/Kg/day
          of oral BCAA throughout the study.

Group B - Pts. in this group were put on a similar restricted protein
          diet as in Group A, but, instead of BCAA supplement, re-
          ceived lactulose sufficient to ensure 2 bowel movements/
          day.

     BCAA were prepared in pellets and manufactured in single doses
each containing 2 g of valine, 1 g of leucine and 1 g of isoleucine
(Table 4).

     The effective absorption of this preparation had been tested
in a small number of patients (four) in which plasma BCAA levels
were measured before and two hours after the administration of a
single dose of 8 g of BCAA.

     Figure 1 shows the rise in plasma concentration of valine,
leucine and isoleucine.

Table 1. Comparison between the two groups of patients:
          clinical findings.

	Group A	Group B
Number of cases	14	14
Drop-outs	5	0
Sex Males	7	13
Females	2	1
Type of anastomosis		
Mesocaval	6	8
Porto-caval	3	6
Months of follow-up	41.7	48.3
Patients with previous multiple serious episodes of HE	5/9	9/14
Age	56	57

Table 2. Comparison between the two groups of patients:
          biochemical findings.

	Group A	Group B
GTP (mU/ml)	13.0+5.2	14.7+6.9
Normotest (% normal)	51.0∓15.4	48.5∓16.2
Cholinesterase (mU/ml)	1503∓532	1393∓384
Albumin (g/dl)	3.63∓0.94	3.57∓0.63
Ammonia (γ/dl)	149.1∓54.1	159.7∓56.2

Table 3. Protocol of the study

	DIET	
	0.5 g/Kg/day	0.8 g/Kg/day
0	30	60 days

Group A + oral BCAA 0.3 g/Kg/day
            (50% valine, 25% leucine, 25 % isoleucine)

Group B + lactulose

During the study the patients were checked every fourteen days
and mental state was assessed by two independent observers. Relatives
of the patients were carefully instructed on the most common signs of
HE and requested to promptly report to our unit any mental or neurological changes.

Routine blood chemistry, ammonia, total and free tryptophan
and plasma amino acids were determined in the post absorptive state
after an overnight fast at the beginning of the study, and after 30
and 60 days.

Blood Chemistry

Blood glucose, urea nitrogen, creatinine, total bilirubin, total
protein, pseudocholinesterase , aspartate transaminase and alkaline
phosphatase activities were colorimetrically assayed using specific
kits (Boehringer, Mannheim). Prothrombin time was measured using a
Clot-timer Carlo Erba 202 A.

Plasma ammonia was determined immediately upon withdrawal
according to the method described by Attili et al.[9] Using this method
normal ammonia levels are 45.5+10.5 (SD) µg/dl and in cirrhotics
without HE, 75.3+15.7 (SD) µg/dl.

Plasma AA. Blood samples were collected in heparinized tubes,
immediately centrifuged at 2000 rpm for 20 min, then stored at -80°C
until assayed.

Once thawed, plasma samples were deproteinized by adding 30
mg of solid sulfosalicylic acid/ml[5] β-hydroxyproline was added as
internal standard to the supernatant obtained by centrifugation at
5,000 rpm for 20 min. The sample was filtered through Whatman Paper
No. 1. Aliquots of 100 microliters were analyzed in an AA-Authomatic
Analyzer, Carlo Erba, Model SA28 M, using lithium buffers to separate glutamine and asparagine.[5] Free tryptophan was assayed employing
the spectrophotofluorimetric technique described by Duggan and
Udenfriend in an ultrafiltrate obtained from 2 ml of plasma centrifuged at 800 g in an Amicon cone 224-CF-50 for 45 min at room
temperature. Using this method, normal values of free tryptophan
are 0.42+0.05 (SD) µmoles/dl.[10]

RESULTS

Five patients in group A dropped out of the study.

One patient in group A and one in group B experienced one
episode of grade II hepatic encephalopathy. Both episodes occurred
during the second month of treatment without evident precipitating
events.

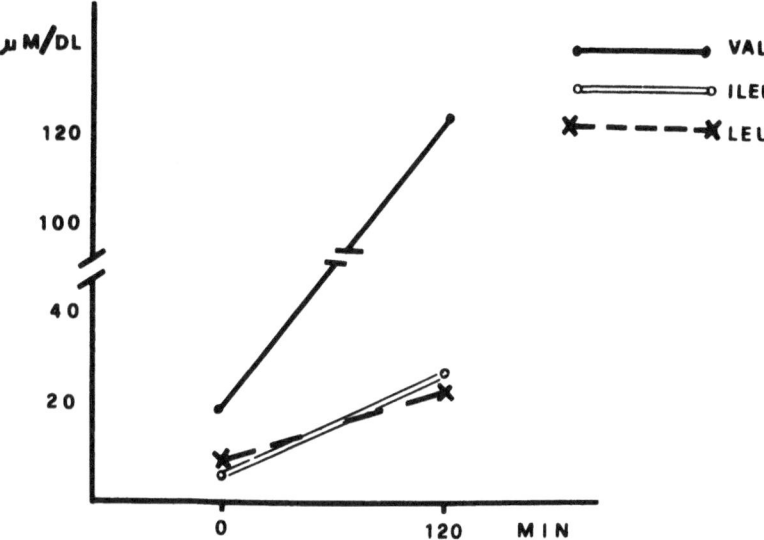

Fig. 1. BCAA plasma rise after one single administration of the
oral supplementation.

Routine blood chemistry as well as liver function tests and
body weight observed in the two groups during the study are reported
in Table 3. No significant differences were observed in any of the
parameters considered after 30 and 60 days with both treatments.

Figures 2 and 3 show the modifications of ammonia, total and
free tryptophan, methionine, BCAA and AAA during the treatment in
the two groups. With the exception of valine supplementation, the
other parameters did not show any modification in either Group A
or B.

DISCUSSION

Because of their metabolic and pharmacological properties BCAA
may be of great benefit in a hypercatabolic condition as in the
case of chronic liver failure.[4] In fact they are known to reduce
degradation and stimulate synthesis of muscular protein, therefore
improving nitrogen balance and reducing AA efflux from muscle.[12]
Given intravenously BCAA were found to reduce plasma aromatic amino
acids and ammonia.[13] Moreover, in our experimental model in dogs,
BCAA have been found to prevent hepatic-like coma induced by intra-
carotideal infusion of phenylalanine and tryptophan.[14] Finally BCAA
infusion may rapidly improve severe HE in man.[8,9]

Oral administration of BCAA has been used in the treatment of
chronic recurrent or persistent HE with controversial results. The
goals of oral BCAA supplementation in the diet of patients with

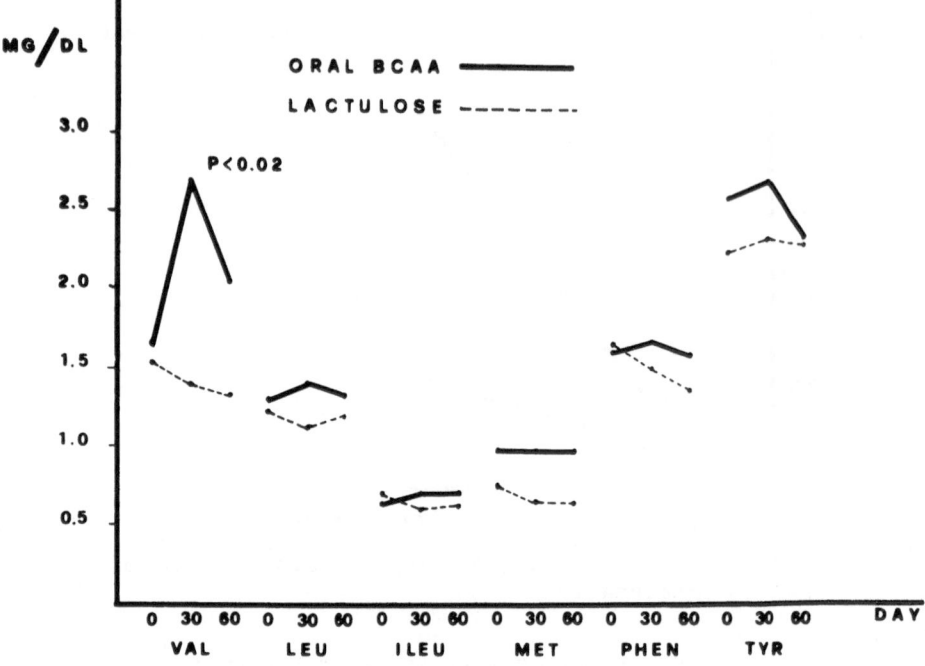

Fig. 2.   Plasma amino acid behavior during the study.

chronic recurrent HE are (a) to prevent recurrent episodes and (b) to give adequate amount of proteins in order to decrease the protein malnutrition present in these patients.

The present study indicates that oral BCAA supplementation may improve protein tolerance and prevent neurological disorders in patients exposed to a high risk of HE. In fact, even though a normal protein intake was allowed (1.1 g/Kg/day) and lactulose not given in the group taking BCAA, the incidence of hepatic encephalopathy during the two months of the study was not greater than in the control group receiving lactulose. On the other hand, the most common index of visceral protein synthesis (i.e. serum albumin and prothrombin activity) as well as the body weight were not apparently affected by oral BCAA supplementation during the 60 days of the study. Also plasma AA profile was not modified in the group taking BCAA.

As summarized in Tables 3, 4 and 5, the studies available in the literature[15,16,17,18] on the use of oral BCAA, give controversial results with regard to the clinical effect as well as to the biochemical findings. In such studies, the profound differences

Table 4. Routine blood chemistry and body weight modifications
during treatment A or B

	0	30	60 days
Group A: oral BCAA			
Bilirubin (mg/dl)	2.1+0.4	1.7+1.0	2.2+0.8
Cholinesterase (mU/ml)	1503+533	1691+436	1474+395
Normotest (% normal)	51+15	59+16	60+12
BUN (mg/dl)	18+5.5	14+6.5	19+20
Albumin (g/dl)	33.63+0.5	3.34+0.4	3.54+0.23
Body weight (Kg)	67+12	67.8+12	68+13
Group B: lactulose			
Bilirubin (mg/dl)	1.9+0.6	2.8+1.1	2.1+0.5
Cholinesterase (mU/ml)	1393+348	1576+435	1544+310
Normotest (% normal)	48+16	45+12	53+21
BUN (mg/dl)	18+6.5	13+10	11+4.6
Albumin (g/dl)	3.57+0.63	2.99+0.56	3.20+0.8
Body weight (Kg)	76+10	76+9	77+10

Table 5. Findings from previous studies on the use of oral
BCAA supplementation

	Number of patients	Type of hepatic encephalopathy
Fischer J. E. 1979	1	Chronic persistent HE
Swart G. R. 1981	8	Previous episodes of HE
Maddrey W. C. 1981	8	Chronic persistent HE
Egberts E. H. 1981	7	Latent HE
Eriksson S. 1981	7	Chronic persistent HE
Ferenci P. 1981	6	Previous episodes of HE
Conn H. O. 1982	14	Chronic recurrent HE
Marchesini G. 1981	1	Chronic persistent HE

in the type of patients, duration of treatment, doses and composition of the mixture used and the associated therapy may well
explain the different results obtained.

In conclusion, this study indicates that oral supplementation
with BCAA may improve protein tolerance and thus prevent HE in
patients with severe liver failure and surgical PSA. Nevertheless
the mechanisms through which BCAA exert their prophylactic effect

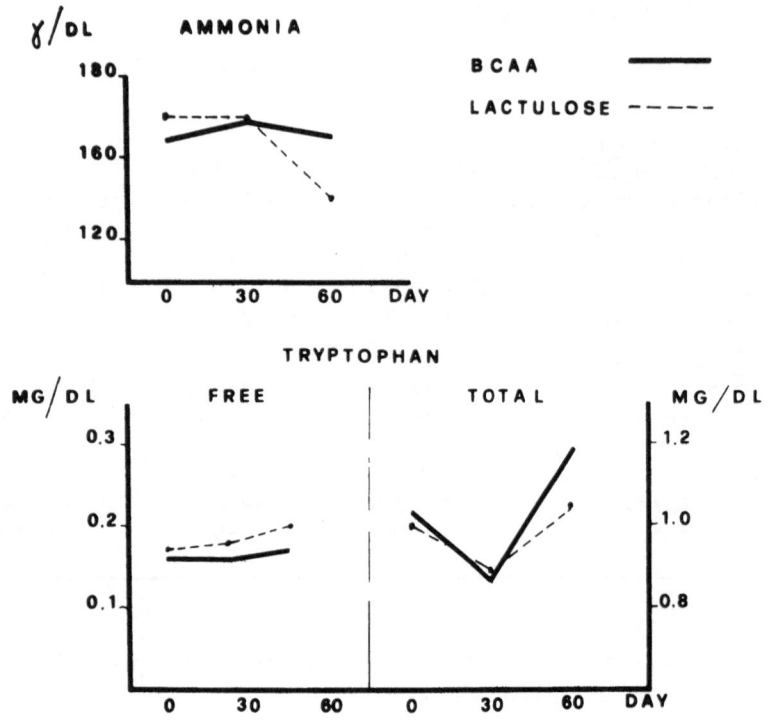

Fig. 3. Ammonia and free tryptophan behavior during the study.

Table 6. Oral BCAA administration in cirrhotic patients

	Dose /g/ day	Composition % Leu	Ileu	Val	Days of treatment	Associated therapy
Fischer J.E.	8.4	33	33	33	Months	Lactulose+Diet
Swart G.R.	14-21-24	40	30	30	15	Lactulose+Diet
Maddrey W.C.	∿ 6		?		7	Lactulose+Diet
Egberts E.H.	0.25/Kg	50	25	25	14	/
Eriksson S.	30	70	20	10	14	Lactul.(3 pts) + Diet
Ferenci P.	10	50	25	25	7	Diet
Conn H.O.	20		?		7	Diet
Marchesini G.	8.4	50	25	25	∿25	Lactulose+Diet

Table 7. Oral BCAA administration in cirrhotic patients

	Effect of hepatic Encephalopathy	Fasting plasma amino acids	Ammonia
Fischer J.E.	Improvement	Correction of Fischer ratio	
Swart G.R.	No episodes (As in controls)	Val ↑ Tir ↓ Try ↓	Stable
Maddrey W.C.	Improvement	Val ↑ Leu ↑ Tir ↓	Stable
Egberts E.H.	Improvement of psychometric tests	Val ↑ Leu ↑ Ileu ↑	Stable
Eriksson S.	No improvement of psychometric tests	No modifications	Stable
Ferenci P.	No episodes	No modifications	Stable
Conn H.O.	No episodes	Correction of Fischer ratio	
Marchesini G.	No improvement	No modifications	Stable

on HE and the nutritional implications of this therapy deserve further investigation.

REFERENCES

1. A. E. Read, S. Sherlock, J. Laidlow, The neuropsychiatric syndromes associated with chronic liver disease and extensive portal-systemic collateral circulation, Q.J. Med. 36: 135 (1967).
2. H. O. Conn and M. M. Lieberthal,"Hepatic Coma Syndromes and Lactulose."The Williams & Wilkins Co. Baltimore (1979).
3. E. Mezey, Liver disease and nutrition, Gastroenterology 74: 770 (1978).
4. A. Cascino, C. Cangiano, V. Calcaterra, F. Rossi Fanelli, and L. Capocaccia, Plasma amino acids imbalance in patients with liver disease, Am. J. Dig. Dis. 23: 591 (1978).
5. J. E. Fischer, J. M. Funovics, A. Aguirre, J. H. James, J. M. Keane, R. I. C. Wesdorp, N. Yoshimura, and T. Westman, The role of plasma amino acids in hepatic encephalopathy, Surgery 78: 276 (1975).
6. J. E. Fischer, H. M. Rosen, A. M. Ebeid, J. H. James, J. M. Flane, and P. B. Soeters, The effect of normalization of plasma amino acids on hepatic encephalopathy in man, Surgery 80: 77 (1976).
7. L. Capocaccia, V. Calcaterra, C. Cangiano, A. Cascino, F.

Fiaccadori, S. Gentile, F. Ghinelli, G. Pelosi, O. Riggio, F. Rossi Fanelli, D. Sacchini, and G. Giunchi, Therapeutic effect of branched chain amino acids in hepatic encephalo-pathy. A preliminary study, in: "Medical and Surgical Pro-blems of Portal Hypertension", M. J. Orloff, S. Stipa, and V. Ziparo, eds., Academic Press, New York (1980).

8. F. Rossi Fanelli, O. Riggio, C. Cangiano, A. Cascino, D. De Conciliis, M. Merli, M. Stortoni, and G. Giunchi (Coordi-nator L. Capocaccia). Branched-chain amino acids vs lactu-lose in the treatment of hepatic coma. A controlled study, Dig. Dis. and Sci. 27: 865 (1982).

9. A. F. Attili, D. Autizi, L. Capocaccia, S. Costantini, and F. Cotta Ramusino, Rapid determination of plasma ammonia using an ion specific electrode, Biochem. Med. 14: 109 (1975).

10. D. E. Duggan and S. Udenfriend, Spectrofluorimetric determi-nation of tryptophan in plasma and of tyrosine and tryptophan in protein hydrolysate, J. Biol. Chem. 223: 313 (1956).

11. H. Freund, H. C. Hoover, S. Atamian, and J. E. Fischer, Infusion of branched chain amino acids in post-operative patients, Am. J. Surg. 190: 18 (1979).

12. F. Rossi Fanelli, M. Angelico, C. Cangiano, A. Cascino, R. Ca-pocaccia, D. De Conciliis, O. Riggio, and L. Capocaccia, Effect of glucose and/or branched chain amino acid infusion in plasma amino acid imbalance in chronic liver failure, J. P. E. N. 5: 414 (1981).

13. F. Rossi Fanelli, H. Freund, R. Krause, A. R. Smith, J. H. James, S. Castorina-Ziparo, and J. E. Fischer, Induction of coma in normal dogs by the infusion of aromatic amino acids and its prevention by the addition of branched chain amino acids, Gastroenterology 83: 664 (1982).

14. H. Freund, N. Yoshimura, and J. E. Fischer, Long-term oral branched chain amino acid therapy in chronic hepatic ence-phalopathy, JAMA 242: 347 (1979).

15. M. Walser and J. R. Williamson, Metabolism and clinical impli-cations of branched-chain amino and ketoacids, Elsevier/North Holland (1981).

16. D. Horst, N. Grace, H. O. Conn, E. Schiff, S. Schenker, A. Vi-teri, D. Law, and C.E. Atterbury, A double-blind randomized comparison of dietary protein and an oral branched chain amino acid (BCAA) solution in cirrhotic patients with chronic portal-systemic encephalopathy, Clinical Research 641A (1982).

17. G. Marchesini, C. Dondi, and M. Zoli, Insuccesso nel trattamento dell'encefalopatia epatica cronica con aminoacidi a catena ramificata per via orale, Il Fegato 27: 51 (1981).

MUSCLE BIOPSY STUDIES ON MALNUTRITION IN PATIENTS WITH

LIVER CIRRHOSIS:

Preliminary results of long-term treatment with a branched-chain
amino acid enriched diet

G. F. Guarnieri, G. Toigo, R. Situlin, G. Pozzato, L.
Faccini, R. Marini, D. Giuntini, S. Parco, A. Lucchesi,
G. Agolini, M. Frezza

Institute of Medical Pathology - University of Trieste,
Italy, Laboratory of Children's Hospital, Trieste, Italy

INTRODUCTION

Protein-calorie undernutrition is common in patients with liver
cirrhosis and may have many causes (Figure 1).[1-7] In recent years
it has become more and more evident that the maintenance of adequate
nutrition is an essential part of the management of these patients,[8]
because malnutrition is positively associated with energy and mortality[7] and may induce severe derangements of liver function.[9,10] It
is obvious that nutritional therapy should minimize the toxicity
arising from protein metabolism while improving the nutritional
state, but it is less clear how this should be done in practice.
Traditional dietary protein restriction can lessen the risk of hepatic
encephalopathy, but often results in chronic protein malnutrition.
Besides, despite careful instruction and considerable effort, it is
often difficult to increase food intake also in cirrhotic patients
on an unrestricted diet because of anorexia, nausea and taste abnormalities (Figure 1).

To treat malnutrition effectively, a preliminary nutritional
assessment is needed. Available techniques enable the clinician to
readily detect the presence of malnutrition and to follow the
response to nutritional therapy. Methods for assessing the nutritional status are: history, physical examination, assessment of dietary
intake, anthropometric measurements, biochemical determinations, immunological assays and studies of body composition.[11-14]

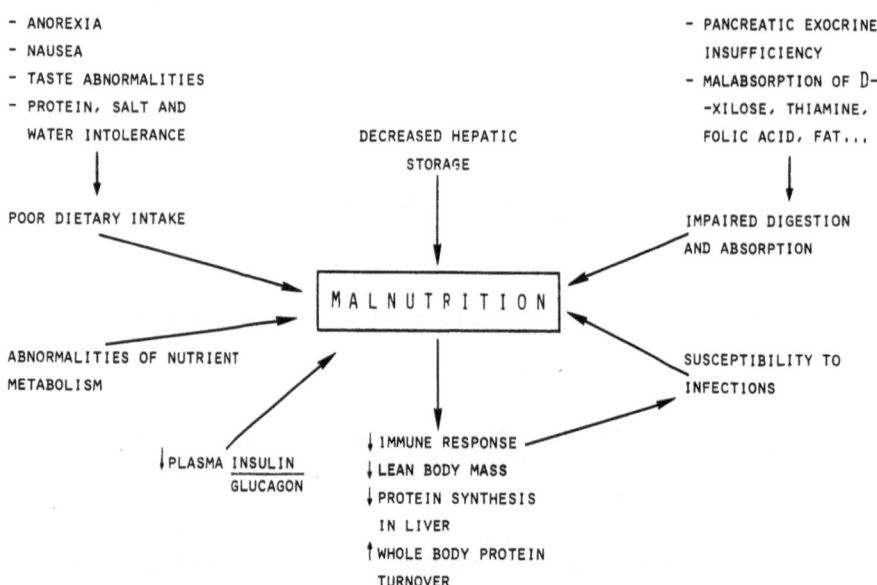

Fig. 1. Principal causes and consequences of malnutrition in liver
         cirrhosis.

        In the study of body composition many techniques are available.[12]
We measure skeletal muscle DNA, RNA and non-collagen alkali-soluble
protein content in muscle specimens obtained through needle biopsy.
[15,16] Skeletal muscle may be considered the largest protein and non-
fat energy store of the body, and changes of muscle protein and
RNA content have been reported in response to undernutrition and
nutrient intake.[17-19] DNA content is considered a stable reference
standard also in malnourished adults, more reliable than fresh or
dry weight or muscle protein content.[20] The RNA:DNA ratio is an
index of cell capacity for protein synthesis and the ASP:DNA ratio
gives the size of the hypothetical muscle cell.[17-19] These direct
tissue analyses "in vivo" allow to overcome the well-known limita-
tions of nitrogen balance techniques[21] in the evaluation of protein
state.

        This report deals with the evaluation of nutritional status in
23 patients with liver cirrhosis by means of anthropometric, biochemical and immunological indices. We also report here the preliminary results, obtained in 8 stable cirrhotic patients, of a
prospective, controlled, randomized study on the effects of long
term diet supplementation with oral amino acids and/or energy on
nutritional status and hepatic encephalopathy. The supplement used
was high in branched-chain and low in aromatic amino acids and may
provide a well tolerated nitrogen source.[8,9,21-27] By this means,
we intended to separately evaluate the effects of amino acids and

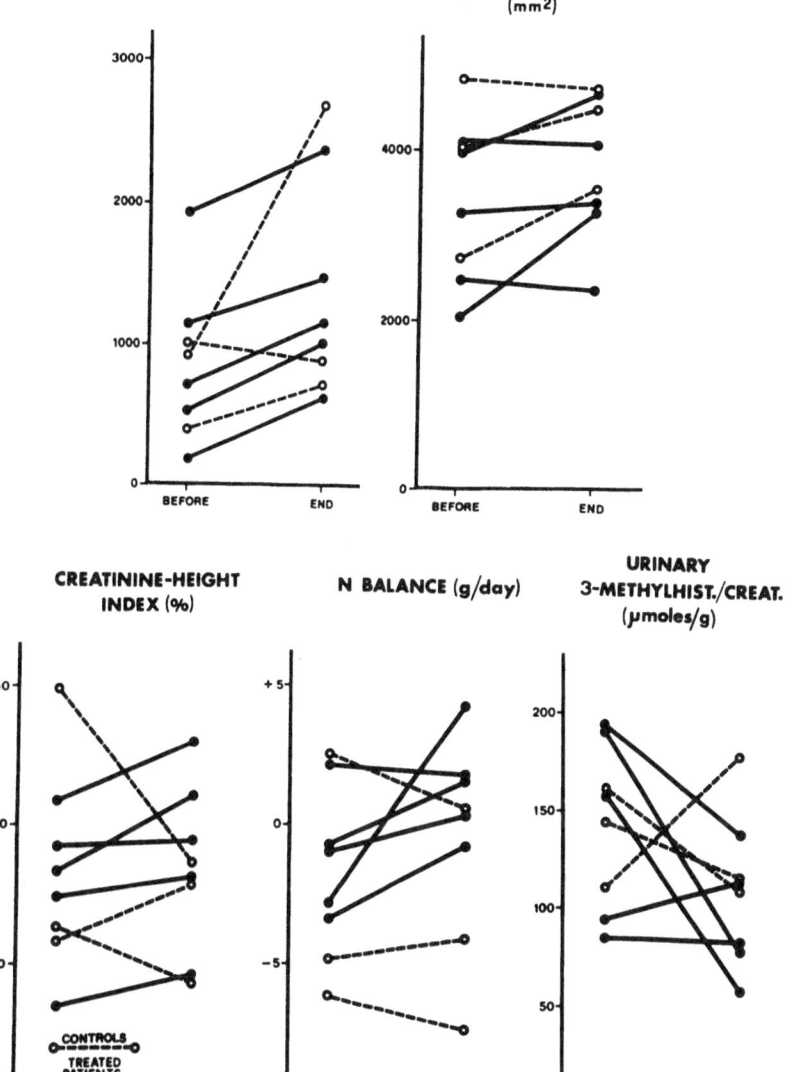

Fig. 2.   Changes of anthropometric indices, creatinine-height index,
           N balance, and urinary 3-methylhistidine:creatinine ratio
           in patients with liver cirrhosis treated with an aminoacid
           and/or energy supplement.

energy. Nitrogen and energy consumption may, in fact, have differential effects on hepatic encephalopathy and nutritional status.
8,28-32

An informed consent was obtained from all the patients prior to admission to the study.

PATIENTS, MATERIALS AND METHODS

The nutritional status was assessed in 23 consecutive patients (14 males) aged 61+8 years (mean $\pm$ S.D.), affected by alcoholic (11 cases), cryptogenic (11 cases) and post-necrotic (1 case) liver cirrhosis. Their laboratory data are summarized in Table 1. Fifteen patients had signs of hepatic encephalopathy during the study and fluid retention was present in 13 of them. Patients with renal insufficiency, diabetes or other metabolic diseases were excluded from the study.

Dietary intake was evaluated by an experienced dietician by means of dietary interviews and food tables.

For the anthropometric measurements of height, weight, triceps (TST) and subscapular (SST) skinfold thickness, and mid-arm muscle circumference (AMC) we used standard techniques and a Lange skinfold caliper.

Blood samples, obtained after an overnight fast, were measured by Technicol Auto-Analyzers for serum glucose, total proteins, calcium, inorganic phosphate, urea nitrogen and creatinine. Cholesterol and triglycerides were determined enzymatically by Boehringer testcombination kits. White cell count and hemoglobin concentration were measured with a Coulter S counter, and the percentage of lymphocytes were determined in a stained blood film. Serum albumin, transferrin, C_3, and C_3 activator were determined in duplicate by radial immunodiffusion (Boehringwerke Partigen). Serum pseudocholinesterase activity was measured by a Boehringer test-combination kit. The response to phytohemagglutinin and PPD was evaluated as previously reported.[12]

Muscle biopsy was performed with Bergström's needle and metabolites were determined as previously reported.[15] Muscle water and lipids were determined according to Bergström. Muscle RNA and DNA were extracted by the method of Schmidt-Tannhauser, as modified by Munro and Fleck. DNA content was determined by the indole method, ASP by the method of Lowry and RNA by UV absorption, corrected for the measured peptide content.[15]

Plasma for amino acid determination was immediately separated, deproteinized with sulphosalycilic acid and analyzed with a Kontron Liquimat III amino acid analyzer. Urinary 3-methyl-histidine content was similarly measured; the reported results are the mean of three consecutive day determinations and are related to creatinine excretion.[14]

Nitrogen balance was performed with standard techniques and

Table 1. Dietary intake, principal laboratory investigations and anthropometric measurements in the patients with liver cirrhosis. Results are expressed as mean +S.D. The percentage of anthropometric values under the 5th percentile[34] is reported in parentheses.

Dietary proteins (g/kg des. wt./day)	0.65 + 0.21
Dietary energy (kcal/kg des.wt./day)	36 + 5
Carbodydrates (% of energy)	63.4 + 4.7
Lipids (% of energy)	29.2 + 2.2
Proteins (% of energy)	7.4 + 2.8
N balance (g/day)	-1.35 + 2.98
AST (U/1)	86 + 47
ALT (U/1)	57 + 39
Alk.phosphatase (U/1)	150 + 64
γ-GT (U/1)	60 + 57
Total bilirubin (mg/dl)	2.43 + 1.63
Prothrombin index	1.34 + 0.16
Glucose (mg/dl)	96 + 31
Urea N (mg/dl)	17 + 7
Creatinine (mg/dl)	1.1 + 0.5
Cholesterol (mg/dl)	169 + 37
Triglycerides (mg/dl)	79 + 25
Hemoglobin (g/dl)	11.7 + 1.4
Ammonium (μg/dl)	89 + 51
Weight	
% desirable (ideal) body wt. (PDW)	106 + 13
% relative body wt. (RBW)	92 + 12
Skinfold thickness	
triceps (TST), mm	7.5 + 5.2 (68%)
subscapular (SST), mm	9.3 + 4.1 (42%)
Arm fat area (AFA), mm^2	895 + 699 (68%)
Arm muscle circ. (AMC), mm	216 + 24 (58%)
Arm muscle area (AMA), mm^2	3781 + 812 (42%)
Creatinine-height I. (%)	82 + 24

corrected for body area nitrogen variations. Fecal and urinary nitrogen was determined with a Coleman nitrogen analyzer. No correction was made for unmeasurable nitrogen losses. The reported balances are the mean of three consecutive day determinations.

The neurologic assessment was performed according to Conn et al.[33] EEG tracings were interpreted by a blinded neurologist.

The second part of our report concerns 8 patients with stable liver cirrhosis who were either unable to ingest an adequate diet,

198 G. F. GUARNIERI ET AL.

or intolerant to an adequate protein intake. Patients had to be
malnourished and to have no more than grade 2 encephalopathy at time
of entry. We also excluded from the study the patients recovering
from an acute episode of encephalopathy or from acute illnesses;
with renal insufficiency; requiring blood or plasma transfusions;
with diabetes or other metabolic diseases; with severe fluid restriction. The patients were hospitalized for the baseline nutritional
and neurologic assessments, performed as reported above. The calorie
content of the basal diet followed by the patients was then reduced
and the patients were randomly supplemented for 100-120 days with
two packages/day of an oral mixture (Hepatic-Aid[R]) containing amino
acids (29 g), carbohydrates and fats (1120 total kcal) or only carbohydrates and fats (1120 total kcal) (Table 2). By this means, in
the 5 treated patients protein + amino acid intake was increased
to 1.2 g/kg and energy intake to 45 kcal/kg. In the 3 controls only
energy intake was increased to 43 kcal/kg (Table 3). The nitrogen
source, high in branched chain and low in aromatic amino acids, was
formulated according to the amino acids compositions of the FO80
parenteral solution.[22] Any previous therapy potentially affecting
the results (diuretics, antibiotics, lactulose, etc.) was maintained
unchanged during the study. The adherence of the patients to the diet
and the treatment, and the grade of encephalopathy were periodically
checked by the dietician and a member of the research staff, who
also made clinical assessments and noted any adverse reactions. The
patients were admitted again to the Hospital at the end of the study
for the complete nutritional and neurologic assessment.

Table 2. Composition of the aminoacid and calorie powder
supplemented to the patients

	Grams	kcalories	Calorie percentage
Amino acids	29	120	10.4
Carbohydrate (maltodextrin, sucrose)	196	784	69.8
Fats (partially hydroge- nated soybean oil)	24.6	216	19.8
Total energy		1,120	
Total nitrogen: approx.	4.5		

Amino acid pattern (g): L-tryptophan 0.24; L-isoleucine
3.28; L-leucine 4.02; L-lysine acetate 3.16; L-methio-
nine 0.36; L-phenylalanine 0.36; L-threonine 1.64; L-
valine 3.06; L-alanine 2.80; L-arginine 2.20; L-histi-
dine 0.88; L-proline 2.92; L-serine 1.82; glycine 3.28.

Table 3 - Nutrient intake in the patients receiving an amino acid and/or energy supplementation. Data are expressed as mean.

	Proteins (and AA) g/kg des.wt./d	Carbohydrate g/kg des.wt./d	Lipids g/kg des.wt./d	Energy kcal des.wt./d
Treated patients (energy + AA)				
Before suppl.	0.75	6.01	1.26	38
During suppl.	1.20	6.90	1.43	45
Controls (energy)				
Before suppl.	0.56	5.80	1.16	36
During suppl.	0.64	7.13	1.34	43

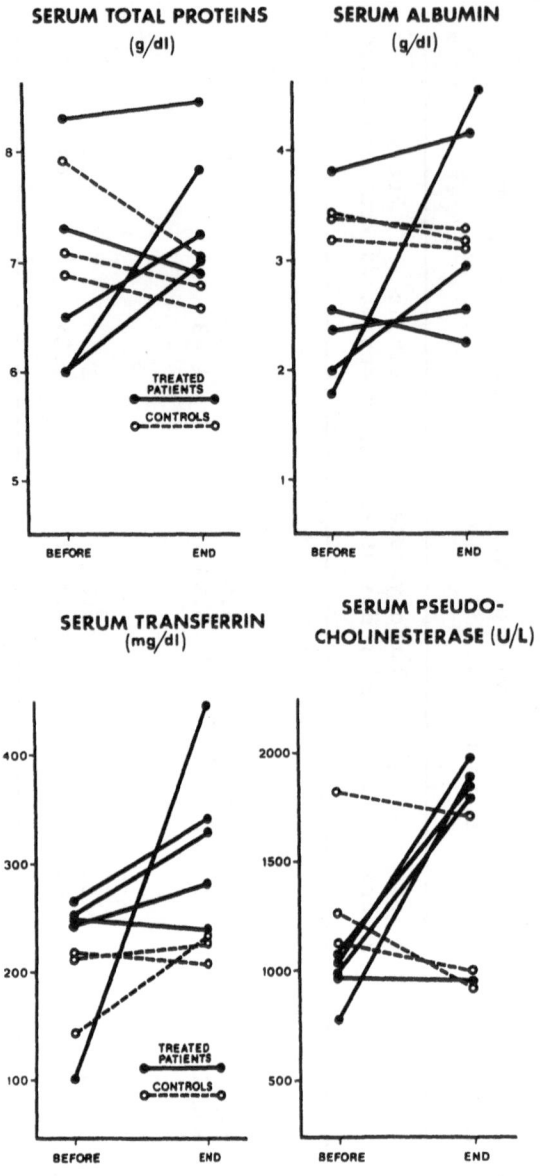

Fig. 3.   Serum protein content in patients with liver cirrhosis
          treated with an amino acid and/or energy supplement.

RESULTS

        The spontaneous dietary protein intake (Table 1) was below
the recommended dietary allowances for healthy people. The mean

dietary energy intake was normal, but the exact energy requirements are not known in these patients. The average corrected apparent nitrogen balance was definitely negative.

The anthropometric indices (Table 1) were frequently under the 5th percentile of a normal population.[34] Also the creatinine-height index was reduced.[11]

Serum protein content (Table 4) was below the normal ranges in the majority of patients.

Also the immune response to PPD and phytohemagglutinin and blood lymphocyte content were lower than in controls (Table 4).

Muscle DNA concentration (Table 5) was significantly increased, whereas muscle ASP content and the RNA:DNA and ASP:DNA ratios were significantly lower than in controls. Some significant correlations (linear regression analysis) of the examined indices are reported in Table 6.

The effects of diet supplementation are reported in Figures 2-4. The examined indices generally improved in the treated patients, whereas inconsistent results were obtained in controls receiving only an energy supplement. Phytohemagglutinin response tended to improve in 4 out of 5 treated patients and to worsen in the three controls. Very limited changes of PPD response were observed.

Serum transaminase content (ALT) decreased in all treated patients from 69 ± 43 to 36 ± 19 U/1, whereas serum alkaline phospha-

Table 4. Serum protein and blood lymphocyte content, and response to PPD (tine test) and phytohemagglutinin in the patients with liver cirrhosis. Results are expressed as mean $\pm$ S.D. The percentage of values under the normal range is reported in parentheses.

	Normal range	Patients
Total proteins, g/dl	6.3-7.8	7.1 ± 0.7 (0%)
Albumin, g/dl	> 3.5	2.9 ± 0.6 (79%)
Transferrin, mg/dl	205-374	169 ± 54 (86%)
Pseudocholinest., U/1	1900-3800	1102 ± 577 (94%)
C_3, mg/dl	100-200	53 ± 19 (100%)
C_3 act., mg/dl	18-40	23 ± 35 (83%)
PPD (% neg.)	53%	62%
Phytohemagglutinin ($\emptyset$ mm)	8.9-14.8	10.2 ± 2.9 (38%)
Blood lymphocytes/mm³	1490-3930	1812 ± 673 (56%)

tase increased in three out of five patients. Slight variations of
flapping and number connection test were observed.

DISCUSSION

Many causes of malnutrition are present in liver cirrhosis
(Figure 1).

In 23 patients with liver cirrhosis we found reduced arm muscle
and fat, urinary creatinine excretion, plasma protein content, immune
response, and muscle RNA:DNA and ASP:DNA ratios. Nitrogen balance
was definitely negative. As expected, total protein determination
is valueless in patients with increased serum immunoglobulin content.
DNA concentration was increased as a consequence of muscle hypo-
trophia. These results suggest that with the reported protein and
energy intake a pattern of protein-calorie undernutrition develops
in cirrhotic patients.

A high prevalence of malnutrition and an impaired immune
response, as well as a relationship among malnutrition, anergy or
mortality rate, have been reported by O'Keefe[7] in patients with
liver cirrhosis. It has also been reported that anergy could be
partly reversed with dietary measures,[7] and adequate nutrition could
improve hepatic function.[9,10] Therefore, nutritional therapy is an
important aspect of management in patients with liver cirrhosis.
Traditional dietary protein restriction, aimed to control the symptoms of hepatic encephalopathy, often negatively affects the nutritional status. Recent studies on whole body protein turnover suggest
that this practice has a limited effect to reduce the load of amino
acids on the liver, because the input of amino acids from endogenous
protein breakdown is much greater than that derived from a diet.[21]
Therefore "it might be more rational to suppress endogenous protein
breakdown and maintain intake at requirement levels, than to restrict
protein intake to level below that required for maintenance".[21] The
diet supplement used in this study, high in energy and in branched-
chain amino acids and low in aromatic amino acids, should achieve
these results without deleterious effects on the mental state.[5,8,9,]
[21-32] The amino acid mixture used in our patients should fulfil
exogenously the demand for branched-chain amino acids. These compounds have an anti-catabolic effect in muscle and, therefore,
improve nitrogen balance and, by minimizing the production of aromatic amino acids and short chain peptides, ameliorate the symptoms
of hepatic encephalopathy.[8,9,22-27,30,31] They also enhance protein
synthesis, including hepatic protein synthesis.[31] The preliminary
results reported here show that in patients receiving this supplement
fat stores, plasma protein content, creatinine-height index, nitrogen
balance, the grade of encephalopathy, and muscle RNA:DNA and ASP:DNA
ratios improved. Urinary 3-methylhistidine:creatinine ratio decreased
in 3 out of 5 patients, suggesting a reduced percent myofibrillar
protein breakdown.[14] An improved response to phytohemagglutinin was

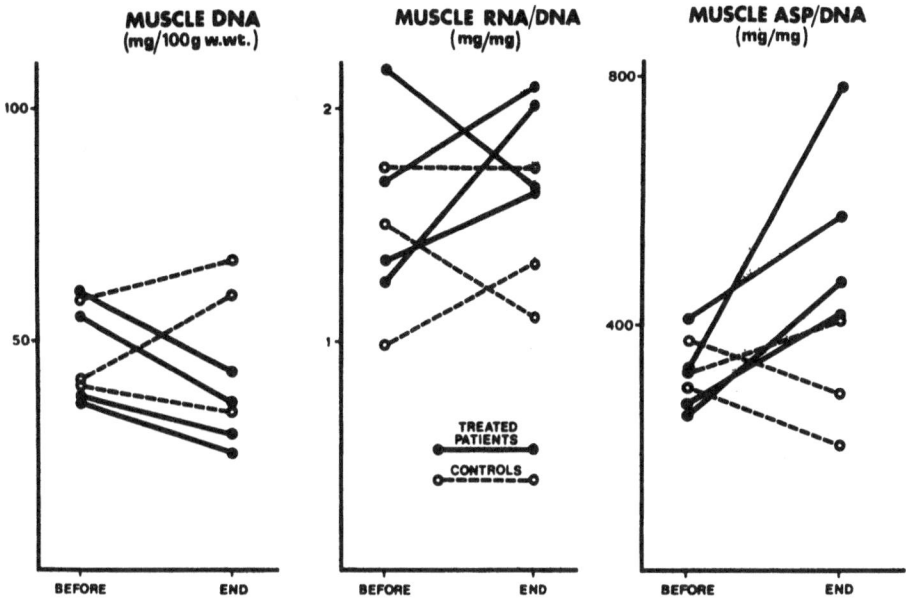

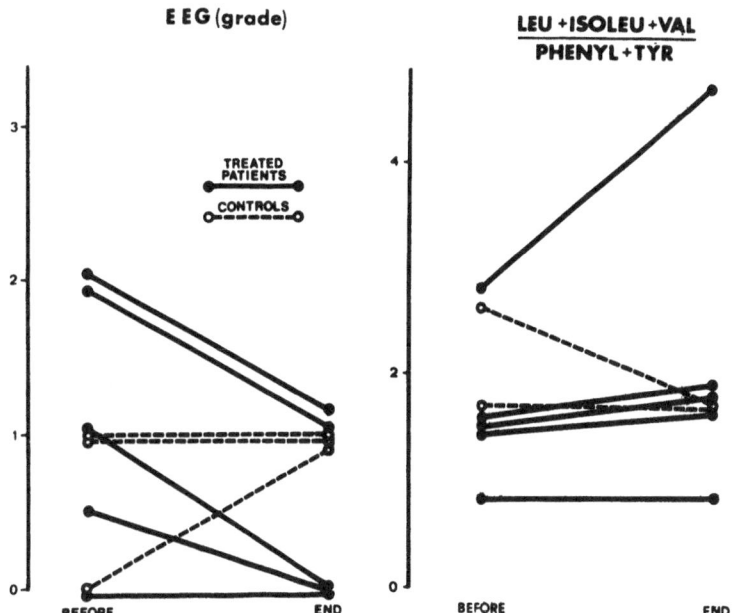

Fig. 4. Muscle DNA content, muscle RNA:DNA and noncollagen alkali-
         soluble proteins (ASP):DNA ratios, EEG grade, and plasma
         branched chain:aromatic amino acid ratio in patients with
         liver cirrhosis treated with an amino acid and/or energy
         supplement.

Table 5. Muscle DNA, RNA, ASP (alkali-soluble proteins),
          water and fat content in muscle biopsy specimens
          of patients with liver cirrhosis. Results are
          expressed as mean + S.D. FFS = fat-free solids.
          The level of significance was evaluated by the
          Student's t-test.

	Controls	Patients	Level of significance
DNA, mg/100 g w.wt.	34+8	44+7	0.005
RNA, mg/100 g w.wt.	77+23	69+17	N.S.
ASP, g/100 g w.wt.	18.0+2.1	16.3+2.0	0.013
RNA/DNA, mg/mg	2.32+0.59	1.56+0.31	0.005
ASP/DNA, mg/mg	554+109	373+77	0.005
Water, g/100 g FFS	301+56	326+53	N.S.
Lipids, g/100 g FFS	25+17	19+19	N.S.

observed only in treated patients. After an overnight fast the plasma
branched-chain to aromatic amino acid ratio did not reveal any
noteworthy trends, as reported also by Eriksson et al.[35] Limited
and inconsistent results were obtained in controls receiving only
an energy supplement. This points out the importance of an increased
nitrogen intake to ameliorate the nutritional status in liver
cirrhosis. The improvement of liver synthesis of plasma proteins,
as well as the decrease of serum ALT, are probably a sign of a general improvement of liver metabolism and function.[9,10,21] An improvement in bone metabolism could be involved in the increased alkaline
phosphatase activity. This increase of plasma protein content with
the treatment suggests that the reduced plasma protein synthesis in
liver cirrhosis is more the consequence of malnutrition than of a
decreased hepatic synthetic capacity, as reported also by O'Keefe.[21]

     In our patients the supplement was well tolerated and we very
seldom observed the side-effects reported by Morgan.[2] Nitrogen balance improved with treatment in our patients, but nitrogen balance
studies have a limited value in the study of protein metabolism in
cirrhotic patients.[21] With the direct muscle tissue analysis and the
determination of plasma proteins synthetized in liver we could,
however, point out the positive effects of the supplement on the
two main sites of protein metabolism, i.e. muscle and liver.

     Positive results on the mental state have been recently obtained
also with short-time nasogastric administration of this supplement
in cirrhotic patients with acute encephalopathy ([26] and G.F. Guar-
neri, unpublished results).

Table 6.   Some significant correlations (p < 0.038 or lower) present in the examined patients.

			r
age	and	muscle water	−0.47
age	and	subscapular sk. th.	−0.46
dietary fats	and	carbohydrates	0.70
dietary fats	and	creatinine−height I.	0.58
dietary fats	and	lymphocytes	0.87
dietary energy	and	lymphocytes	0.99
relative body wt.	and	triceps sk. th.	0.52
relative body wt.	and	subscapular sk. th.	0.78
relative body wt.	and	arm muscle circum.	0.66
relative body wt.	and	arm muscle area	0.67
relative body wt.	and	arm fat area	0.58
subscapular sk. th.	and	triceps sk. th.	0.84
subscapular sk. th.	and	arm fat area	0.86
arm muscle area	and	phytohemagglutinin	0.53
albumin	and	pseudocholinester.	0.58
albumin	and	prothrombin index	−0.70
C_3	and	C_3 activator	0.66
C_3 activator	and	prothrombin index	−0.64
PPD	and	C_3	0.51
PPD	and	C_3 activator	0.63
AST (SGOT)	and	C_3	−0.66
muscle RNA	and	muscle DNA	0.51
muscle RNA/DNA	and	lymphocytes	0.87
muscle ASP	and	arm muscle area	0.66

We conclude that poor nutritional status and muscle wasting often occur in patients with liver cirrhosis, and periodic nutritional assessment and monitoring of dietary intake are important aspects in the treatment of these patients. Many nutritional and metabolic abnormalities can be reversed with long-term administration of an energy and branched-chain amino acid enriched diet, without any worsening of the encephalopathy. The determination of protein and nucleic acid content in muscle biopsy specimens enables the clinician to directly study muscle protein metabolism in humans.

ACKNOWLEDGEMENTS

Many thanks are due to Ms. Maria Crevatin, R.N., for the valuable assistance in the care of the patients.

The Authors thank Miss Luisella Vici for secretarial assistance. This work was supported in part by a grant from M.P.I.

REFERENCES

1. A. G. Morgan, J. Kelleher, B. E. Walker, and M. S. Losowsky,
   Nutrition in cryptogenic cirrhosis and chronic aggressive
   hepatitis, Gut 17: 113 (1976).
2. M. Y. Morgan, Enteral nutrition in chronic liver disease, Acta
   Chir. Scand. suppl. 507: 81 (1981).
3. R. A. Quercia, Malnutrition and nutritional support in hepatic
   failure, Nutr. Supp. Serv. 1: 22 (1981).
4. E. Mezey, Liver disease and nutrition, Gastroenterology 74: 770
   (1978).
5. N. McIntyre and M. Y. Morgan, Nutritional aspects of liver
   disease, in: "Liver and Biliary Disease," R. Wright, K. G.
   M. M. Alberti, S. Karran, G. H. Millward-Sadler, eds., W. B.
   Saunders Co. Ltd., London, Philadelphia, Toronto (1979).
6. F. Fiaccadori, F. Ghinelli, G. Pedretti, G. Pelosi, D. Sacchini,
   and G. Spadini, Negative nitrogen balance in cirrhotics (A
   correct therapeutic approach), La Ricerca Clin. Lab. 11: 259
   (1981).
7. S. J. O'Keefe, A. R. El-Zayadi, T. E. Carraher, M. Davis, and
   R. Williams, Malnutrition and immuno-incompetence in patients
   with liver disease, Lancet ii: 615 (1980).
8. P. D. Wright, Intravenous feeding in liver disease, Acta Chir.
   Scand. suppl. 507: 102 (1981).
9. H. Freund, N. Yoshimura, and J. E. Fisher, Chronic hepatic encephalopathy. Long-term therapy with a branched-chain amino-
   acid-enriched elemental diet, J.A.M.A. 242: 347 (1979).
10. C. M. Leevy and F. Smith, Nutritional factors in alcoholic
    liver disease in man, in: "The Liver and its Disease," F.
    Schaffner, S. Sherlock, C. M. Leevy, eds., George Thieme
    Publishers, Stuttgart (1976).
11. G. L. Blackburn, B. R. Bistrian, B. S. Maini, H. T. Schlamm,
    and H. F. Smith, Nutritional and metabolic assessment of
    the hospitalized patients, J. Parent. Ent. Nutr. 1: 11(1977).
12. G. F. Guarnieri, L. Faccini, T. Lipartiti, F. Ranieri, F. Span-
    garo, F. Berquier-Vidali, A. Raimondi, D. Giuntini, G. Toigo,
    and F. Dardi, Simple method for nutritional assessment in
    hemodialyzed patients, Am. J. Clin. Nutr. 33: 1598 (1980).
13. R. L. Weinsier, E. M. Hunker, C. L. Krumdieck, and C. E. But-
    terworth, Hospital malnutrition. A prospective evaluation
    of general medical patients during the course of hospita-
    lization, Am. J. Clin. Nutr. 32: 418 (1979).
14. P. Milewski, I. Holbrook, and M. Irving, Urinary 3-methylhisti-
    dine: creatinine ratio in patients on long-term parenteral
    nutrition, J. Parent. Ent. Nutr. 4: 286 (1980).
15. G. F. Guarnieri, G. Toigo, R. Situlin, L. Faccini, U. Coli,
    S. Landini, G. Bazzato, F. Dardi, and L. Campanacci, Muscle
    biopsy studies in chronically uremic patients. Evidence for
    malnutrition, Third Intern. Congr. on Nutrition and Metabo-
    lism in Renal Disease, Marseille, September 1-4, in press

in Kidney Intern. (1982).

16. G. F. Guarnieri, G. Toigo, R. Situlin, L. Faccini, R. Rustia,
     and F. Dardi, Muscle cathepsin D activity, and RNA, DNA and
     protein content in maintenance hemodialysis patients, Intern.
     Symp. on "Proteases: potential role in health and disease",
     Würzburg, October 17-20, Plenum Publishing Co., in press
     (1982).
17. D. J. Millward and J. C. Waterlow, Effect of nutrition on
     protein turnover in skeletal muscle, Fed. Proc. 37: 2283
     (1978).
18. J. C. Waterlow, P. J. Garlick, and D. J. Millward, The effects
     of nutrition and hormones on protein turnover in muscle,
     in: "Protein Turnover in Mammalian Tissues and in the Whole
     Body," Elsevier/North Holland Biomedical Press, Amsterdam
     (1978).
19. E. S. Ogata, S. K. H. Foung, and M. A. Holliday, The effect of
     starvation and refeeding on muscle protein synthesis and
     catabolism in the young rat, J. Nutr. 108: 759 (1978).
20. G. A. O. Alleyne, R. W. Hay, D. I. Picou, J. P. Stanfield, and
     R. C. Whitehead, "Protein-Energy Malnutrition,"Edward
     Arnold Publisher, Meidenhead (1977).
21. S. J. D. O'Keefe, R. R. Abraham, M. Davis, and R. Williams,
     Protein turnover in acute and chronic liver disease, Acta
     Chir. Scand. suppl. 507: 91 (1981).
22. J. E. Fischer and R. H. Bower, Nutritional support in liver
     disease, Surg. Clin. North America 61: 653 (1981).
23. D. B. A. Silk, Malnutrition in liver disease and its relation-
     ship to hepatic encephalopathy, Acta Chir. Scand. suppl.
     507: 106 (1981).
24. D. Horst, N. Grace, H. O. Conn, E. Schiff, S. Schenker, A.
     Viteri, D. Law, and C. E. Atterbury, A double-blind rando-
     mized comparison of dietary protein and an oral branched
     chain amino acid (BCAA) solution in cirrhotic patients with
     chronic porta-systemic encephalopathy (PSE), in "Hepatic
     Encephalopathy in Chronic Liver Failure," L. Capocaccia,
     J. E. Fischer, and F. Rossi-Fanelli, eds., Plenum Press,
     New York,
25. K. Von Schäfer, M. B.Winther, M. Ukida, H. Leweling, H. J.
     Reiter, and J. C. Bode, Influence of an orally administered
     protein mixture enriched in branched chain amino acids on
     the chronic hepatic encephalopathy (CHE) of patients with
     liver cirrhosis, Z. Gastroenterologie 19: 356 (1981).
26. P. P. Keohane, H. Attrill, O. Grimble, R. Spiller, and D. B.
     A. Silk, Nutritional support of malnourished encephalopathic
     cirrhotic patients using a specially formulated enteral diet,
     Gastroenterology 82: 1098 (1982).
27. F. Rossi-Fanelli, M. Angelico, C. Cangiano, A. Cascino, R. Ca-
     pocaccia, D. DeConciliis, O. Riggio, and L. Capocaccia,
     Effect of glucose and/or branched chain amino acid infusion
     on plasma amino acid imbalance in chronic liver failure,

J. Parent. Ent. Nutr. 5: 414 (1981).

28. G. H. Anderson and L. M. Blendis, Plasma neutral amino acid
     ratios in normal man and in patients with hepatic encepha-
     lopathy: correlations with self-selected protein and energy
     consumption, Am. J. Clin. Nutr. 34: 377 (1981).

29. C. Walker, W. Peterson, and R. Unger, Blood ammonia levels in
     advanced cirrhosis during therapeutic elevation of the
     insulin:glucagon ratio, N. Engl. J. Med. 291: 168 (1974).

30. G. Marchesini, M. Zoli, C. Dondi, G. Bianchi, M. Cirulli, and
     E. Pisi, Anticatabolic effect of branched-chain amino acid-
     enriched solutions in patients with liver cirrhosis, Hepa-
     tology 2: 420 (1982).

31. H. R. Freund and J. E. Fischer, Hepatic failure, in: "Nutrition
     and the Surgical Patient," G. L. Hill, ed., Churchill Living-
     stone, Edinburgh, London, Melbourne, New York (1981).

32. H. N. Munro, Energy and protein intakes as determinants of ni-
     trogen balance, Kidney Internat. 14: 313 (1978).

33. H. O. Conn, C. M. Leevy, Z. R. Vlahcevic, J. B. Rodgers, W. C.
     Maddrey, L. Seeff, and L. L. Levy, Comparison of lactulose
     and neomycin in the treatment of chronic portal-systemic en-
     cephalopathy. A double blind controlled trial, Gastroentero-
     logy 72: 573 (1977).

34. A. R. Frisancho, New norms of upper limb fat and muscle areas
     for assessment of nutritional status, Am. J. Clin. Nutr. 34:
     2540 (1981).

35. A. P. Eriksson, and J. Wahren, Failure of oral branched-chain
     amino acids to improve chronic hepatic encephalopathy, J.
     Parent. Ent. Nutr. 5: 355 (1981).

THE ROLE OF MUSCLE PROTEIN CATABOLISM IN THE PLASMA AMINO ACID PROFILE OF CIRRHOTICS (*)

M. Zoli, G. Marchesini, G. P. Bianchi, C. Dondi, A. Melli,
S. Cassarani, V. Bua
Istituto di Patologia Medica 1, Università di Bologna
Bologna, Italy

Patients with liver cirrhosis have peculiar abnormalities in plasma amino acid concentrations: increased aromatic amino acids, methionine and free tryptophan, and decreased branched-chain amino acids.[1,2] Increased breakdown of lean body mass was suggested as a mechanism by which aromatic amino acids may accumulate in the general circulation.[3] A complete evaluation of myofibrillar protein degradation may be achieved by simultaneous assessment of daily 3-methylhistidine and creatinine in urine.[4] In previous studies an increased myofibrillar protein catabolic rate was demonstrated in patients with liver cirrhosis with and without muscle wasting.[5]

The present study was undertaken to evaluate the role of increased muscle protein catabolism on plasma levels of different amino acids which are altered in patients with liver cirrhosis.

Patients and Methods

Twenty-five patients with cirrhosis, aged 19-72 years (median 56), without ascites and without clinical signs of encephalopathy, and 15 healthy controls, are the subjects of the present report. They were put on a meat-free diet for 4 days. On the last 2 days fasting plasma amino acids[6] and the urinary excrection of 3-methylhistidine and creatinine[5] were measured. The myofibrillar protein catabolic rate (MPCR) was calculated as well.[4] Data in the text and in the Table are expressed as mean $\pm$ SEM of the mean value of individual subjects obtained during the 2 consecutive days.

(*)Paper selected for publication

Results and Discussion

In controls, MPCR, which estimates the percentage turnover per day of myofibrillar protein, was 0.81 ± SE 0.08 %/day. In 12 patients with cirrhosis MPCR was > 2SD above mean control rates, while in 13 it was normal. No clear-cut differences in liver function tests were present between the 2 groups.

Plasma amino acid values in the 2 groups of cirrhotics divided on the basis of their MPCR are reported in the Table. Both phenylalanine and tyrosine were significantly increased in subjects with high MPCR, compared to patients with normal MPCR and to controls. An overall correlation was present in cirrhotics between MPCR and fasting phenylalanine (r=0.647) or tyrosine levels (r=0.587).

These data confirm that muscle protein catabolism is increased in cirrhosis.[7] In these subjects "catabolic" stimuli are likely to release large amounts of amino acids from the lean body mass. They flood the failing liver, which is unable to metabolize large amounts of substrates.

Our data support a role of muscle protein catabolism in the increased levels of phenylalanine and tyrosine, which frequently occur in patients with cirrhosis.

Table 1. Plasma amino acids in control subjects and in cirrhotic patients with normal or increased MPCR (means ± SEM in nmol/ml)

	Controls	Cirrhotics with normal MPCR	Cirrhotics with high MPCR
Phenylalanine	69±8	69±5	89±8[b]
Tyrosine	74±8	90±6	119±9[a,b]
Valine	278±20	220±19[a]	196±18[a]
Isoleucine	80±6	55±4[a]	59±4[a]
Leucine	150±12	113±6[a]	98±6[a]
Total tryptophan	63±5	47±4[a]	45±4[a]
Free tryptophan	5.5±0.5	6.5±0.6	6.3±0.8
Methionine	25±9	30±2	36±5

[a] Significantly different from controls: p<0.05 or less.

[b] Significantly different from the corresponding value of cirrhotics with normal MPCR: p<0.05 or less.

REFERENCES
1. J. E.Fischer, J. M. Funovics, A. Aguirre, J. H. James, J. M.
    Keane, R. I. C. Wesdorp, N. Yoshimura, and T. Westman, The
    role of plasma amino acids in hepatic encephalopathy, Surgery,
    78: 276 (1975).
2. H. M. Rosen, N. Yoshimura, J. M. Hodgman, and J. E. Fischer,
    Plasma amino acid patterns in hepatic encephalopathy of
    differing etiology, Gastroenterology, 72: 483 (1977).
3. H. N. Munro, J. D. Fernstrom, and R. J. Wurtman, Insulin,
    plasma amino acid imbalance, and hepatic coma, Lancet, 1:
    722 (1975).
4. R. O. McKeran, D. Halliday, P. Purkiss, and P. Royston, 3-Me-
    thylhistidine excretion as an index of myofibrillar protein
    catabolism in neuromuscular disease, J. Neurol. Neurosurg.
    Phych. 42: 536 (1979).
5. M. Zoli, G. Marchesini, C. Dondi, G. P. Bianchi, and E. Pisi,
    Myofibrillar protein catabolic rates in cirrhotic patients
    with and without muscle wasting, Clin. Sci. 62: 683 (1982).
6. G. Marchesini, G. Forlani, M. Zoli, A. Angiolini, M. P. Scola-
    ri, F. B. Bianchi, and E. Pisi, Insulin and glucagon levels
    in liver cirrhosis: relationship with plasma amino acid
    imbalance of chronic hepatic encephalopathy, Dig. Dis. Sci.
    24: 594 (1979).
7. G. Marchesini, M. Zoli, A. Angiolini, C. Dondi, F. B. Bianchi,
    and E. Pisi, Muscle protein breakdown in liver cirrhosis
    and the role of altered carbohydrate metabolism, Hepatology
    1: 294 (1981).

PLASMA PROLACTIN IN LIVER CIRRHOSIS [*]

L. Demelia and A. Solinas

Istituto di Medicina Interna, Cattedra di Patologia
Speciale Medica II, Università di Cagliari
Cagliari, Italy

INTRODUCTION

Increased basal Prolactin (PRL) levels have been reported in patients with hepatic cirrhosis of mainly alcoholic etiology. These high levels have been correlated to conditions secondary to liver cirrhosis such as hypogonadism and feminization other than to a direct action of alcohol at pituitary level.

It has recently been suggested that PRL assay may be a useful marker of Portal Systemic Encephalopathy (PSE).[3] In fact, it is known that dopamine is a physiological PRL inhibiting factor. Fischer et al.[4] suggest that the presence of "weak or false" neurotransmitters and the reduction of dopamine or norepinephrine in the CNS are fundamental in the genesis of PSE. Therefore, the modified dopaminergic tone could explain the altered cerebral neuroendocrine control and, particularly, the PRL secretion.

The present study was carried out to investigate basal PRL levels and those after stimulation and inhibition tests in cirrhotic subjects.

MATERIALS AND METHODS

Patients

Three groups of patients were included in this study. Group C comprised 20 patients affected by liver cirrhosis, of these 14

---

[*]Paper selected for publication

were males and 6 females, aged between 32 and 68 years (mean age 49 years). The diagnosis was post-necrotic HBs Ag positive cirrhosis in 12 patients and alcoholic cirrhosis in 8. None of these subjects had evidence of PSE and no clinical or endoscopic signs of portal hypertension were seen. The group PSE included 14 cirrhotic patients, 11 males and 3 females, aged between 34 and 65 years (mean age 53 years). Seven of these patients had post-necrotic HBs Ag positive liver cirrhosis and 7 alcoholic cirrhosis. All the subjects in this group presented clinical and/or endoscopic symptoms of portal hypertension and of hepatic encephalopathy (stage 1-2 according to Trey et al.[5]). The group PSE-PCA included 6 patients, all were males, aged between 40 and 60 years (mean age 45 years), affected by liver cirrhosis with surgical porto-caval shunt. All the patients in this group had clinical signs of hepatic encephalopathy (stage 3-4).

Moreover, 16 healthy controls (N) were studied. Twelve were males and 4 females, aged between 32 and 65 years (mean age 42 years). All subjects had normal renal function and none was taking drugs which alter PRL secretion.

PRL Assay

Blood samples were drawn at 8.00 a.m. after 12 hours fasting and bed-rest. Plasma was immediately separated and frozen at -20°C till the time of assay. PRL (ng/ml) was assayed using a RIA method with double antibody technique (Diagnostic Products Corporation - Medical Systems, Italy). Intraassay variation was less than 5% and interassay variation was less than 6%.

TRH stimulation test

Six patients from group PSE, 3 males and 3 females, and 6 controls were studied. It is known that TRH is involved in the regulation of PRL secretion and is a potent PRL releasing factor. For the stimulation test, 400 µg TRH (Biodata, Serono, Italy) were given as an intravenous bolus. The test began at 8.30 a.m. after all-night fasting and bed-rest. A catheter was placed into an antecubital vein at least one hour before the test was started, and kept open by slow infusion of 0.9% NaCl. Blood was drawn at -30, 0, 15, 30, 45, 60, 90, 120 and 180 min.

Propranolol - L - Dopa test

Three days after having completed the TRH test, the same patients underwent the Propranolol - L-Dopa inhibition test. They received 40 mg orally Propranolol (Inderal, ICI-Pharma, Italy) at 6.30 a.m. At 8.30 a.m. they received orally 500 mg of L-Dopa (Larodopa, Roche, Italy). Blood was drawn 30 and 15 min before L-Dopa administration and 30, 60, 90, 120, 180 and 300 min after the beginning of the test.

STATISTICAL ANALYSIS

All values are expressed as mean $\pm$ S.E.M. The statistical significance of the results was evaluated using the Student's t test.

RESULTS

The cirrhotic subjects of group PSE-PCA showed markedly higher PRL levels (44.8 $\pm$ 5.2 ng/ml) than groups: PSE (18.1 $\pm$ 3.3; P<0.001); C (12 $\pm$ 0.9; P<0.001) and group N (10.7 $\pm$ 1.4; P<0.001). The PSE cirrhotic subjects also had increased PRL levels (P<0.05) when compared with cirrhotics without PSE and normal subjects (Fig. 1).

After Propranolol + L-Dopa administration, cirrhotic subjects showed normal PRL inhibition without significant difference from normal subjects (Fig. 2).

After TRH stimulation, one cirrhotic patient showed a normal response; three a low response with a mean peak (54 $\pm$ 3 ng/ml) which was significantly lower than normal (111 $\pm$ 5; P<0.001). Two cirrhotic patients showed a significantly higher TRH response (mean peak: 160 $\pm$ 20 ng/ml; P<0.001) than normal (Fig. 3).

DISCUSSION

The increased PRL levels in PSE subjects, particularly in those with surgical porto-caval shunt, confirm the relationship between altered PRL secretion and modified neuroendocrine control at CNS level. The altered aminoacid pattern in the CNS in cirrhotic PSE subjects induces reduced catecholamine concentration in the CNS with increased serotonin, GABA and presence of octopamine and phenylethanolamine.[6,7] It is known that decreased dopaminergic and an increased serotonin tone stimulates PRL secretion. Thus, an increase in PRL incretion may be expected in PSE. Our results are in agreement with the proposal of McClain et al.[3] that plasma PRL is correlated with the stage of PSE and can be considered a useful marker of such a condition. Moreover, it does not seem that increased PRL levels should always suggest the use of dopamine agonists, since even the cirrhotics with PSE and normal basal PRL levels showed a normal response to Propranolol + L-Dopa.

Also the hyperestrogenism in cirrhotic patients may influence the hyperprolactinemia. In fact, it is known that estrogens exert an antidopaminergic action at hypothalamic level, other than their direct effect on the adeno-hypophysis.[8]

The PRL pattern after L-Dopa inhibition test, could be secondary to increased cerebral dopamine levels. Indeed it is known that L-Dopa crosses the blood-brain barrier and is decarboxylated to dopamine in CNS. The dopamine action could be further enhanced by

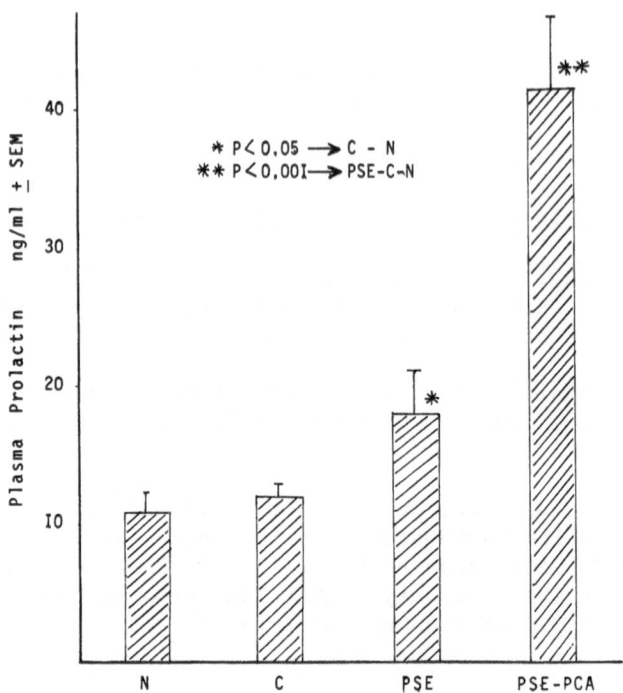

Fig. 1.   Fasting plasma prolactin levels in subjects studied: N =
          normal controls; C = cirrhotics without PSE; PSE = cirrho-
          tics with portal-systemic encephalopathy; PSE-PCA = cirrho-
          tics with PSE and surgical porto-caval anastomosis.

the previous administration of β-blockers, since the noradrenergic
pathway play a stimulatory role in PRL estrogen-induced release.

     The different PRL responses to TRH stimulation seen in our
patients are more difficult to explain. Some authors[9,10] have
reported significantly increased PRL levels after TRH stimulation
in cirrhotic patients, when compared to the normal range. These
authors hypothesized a serotonin and estrogen influence in this
response. Conversely, we observed a low PRL response to TRH in 3
out of 6 cirrhotic patients with PSE. A similar pattern was interpreted by Van Thiel et al.[11] as due to independent PRL secretion
by PRL-secreting microdenomas. However, it should be pointed out
that basal PRL levels were within the normal range in all six
patients.

     In conclusion, it seems that altered PRL secretion in patients
with liver cirrhosis and PSE is indicative of serious multifactorial
hypothalamo-hypophyseal damage. The main factor in producing this
damage seems to be the cerebral aminoacid imbalance present in
these patients.

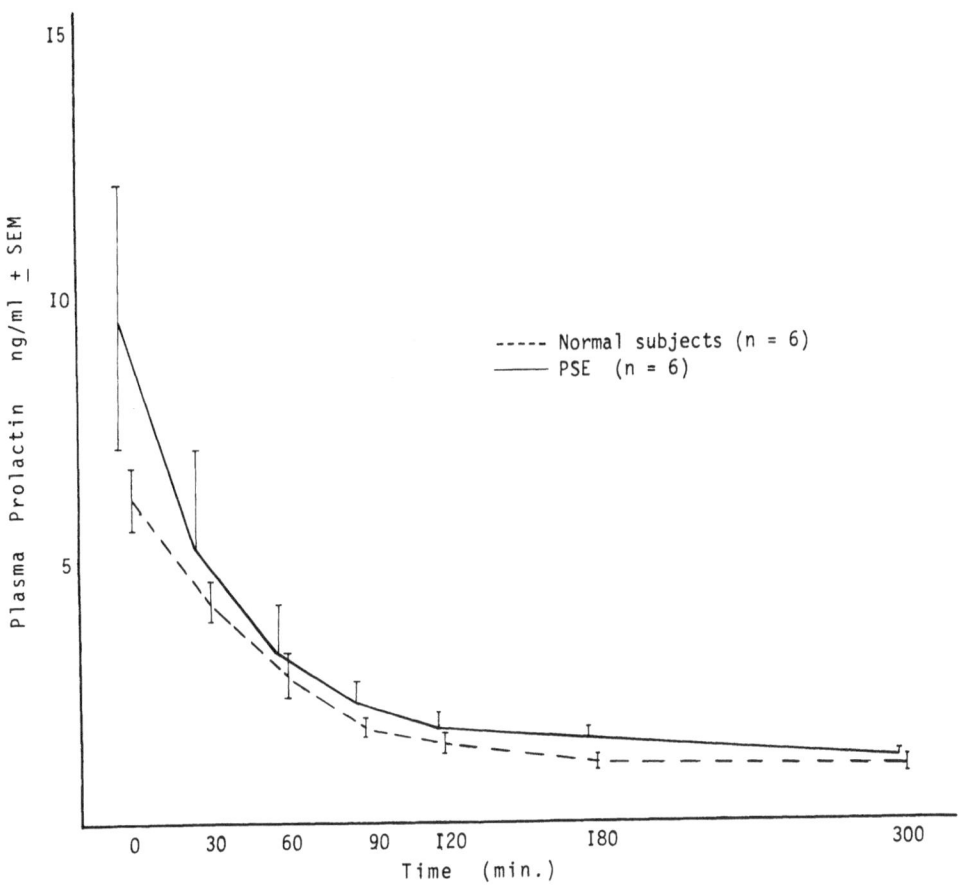

Fig. 2. Behavior of plasma prolactin levels in six normal controls
and six cirrhotic patients with PSE after propranolol +
L-Dopa suppression test.

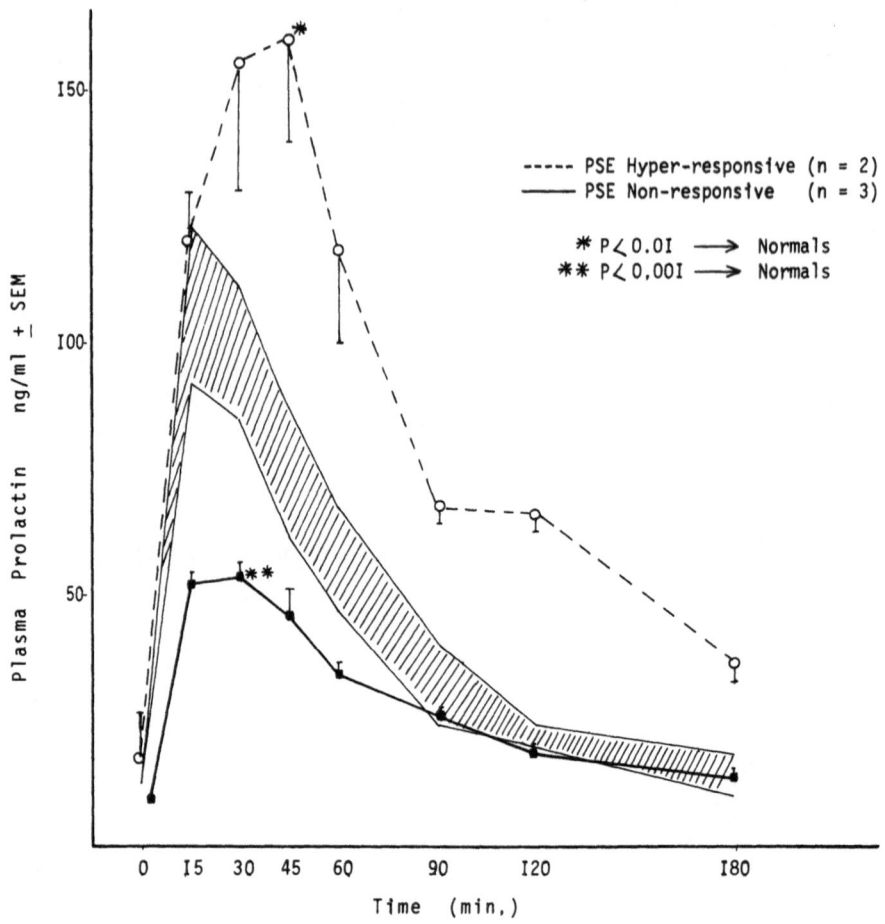

Fig. 3. Behavior of plasma prolactin levels in five cirrhotic patients after TRH stimulation test. Shaded area represents
the normal range.

ACKNOWLEDGEMENTS

    We wish to thank Ms. Maria Cristina Lai for excellent technical
assistance and Ms. Maria Rosa Crisponi for typing the manuscript and
performing the artwork.

REFERENCES

1. D. H. Van Thiel, J. S. Gavaler, R. Lester, D. Lynn Loriaux,and
    G. D. Braunstein, Plasma estrone, prolactin, neurophysin and
    sex steroid-binding globulin in chronic alcoholic men,
    Metabolism 24: 1015 (1975).

2. M. Bahnsen, C. Glyyd, S. G. Johnsen, P. Bennett, S. Svenstrup, S. Micic, O. Dietrichson, L. B. Svendsen,and U. A. Brodthagen, Pituitary-testicular function in patients with alcoholic cirrhosis of the liver, Eur. J. Clin. Invest. 11, 473 (1981).

3. C. G. McClain, J. P. Kromhout, M. K. Elson,and D. H. Van Thiel, Hyperprolactinemia in portal systemic encephalopathy, Dig. Dis. Sci. 26: 353 (1981).

4. J. E. Fischer and R. J. Baldessarini, False neurotransmitters in hepatic failure, Lancet 2: 75 (1971).

5. C. Trey, D. G. burns, and S. J. Saunders, Treatment of hepatic coma by exchange blood transfusions, New Eng. J. Med. 274: 473 (1966).

6. J. H. James, B. Jeppsson, V. Ziparo, and J. E. Fischer, Hyperammonaemia, plasma aminoacid imbalance, and blood-brain aminoacid transport: an unified theory of portal-systemic encephalopathy, Lancet 2: 772 (1979).

7. F. Rossi-Fanelli, H. Freund, R. Krause, A. R. Smith, J. H. James, S. Castorina-Ziparo, and J. E. Fischer, Induction of coma in normal dogs by the infusion of aromatic amino acids and its prevention by the addition of branched-chain amino acids, Gastroenterology 83: 664 (1982).

8. A. G. C. Bauer, W. J. De Greef, F. H. De Jong, J. H. P. Wilson, and S. W. J. Lamberts, Hyperprolactinemia of portal hypertension in rats, Gastroenterology 82: 179 (1982).

9. A. Zanoboni and W. Zanoboni-Muciaccia, Gynaecomastia in alcoholic cirrhosis, Lancet 1: 876 (1975).

10. A. E. Panerai, F. Salerno, M. Manneschi, D. Cocchi, and E. Müller, Growth hormone and prolactin responses to thyrotropin releasing hormone in patients with severe liver disease, J. Clin. Endocrinol. Metab. 45: 134 (1977).

11. D. H. Van Thiel, C. J. McClain, M. K. Elson, M. J. McMillan, and R. Lester, Evidence for autonomous secretion of prolactin in some alcoholic men with cirrhosis and gynecomastia, Metabolism 27: 1778 (1978).

SHORT-TERM BRANCHED CHAIN AMINO ACID PARENTERAL NUTRITION IN LIVER
CIRRHOSIS: A DOSE-RELATED EFFECT ON PLASMA AMINO ACIDS AND NITROGEN
BALANCE *

E. Rocchi, P. Gibertini, M. Cassanelli, A. Pietrangelo,
G. Casalgrandi and E. Ventura

Clinica Medica III, University of Modena, Modena, Italy

INTRODUCTION

Selective amino acid solutions and particularly branched chain
amino acids (BCAA) or their keto-analogues have been successfully
employed in treatment of hepatic encephalopathy,[1,2] despite their
pathophysiological role is still debated.[3] Previous studies have
documented their beneficial effects in ameliorating the neutral
amino acid (NAA) pattern;[1,4] but few data concerning the nitrogen
balance are available in chronic and severe liver disease, where
both hepatic and muscular utilisation of amino acids result impaired.[5]

This study is aimed to investigate the amino acid metabolism
and particularly the nitrogen balance over a five days period of
parenteral nutrition with different doses of BCAA as compared with
balanced amino acids (BCAA) in liver cirrhosis.

MATERIAL AND METHODS

Twenty nine adult inpatients with documented liver cirrhosis,
without encephalopathy, took part in this study after an informed
consent was obtained. They were maintained during a 3 day base
period on an oral standard diet (30 Kal.Kg^{-1}.day^{-1}), containing
carbohydrates and lipids, with parenteral supplementation of commercially available balanced amino acid solution (Isopuramin$^{(R)}$
Stholl, Modena, Italy) at doses of 0.5 g . Kg^{-1}. day^{-1} plus glucose
(50% of daily carbohydrate allowance). On the 4th day the patients
were divided in 3 groups (A, B and C), as presented in Table 1.

---

*Paper selected for publication.

Table 1. Patients and protocol.

Group	Treatment (5 days)	N.	Age,yrs ($\bar{X}\pm$SD)	Sex M	Sex F	Etiology of liver disease	
A	B C A A : 0.5 g.Kg^{-1}.day^{-1}	12	54 $\pm$ 10	9	3	alcoholic postnecrotic cryptogenic	7 4 1
B	B C A A : 1.0 g.Kg^{-1}.day^{-1}	7	48 $\pm$ 9	6	1	alcoholic postnecrotic cryptogenic	4 1 2
C	B A A : 0.5 g.Kg^{-1}.day^{-1}	10	49 $\pm$ 8	9	1	alcoholic postnecrotic cryptogenic	4 4 2

B C A A: branched chain amino acids; B A A: balanced amino acids.

They all received the same oral diet of the basal period and a parenteral supplementation of BCAA (leucine, isoleucine and valine BS 692 Boehringer Biochemia Robin, Milan Italy) as the only source of nitrogen (group A and B) or continued the same basal protocol (C).

Venous blood samples for plasma amino acid profiles were taken in the 14 h fasting patients on the 3rd basal day, 3rd and 5th day of the treatment. Daily nitrogen intake and urinary output (from urea, uric acid and creatinine) were calculated over the same days. Plasma amino acids were detected by an automatic Kontron AA Analyzer Liquimat III operating with programmed temperature, lithium citrate buffers and equipped with a Kontron Computing Integrator. Urea nitrogen, uric acid and creatinine in urine were determined by colorimetric-enzymatic combination kits (Boehringer Mannheim, West Germany).

Statistical comparisons (before vs after) were performed using Student's t test pair data analysis.

RESULTS AND DISCUSSION

The results are summarized in Figures 1, 2 and 3.

Figure 1 presents the plasma amino acid profiles in the treated groups at the end of the basal period and after 5 days of parenteral nutrition with the different protocols. The amino acid values are expressed as mean percent deviation from the mean normal values in our laboratory (sketched line of 100%).

In group C (protocols) treated with BAA only citrulline and arginine seem significantly reduced while essential and NAA result unaffected by such balanced solutions.

In group A treated with 0.5 g of BCAA we observed a significant increase of leucine and isoleucine ($p < 0.02$) and a decrease of threonine and lysine ($p < 0.02$) among the essential amino acids.

As regarding the nonessential ones a slight reduction of taurine, cystine, ornithine and histidine, and more marked of citrulline, arginine and alpha-aminobutyric acid were recorded. The BCAA significantly increase while the aromatic amino acids (AAA) decrease. In group B treated with 0.1 g of BCAA we observed almost the same variations among the NAA as previous one, with the exception of slight increase of several amino acids, AAA included.

Figure 2 shows the results of the different treatment on some amino acid ratios which are considered to be meaningful in the pathophysiology of hepatic encephalopathy (BCAA to AAA, total tryptophan (TRP) to NAA sum)[6,7] or of alcoholism, as alpha-aminobutyric acid (AANB) to leucine.[8,9] None of these parameters was significantly

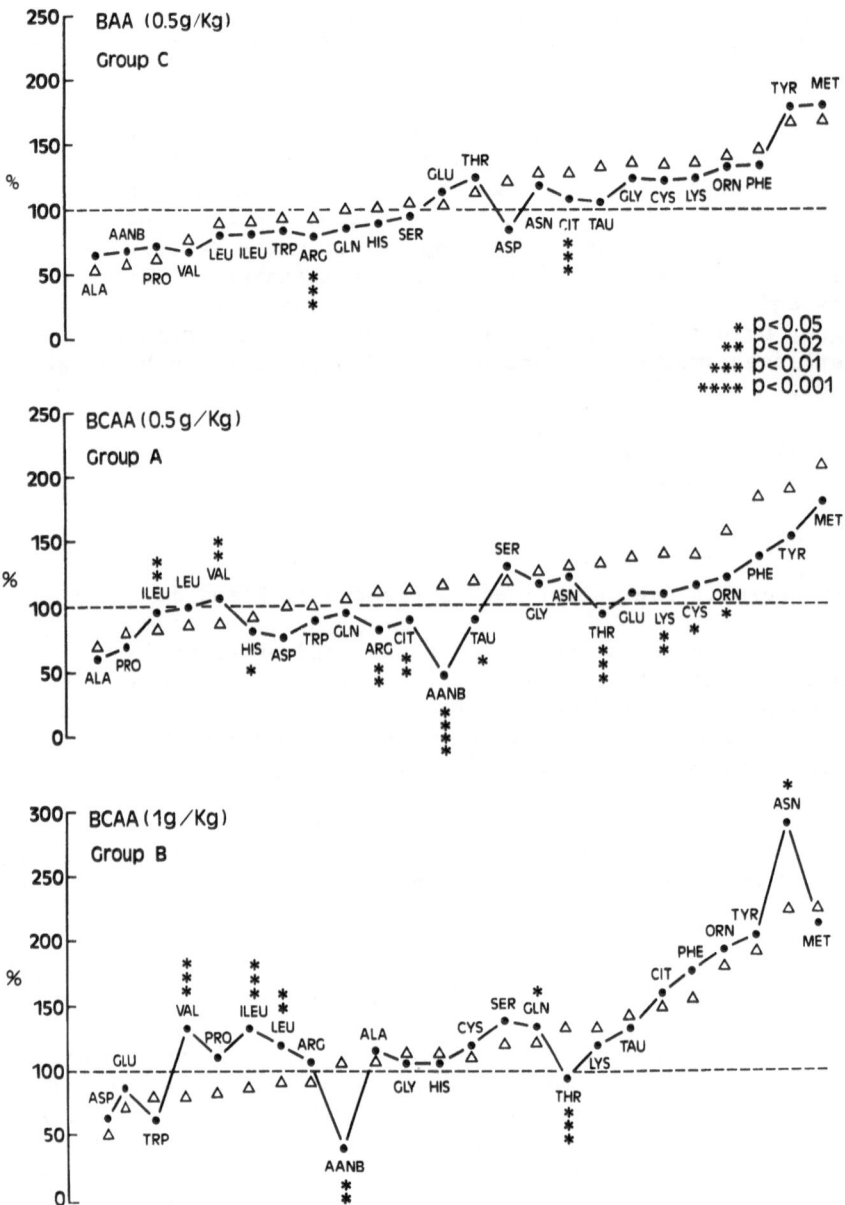

Fig. 1.   Mean plasma levels of amino acids with standard diet (●) and after 5 days (▼) of treatment with balanced (BAA) or branched chain amino acids (BCAA) at different doses in liver cirrhosis. Deviation from normal values (100%). Statistical comparison: t test pair data analysis.

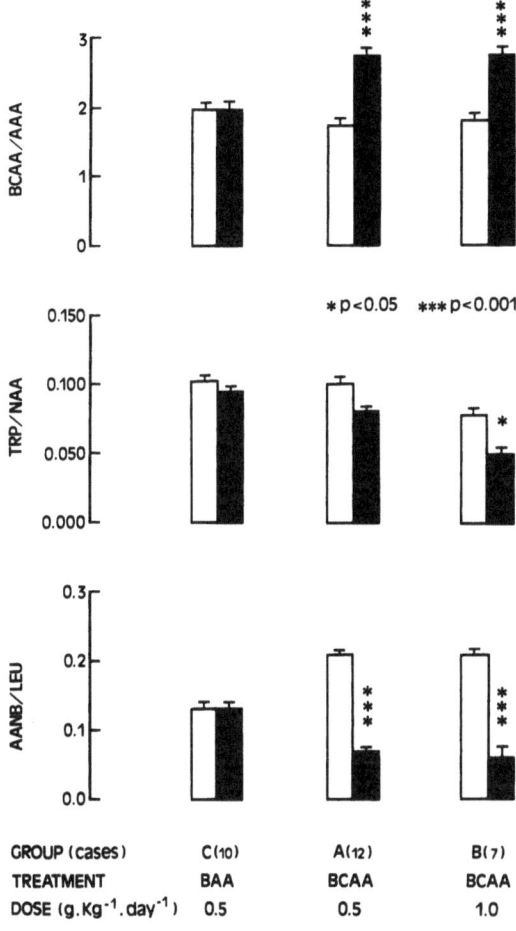

Fig. 2.   Plasma amino acid ratio ($\bar{X}$ + SEM) before ($\square$) and after
($\blacksquare$) 5 days of treatment with balanced (BAA) or branched
chain amino acids (BCAA) at different doses in liver
cirrhosis. Statistical comparison: t test pair data
analysis.

affected by the nutritional support with BAA (group C). On the
contrary the BCAA at 0.5 and 1.0 g . Kg^{-1} doses obtained a significant increase of the BCAA to AAA ratio, which is pathologically
reduced in the basal state.

A decrease of TRP/NAA after the BCAA treatments was obtained
as well, and this might suggest a depression of the central seroto-
ninergic pathways.[7] The AANB to leucine ratio results positively
reduced ($p < 0.001$ and $p < 0.01$) only in the BCAA treated groups A
and B.

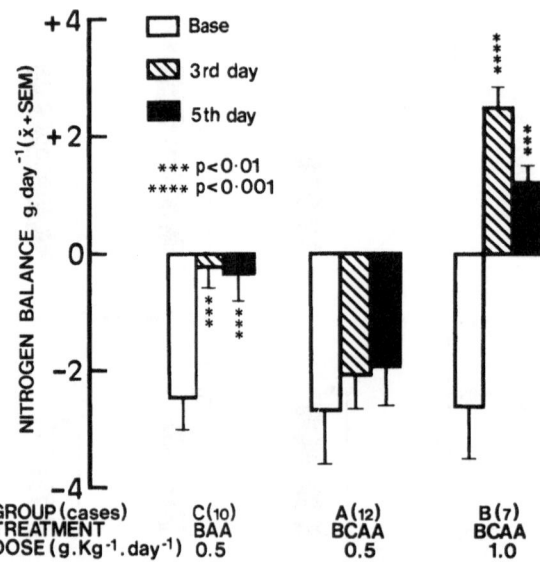

Fig. 3. Variations of the nitrogen balance before (base) and after
         3 and 5 days of treatment with balanced (BAA) or branched
         chain amino acids (BCAA) at different doses in liver cir-
         rhosis. Statistical comparison: t test pair data analysis.

        Figure 3 presents the nitrogen balance before, during and after
the treatments. Despite the lack of complications our cirrhotic
patients presented a negative nitrogen balance in the basal state.
This remains unchanged after 0.5 g of BCAA, slightly improves with
0.5 g of BAA and shows an impressive positivisation during and after
1.0 g.Kg^{-1} of BCAA.

        We have employed low doses of BAA because a presumed poor intol-
erance in cirrhotic patients. Notwithstanding this no negative
influence on their ratios was observed. Moreover 0.5 g.Kg^{-1} of BAA
seem to significantly improve the nutritional status in a resting
condition and for a few days. On the contrary 0.5 g of BCAA, usually
employed in the hepatic encephalopathy, even if a significant improvement of NAA plasma profiles is gained. Also the AANB to leucine
ratio, which is considered a specific empirical marker of alcoholism,
not dependent on nutritional influences,[8,9] results significantly
reduced by BCAA infusions and mainly in group A were a higher incidence of alcoholism was recorded.

        The present study confirms a poor correlation between amino
acid pattern and nutritional status as shown by Weber,[10] as in the
control group (C) amino acid profiles remain unchanged, while the

nitrogen balance improves. In group A the plasma amino acid improvement coexists with a persistently negative nitrogen balance. Doubled amounts of BCAA obtain the same results on plasma amino acids, but are followed by an impressive amelioration of the nitrogen balance. For this reason a dose of 1.0 g.Kg^{-1}.day^{-1} of BCAA seems highly recommended in the short term nutrition support of severe disease as well as in the hepatic encephalopathy treatment.

Acknowledgement

The authors are grateful to Prof. R. Bernardi (Boehringer Biochemia Robin, Milan, Italy) for generously providing the branched chain amino acid solutions and the laboratory analytical kits.

REFERENCES

1. J. E. Fischer, Amino acids in hepatic coma, Dig. Dis. Sci. 27: 97 (1982).
2. L. Capocaccia, V. Calcaterra, C. Cangiano, A. Cascino, F. Fiaccadori, S. Gentile, F. Ghinelli, G. Pelosi, O. Riggio, F. Rossi Fanelli, D. Sacchini, and G. Giunchi, Therapeutic effect of branched chain amino acids in hepatic encephalopathy: a preliminary study, in: "Medical and Surgical Problems of Portal Hypertension",Serono Symposium No. 34, M. J. Orloff, S. Stipa and V. Ziparo, eds., Academic Press, London and New York (1980).
3. L. Zieve, The mechanism of hepatic coma, Hepatology 1: 360 (1981).
4. H. Freund, N. Yoshimura,and J. E. Fischer, Chronic hepatic encephalopathy: long term therapy with a branched chain amino acid-enriched elemental diet, JAMA 242: 347 (1979).
5. E. Rocchi, P. Gibertini, F. Farina, M. Cassanelli, A. Pietrangelo, and C. Casalgrandi, Plasma glucose, insulin and neutral amino acids in response to prolonged glucose and selective amino acid infusion in liver cirrhosis, Med. Chir. Dig. in press.
6. J. E. Fischer and R. J. Baldessarini, Pathogenesis and therapy of hepatic coma, in: "Progress in Liver Disease," H. Popper and F. Shaffner, eds., Grune and Stratton, New York and London (1976).
7. A. Cascino, C. Cangiano, V. Calcaterra, F. Rossi Fanelli,and L. Capocaccia, Plasma amino acids imbalance in patients with liver disease, Am. J. Dig. Dis. 23: 591 (1978).
8. S. Shaw and C. S. Lieber, Plasma amino acid abnormalities in the alcoholic. Respective role of alcohol, nutrition and liver injury, Gastroenterology 74: 677 (1978).
9. S. Calandra, E. Ventura, M. L. Zeneroli,and E. Rocchi, Effects of alcohol on plasma amino acids, in: "Metabolic Effect of Alcohol,"P. Avogaro, C. R. Sirtori and E. Tremboli, eds., Elsevier Biochemical Press, North Holland (1980).

10.   F. L. Weber and J. B. Reiser, Relationship of plasma amino acids
      to nitrogen balance and portal-systemic encephalopathy in
      alcohol liver disease, Dig. Dis. Sci. 27: 103 (1982).

NUTRITIONAL EFFECTS OF BRANCHED-CHAIN KETOANALOGUES IN CHRONIC HEPATIC AND RENAL FAILURE: A PRELIMINARY REPORT [*]

F. Fiaccadori[*], L. Borghi[**], G. Elia[**], F. Ghinelli[*], A. Montanari[**], A. Novarini[**], G. Pedretti[*], G. Pelosi[*], D. Sacchini[*] and A. Borghetti[**]

[*]Cattedra di Malattie Infettive, Università di Parma and [**]Istituto di Semeiotica Medica, Università di Parma Parma, Italy

INTRODUCTION

Patients with chronic renal failure (CRF) and with liver cirrhosis (LC) show a severe impairment of nitrogen metabolism[1] which is characterized by a quantitative (i.e. catabolic state, negative nitrogen balance) and qualitative (i.e., modified amino acid profile) imbalance. Restriction of dietary proteins has frequently been used in the treatment of both diseases. It was recently reported that branched chain ketoanalogues (BCKA) might also provide a useful tool in the management of CRF[2] as well as LC.[3] The aim of the present investigation was to establish whether a restricted diet supplemented by oral BCKA might be more efficacious than a protein restricted diet alone in the treatment of patients presenting both CRF and LC with recurrent hepatic encephalopathy (HE). The effect of the two protocols were ascertained by the assessment of nitrogen balance and intracellular muscle composition.

MATERIALS AND METHODS

Five patients (sex, age and diagnosis are given in Table 1) with LC and CRF (both biopsy proven) and showing a negative nitrogen balance (NB) prior to the onset of the investigation, were studied for a 4-month period. For the first 2 months (period 1) patients were kept on a protein restricted diet (0.5 g/kgBW/day) without BCKA supplementation (Table 2); for the following 2 months (period 2)

(*) Paper selected for publication.

patients received the same diet supplemented by oral administration
of BCKA, in an amount equivalent to 20 g proteins. The ketoacid
analogues of valine (40%), leucine (30%) and isoleucine (30%) were
supplied by Boehringer-Biochemia Robin as Ca salts, under the trade
name of BS 704 (Table 2). Throughout the study, the neurologic status
of the patients was assessed daily by means of neuroclinical tests
(asterixis, Reitan test, star construction test) and EEG was recorded
weekly. Liver function tests (albuminemia, prothrombin activity, p-
cholinesterase, venous blood ammonia) and renal function tests (BUN,
GFR, serum and urine Na and K) were carried out before, during and
at the end of the investigation. Total potassium losses, evaluated
for 20 consecutive days in each period, were calculated by adding
the measured urinary amount to that lost with the faeces (considered
stable and equal to 5 mM/day). Nitrogen balance (NB), assessed by
the Kjeldahl method, was determined 10 times during period 1 and 10
times during period 2: the latter parameter was calculated as the
difference between the daily intake of nitrogen and the loss in urine
and faeces: skin, sweating and desquamation losses were not taken
into account. At the end of each period, a biopsy specimen of the
femoris quadriceps muscle was performed, as described by Bergstrom,[4]
in order to determine the tissue composition of water, electrolytes

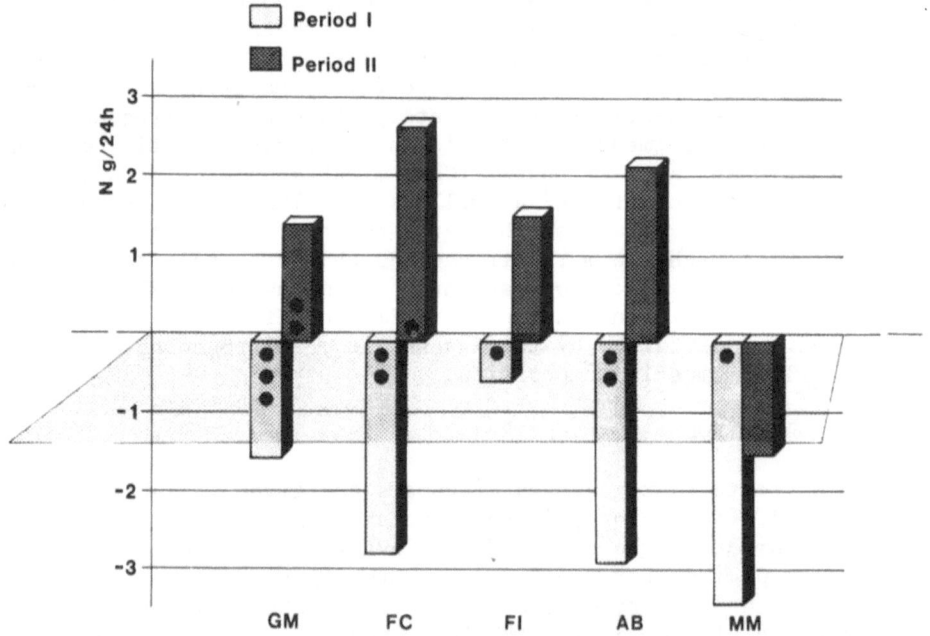

Fig. 1.   N balance in period 1 (two months without ketoacid supple-
          mentation) and in period 2 (two months with ketoacid sup-
          plementation). Mean of 10 determinations for each period.
          ● indicates HE episodes.

Table 1. Clinical details of the patients

Patient	Sex	Age	Diagnosis (liver and kidney biopsies)
G.M.	M	42	Post-necrotic LC (ascites, HE) Mesangioproliferative Glomerulonephritis
F.C.	M	55	Post-necrotic LC (ascites, HE) Mesangioproliferative Glomerulonephritis
F.I.	F	66	Alcoholic LC (HE) Mesangial Glomerulonephritis
A.B.	F	58	Alcoholic LC (HE) Mesangioproliferative Glomerulonephritis
M.M.	M	55	Alcoholic LC (HE) Chronic Pyelonephritis

LC: liver cirrhosis; HE: hepatic encephalopathy.

and nitrogen. The following parameters were evaluated in muscle: total, extra- and intracellular water (respectively, TW, ECW, ICW) expressed in g/kg FFDS (fre-fat-dry solid); sodium (Na_m), chloride (Cl_m), potassium (K_m), magnesium (Mg_m), phosphorus (P_m), expressed in mM/kg FFDS; alkali soluble protein nitrogen (ASPN), as g/kg/FFDS; intra- and extra-cellular K concentration K_i/K_e.[5-8]

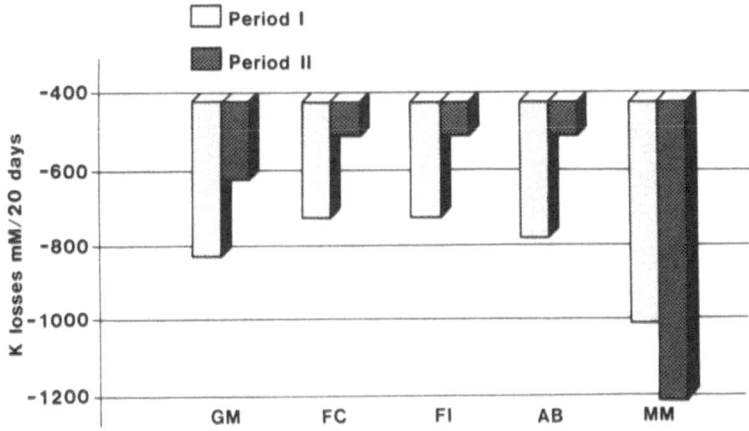

Fig. 2. Cumulative K losses (20 days) in period 1 (two months without ketoacid supplementation) and period 2 (two months with ketoacid supplementation).

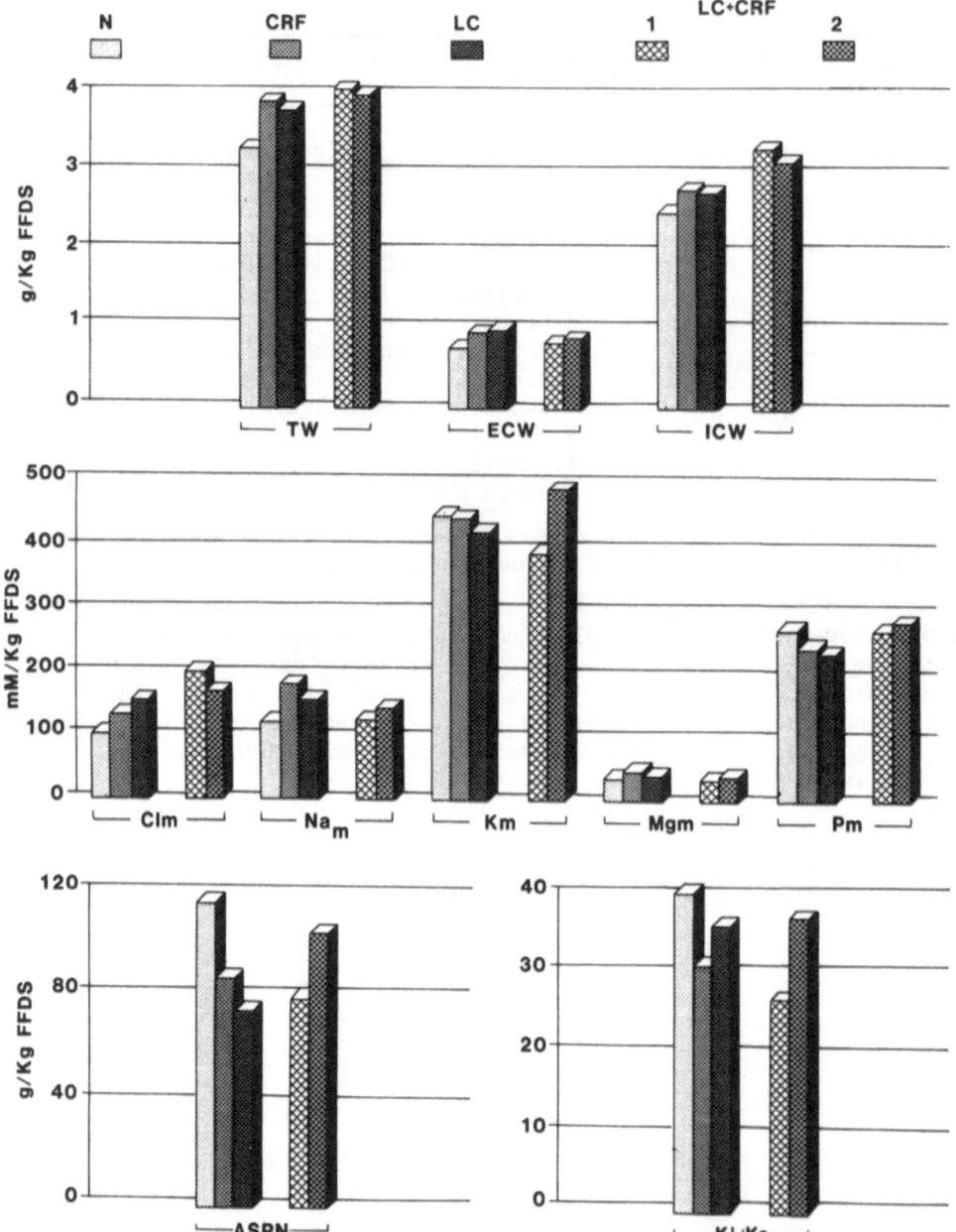

Fig. 3. Muscle composition (needle biopsy) in patients with CRF(24), LC(21)and LC + CRF (5, period 1 and 2). Changes induced by dietary supplementation with BCKA in 5 patients with associated LC and CRF.

Table 2. Diet schedules used in the treatment of 5 patients
          presenting liver cirrhosis with recurrent hepatic
          encephalopathy and chronic renal failure

___

Period 1 (2 months)

Diet schedule

Intake kg. B.W./day	Range
K calories 30-35	1800-2685
Proteins (g) 0.5	30-45
Sodium mM 1.0-1.5	60-112
Potassium mM 0.5-1.5	30-112
Phosphorus mM 0.3-0.6	18-45
Magnesium mM 0.1-0.2	6-15

Period 2 (2 months)

The same diet schedule as period 1 plus oral supplementation
with:

    BCKA   20 g protein equivalents:
    KIVA   40%
    KICA   30%
    KMVA   30%
    (BS   704 Boehringer-Biochemia-Robin)

___

RESULTS

     The hepatic and renal function indexes of the 5 patients showed
no significant change during the two study periods. Furthermore,
blood urea nitrogen levels remained unchanged in all patients following BCKA treatment. Of significance was the observation that none
of the patients gained weight.

     No modification in NB occurred by the end of period 1, whereas
a positive NB was achieved in 4 out of 5 patients during oral BCKA
supplementation. In one remaining patient, NB became less negative
(Fig. 1). As far as concerns the incidence of HE during the two
periods, 9 episodes of HE were recorded during period 1 and 3 during
period 2 (Fig. 2). Figure 2 shows K losses during the two periods:
in the second period the loss of K was less marked in 4 patients,
while a slight rise was observed in the one remaining.

     At the end of period 1, i.e. after protein restricted diet
alone, muscle cell composition was very similar to that observed in

earlier studies (Fig. 3) on 21 cases of LC and 24 cases of CRF (unpublished data); K_m, the K_i/K_e ratio and ASPN were lower than normal.
The most important changes observed at the end of period 2, i.e.,
after treatment with BCKA, concern the return to normal of K_m, ASPN
and the K_i/K_e ratio. ASPN findings analyzed by Student's t test
for paired data revealed statistically significant changes (Fig. 3).

CONCLUSIONS

The lower incidence of HE and the less severe loss of K during
BCKA treatment observed in the present investigation represent reliable indexes of clinical and metabolic improvements, while the
positive NB obtained in 4 out of 5 patients, together with unchanged
BUN levels, in the absence of weight gain may be considered evidence
of the efficacy of BCKA as an anabolic agent.

Analysis of the intracellular parameters determined at the end
of each treatment period strongly suggests that the intracellular
abnormalities observed may be partly corrected by a diet well balanced
in calories and proteins and supplemented with BCKA. In fact ASPN, K_m
and the K_i/K_e ratio which are closely related to the cellular metabolic and nutritional status, improved in 4 out of 5 patients treated
with BCKA supplementation.

In conclusion, the present data suggest that the favourable
effect of dietary supplementation with BCKA upon recurrent HE in
patients with associated chronic liver disease and organic renal
failure may be attributed to the restoration of the cellular protein
and K contents, which, in turn, probably correct the lack of intracellular metabolic energy.

REFERENCES

1. J. H. Close, The use of amino acid precursors in nitrogen ac-
    cumulation disease, N. Engl. J. Med. 290: 663 (1974).
2. M. Walser, Ketoacids in the treatment of uremia, Clin. Nephr.
    3: 180, (1975).
3. W. C. Maddrey, F. L. Weber, A. W. Coulter, C. M. Chura, N. P.
    Chapanis, and M. Walser, Effects of ketoanalogues of essen-
    tial aminoacids in portal-systemic encephalopathy, Gastro-
    enterology 71: 190 (1976).
4. J. Bergstrom, Muscle electrolytes in man, Scand. J. Clin. Lab.
    Invest. 14 Suppl. 68: 1 (1962).
5. E. Cotlove, Determination of the true chloride content of bio-
    logical fluids and tissues. II Analysis by simple, non
    isotopic methods, An. Chem. 35: 101 (1963).
6. M. W. Bradbury, C. R. Cleeman, H. Bagdoyan, and A. Berberian,
    The calcium and magnesium content of skeletal muscle, brain
    and cerebrospinal fluid as determined by atomic absorption
    plane photometry, J. Lab. Clin. Med. 71: 884 (1968).

7. P. S. Chen, T. Y. Toribara, and H. Warner, Microdetermination of
    phosphorus, An. Chem. 28: 1756 (1956).

8. O. H. Lowry, N. J. Rosebrough, L. Farr, and R. J. Randall, Protein
    measurement with the folin phenol reagent, J. Biol. Chem.
    193: 265 (1951).

SECTION 3

ASSESSMENT AND EVALUATION OF HEPATIC ENCEPHALOPATHY

SUMMARY OF THE CONTRIBUTIONS:

ASSESSMENT AND EVALUATION OF HEPATIC ENCEPHALOPATHY

By the Editors

An entire morning was devoted to the assessment and evaluation of hepatic encephalopathy. Chairmen of the Round Table were G. Giunchi, M. D. and L. Zieve, M.D. The panelists were F. Balsano, M. D., L. Capocaccia, M. D., P. Gentilini, M. D., L. Pagliaro, M. D., E. Pisi, M. D., and E. Ventura, M. D.

For the sake of clarity the Editors have decided to present a compendium of what was debated and substantially agreed upon by the participants in the Round Table as well as by the audience on the following points:

- TERMINOLOGY AND DEFINITION
- DIAGNOSIS AND EVALUATION
- LATENT OR COVERT ENCEPHALOPATHY
- CLINICAL PATTERNS.

TERMINOLOGY AND DEFINITION

Various terms have been coined in the past to define the neuro-psychiatric disorders associated with acute or chronic liver failure, each stressing different aspects of the syndrome. Portal-systemic encephalopathy (PSE), hepatic encephalopathy and hepatic coma are among the more common terms encountered. The term PSE emphasizes the importance of the diversion of portal blood from the liver and is derived from the evidence that after portacaval shunt cirrhotic patients usually become more prone to develop encephalopathy. However, mild to severe encephalopathy may occur in cirrhotic patients independently of the presence of large portal blood shunting, i.e., surgically constructed shunts. In reality, shunting may occur, but it is blood flowing through a liver which does not process blood

239

presented to it, because of hepatocyte failure. The blood flows past
the hepatocytes unprocessed. Encephalopathy is precipitated in most
cases of cirrhosis by events such as gastrointestinal bleeding, renal
failure, sepsis, drugs affecting CNS, etc. which do not usually
induce severe mental disorders in patients with normal hepatic function. However, the encephalopathy observed in fulminant hepatitis is
undoubtedly dependent upon acute liver failure. Thus, failing liver
represents the main factor and the "condition sine qua non" encephalopathy requires. Hepatic coma is undoubtedly a better term, but
while it may well be used to define most severe stages, it may not
be adopted for mild or moderate encephalopathy. "Hepatic encephalopathy", although it does not include all the pathogenetic mechanisms
of encephalopathy, is the term which better links the failing liver
to the neurological disorders and should therefore be more widely
adopted. Physicians studying these patients would then be using a
common language.

In conclusion, hepatic encephalopathy (HE) can be defined as
a disorder of mentation, neuromuscular function, and consciousness
occurring in patients with either acute or chronic liver disease.

DIAGNOSIS AND EVALUATION

The diagnosis of HE is usually based on clinical, instrumental
and laboratory criteria, but because of their poor specificity and
sensitivity no one of these criteria alone is sufficient in the
large majority of cases to enable a correct diagnosis to be made.
Another problem encountered in the diagnosis of HE is patient's
cooperation and severity of the neurological disorders. In fact,
the diagnostic approach to a patient with mild HE may be quite
different from that in a patient with severe HE.

Clinical Criteria

The clinical history is of primary importance. A long history
of liver disease will usually indicate that encephalopathy is of
"hepatic" origin. The only exception to this rule is the severe
encephalopathy complicating fulminant hepatic failure, the clinical
picture of which, however, is rather specific, and a careful epi-
demiological inquiry will invariably reveal the etiologic factor
(viral, toxic, etc.). It is also important to inquire about events
known to favor or precipitate HE (G.I. bleeding, sepsis, overdiuresis, protein load, etc.).

Physical examination of the patient will also provide useful
information in the diagnosis of HE. The presence of jaundice, hepa-
tosplenomegaly, ascites, spiders nevi, erythema palmare, gynecomastia and lean body mass wasting may reveal the underlying liver
disease. A careful neuropsychiatric examination should always be
carried out in order to evaluate the patient's sense of space and

time, behaviour, sleep rhythm, tendon reflexes and fluency of speech.
The presence of flapping tremor and other extra-pyramidal signs should
also be sought. Finally, if the patient is unconscious, his responsiveness to acoustic and/or painful stimuli should be checked. This
neurological assessment should allow the physician to establish the
grade of HE at the patient's bedside. Common criteria to grade HE
are mandatory if patients studied by different investigators, or
efficacy of new treatments, are to be assessed. The terminology for
the grading of HE agreed upon by the participants at the Round Table,
as well as by the audience, is given in Table 1.

Instrumental and Laboratory Criteria

The following section deals with the specificity and sensitivity of the instrumental and laboratory parameters currently used in
the assessment of HE.

As far as concerns instrumental tools, EE-graphy is probably
the most widely-used. While the EE-gram is constantly altered in HE,
a progressively slower rhythm being observed from grade 1 to grade 4,
the only specific pattern is that characterized by the presence of
triphasic waves. Unfortunately, however, triphasic waves are not
always present on the EEG recorded in patients with HE. Thus, conventional EEG lacks specificity and sensitivity, and its contribution
to the diagnosis and grading of HE is of little use.

The use of power spectra may help to improve the evaluation of
the EEG. Power spectra which depend upon the duration and amplitude
of EEG waves provide an extremely sensitive method of enabling even
slight abnormalities in EEG to be detected. The EEG power spectra
are still under investigation, and their usefulness in the diagnosis
and grading of HE remains to be proven.

Psychometric testing may also prove useful in the assessment of
HE. A series of different tests may be used, including verbal abilities, visual memories, memory, intellectual concentration and
attention, motive performance and reaction time. Psychometric tests,
while not showing modifications specific for HE, have been found to
be extremely sensitive, particularly in revealing minimal changes
characteristic of latent HE (see next chapter). Visual and/or audi-
tive-evoked potentials have recently been proposed to reveal and
quantify the neurological changes in HE. The evoked potentials (the
electrical manifestations of the brain response to a photic or
acoustic stimulus) were first employed to detect demyelinizating
diseases of the visual and/or acoustic system(s), and more recently
to study Parkinson's disease and the effects of psychotropic drugs
upon brain inasmuch as they also reflect neurotransmitter-mediated
neuron activity. A good correlation between the alteration of evoked
potentials and degree of HE has been reported. If these data are
confirmed, evoked potentials may well provide a useful tool in the
diagnosis.

Changes in blood ammonia, plasma amino acids, free tryptophan and CSF amino acids and glutamine represent the most useful and characteristic biochemical markers in HE.

The role played by each of these tests in formulating the diagnosis of HE depends on its specificity and sensitivity, but it is also clearly related to the technical aspects of the analytical procedures. Blood ammonia, for instance, which is easily measured, cannot be considered the test of choice because of its poor correlation with HE. Plasma amino acids are altered in most patients with HE, but a one-to-one correlation with HE is not present. Plasma-free tryptophan is always increased in HE and shows a good correlation with the degree of mental impairment. However, the procedure to measure free tryptophan is rather time-consuming and, furthermore, the instrument required (fluorimeter) may not always be available. CSF glutamine, undoubtedly the most sensitive and specific test, is constantly increased in HE, showing an extremely good correlation with the degree of encephalopathy. Glutamine may easily be determined with the same procedure as that used for ammonia after enzymatic or chemical deamination. The use of this test in the follow-up of patients is, however, limited since it is unethical to repeatedly collect samples. CSF amino acids are promising, but sufficient data do not exist as yet. The same can be said for CSF homovanillic acid and 5-hydroxy indoleacetic acid.

Despite the poor specificity of the various diagnostic criteria examined, possibly with the exception of CSF glutamine, diagnosis of HE can be made. In fact, correct evaluation of all clinical, instrumental and laboratory data allows the physicians to make correct diagnosis of HE and precise grading of the mental state of the patient.

LATENT OR COVERT ENCEPHALOPATHY

The problem of latent or sub-clinical HE has emerged due to the observation that EEG, visual or acoustic-evoked potentials, recordings and psychometric test performance do not fall within normal limits in a large number (up to 60%) of cirrhotic patients without clinical evidence of encephalopathy.

EEG is usually normal in patients in grade O HE. Using EEG power spectra, however, about 30% of patients with latent HE show a slight increase in delta-waves. Similar results are obtained using acoustic or visual-evoked potentials. Psychometric testing has been shown to be the most sensitive means for detecting latent encephalopathy. Using only one simple test (Reitan, part A, number connection test), scores in 33% of cirrhotics in grade O HE are well above the normal range. If multiple psychometric tests, including the evaluation of intellectual and amnestic function, attention, psychomotor function and personality are carried out simultaneously and appropriately evaluated, taking into consideration their interdependence, the percentage of patients without signs of HE, but with tests not comprised within normal limits, increases to 60%. This high rate of abnormalities demonstrates that latent HE is not merely a problem of patient classification but rather is of considerable importance. A number of these patients are still actively involved in a profession requiring a perfect neuropsychiatric equilibrium. Thus, the real clinical impact of these tests is far from being proven.

CLINICAL PATTERNS

The last topic discussed in the Round Table was the different clinical pattern of HE. To recognize that HE may present with varying clinical patterns and to precisely define them is not only a problem of semantics.

Well-defined groups of patients are extremely important when comparing studies carried out by different investigators in different countries. Too often, indeed, strikingly different results of therapeutic trials are the result of gross differences in patient classification.

The wide range of clinical patterns with which HE may present may be identified according to pathogenetic or chronological criteria.

Although our knowledge of the pathogenesis of HE has improved considerably over the last ten years, much remains to be elucidated. Thus, pathogenetic criteria should not be used to identify the clinical patterns of HE. A chronological criterion would appear to be more suitable in this respect. According to this criterion, HE may be classified as acute or chronic. Acute HE may ensue in a patient with acute (viral or toxic), massive liver necrosis (Acute Encephalopathy) or in a cirrhotic patient with long-standing liver disease (Acute Episodic Encephalopathy). In these latter cases the acute episode may be precipitated by a known event (G.I. bleeding, sepsis, renal failure, etc.), and is usually reversed by specific treatment after which dietetic restriction or prophylactic treatment may not be necessary.

In a patient with chronic liver disease (failure), the course of HE may also be chronic. It may be characterized either by frequent recurrences or prolonged persistence of clinical symptoms. A protein-restricted diet and suitable treatment may still be sufficient to regulate these symptoms during intervening periods (Chronic Recurrent Encephalopathy). When HE becomes permanent and unresponsive to treatment, frequent neurological abnormalities resembling those seen in Wilson's disease or myelopathy may develop (Chronic Permanent Encephalopathy). This latter pattern may slowly develop as such or follow Chronic Recurrent Encephalopathy.

In conclusion, four main clinical patterns of HE have been identified and characterized:

1. Acute Encephalopathy

A single episode with acute onset and a short, intense course, occurring typically in acute fulminant viral or toxic hepatitis.

2. Acute Episodic Encephalopathy

One or more episodes occurring in patients with chronic liver disease and precipitated by specific factors. Intervening periods without overt manifestations and not requiring particular diet or treatment.

3. Chronic Recurrent Encephalopathy

Frequent recurrences or prolonged persistence of manifestations. During the intervening periods, symptoms may be controlled with diet and therapy.

4. Chronic Permanent Encephalopathy

May or may not follow the above variant. Symptoms are permanent and unresponsive to treatment. Neurological abnormalities resembling those observed in Wilson's disease and/or myelopathy are often present.

VISUAL EVOKED POTENTIALS IN THE QUANTITATIVE ASSESSMENT

OF PORTAL-SYSTEMIC ENCEPHALOPATHY AND ITS PRECLINICAL STAGE

M.L. Zeneroli, G. Pinelli, C. Gollini, P. Ricci, A. Penne,
E. Messori* and E. Ventura

Istituti di Clinica Medica III e di Clinica Oculistica*
Università di Modena, 41100 Modena, Italy

INTRODUCTION

The monitoring of the cerebral dysfunctions of patients with
hepatic encephalopathy (HE) due to liver cirrhosis or to fulminant
hepatic failure is still empirical and imprecise.

We believe that an intensive care liver unit for treatment of
these patients would require an objective method of evaluation, which
should (1) not induce tolerance, (2) not be time-consuming in performance, (3) be easily understood and applied by every component of
the staff and finally (4) be sensitive enough to evidentiate and to
grade both the latent stage of encephalopathy and the clinically manifested coma.

Of the wide variety of tests so far proposed (for review[1]),
EEG fails in points 2, 3 and 4; psychometric tests fail in points
1, 2 and 3. Portal systemic index generates an integrated number
derived from the summation of a quantitative measurement of ammonia
plus a semiquantitative evaluation of EEG mixed up with numbers
coming from subjective evaluation of mental status, of asterix and
from trail-making tests which fail in points 1 to 4 and which are
influenced by age and education of patient. The most appropriate
and objective test so far proposed is the reaction time test[2] which
is valuable in assessing mental state in the early stages of HE, but
not suitable for evaluating the later stages.

Herein we report our preliminary study carried out in order to
determine whether visual evoked potential (VEP) recordings could be
a valuable technique in the assessment of the mental state of HE in
liver cirrhosis.

245

NEUROPHYSIOLOGICAL AND EXPERIMENTAL BASES OF THE VEP TECHNIQUE

A visual evoked potential is an electrical manifestation of the brain's response to a photic stimulus. Through the visual area, the stimulus elicits post-synaptic potential changes of subcortex and cortex neurons which can be recorded from the scalp. By recording the EEG during sequential photic stimulation with the technique of computer signal averaging, average VEP waveforms can be detracted from the background random brain-wave activity and artifacts.

VEPs, first utilized in detecting abnormalities of visual system and in demyelinizating diseases of visual system such as multiple sclerosis, are now proposed in the evaluation of Parkinson's disease and in studying the brain effect of psychotropic drugs (for review[3,4].) This because depolarization and hyperpolarization of neurons expressed in the VEP pattern reflect neurotransmitter changes at the neuronal levels.[5]

In our hands, VEPs have proved a reliable method in the evaluation of HE in rats with galactosamine-induced fulminant hepatic failure,[6] as they have for rabbit by another author.[7] Changes in VEP pattern during HE have proved different from other kinds of coma[8] and from unconscious states induced by drugs.[7] Moreover VEPs have generated useful information in the identification of factors leading to HE.[9]

On the basis of this experience it seemed likely that the VEP method can satisfy points 1, 2 and 3 and possibly 4.

PERSONAL EXPERIENCE IN HE DUE TO LIVER CIRRHOSIS

It is well known that VEP patterns are critically dependent on many recording parameters that must be kept constant during experiments. For this reason normal results from one laboratory are not fully applicable to another when apparatus and recording conditions are different.[3]

After preliminary experiments we chose the following working conditions. VEPs were recorded in a dark, electrically shielded Faraday room by the use of two electrodes applied to the scalp with collodium: active electrode in Oz, reference electrode in Fz. Energy of lamp was 1 J, stimulation frequency 1 Hz. Pupils were fully dilated with phenylephrine and tropicamide and VEPs were recorded with patients having closed eyes. 64 responses to the signal were averaged by an Ortec Averager.

VEPs recorded in ten normal subjects of both sexes with ages ranging between 32 and 45 years showed a pattern constantly characterized by the appearance of negative and positive waves labelled N_1, P_1, N_2, P_2 and N_3 as shown in Figure 1. Values of amplitudes

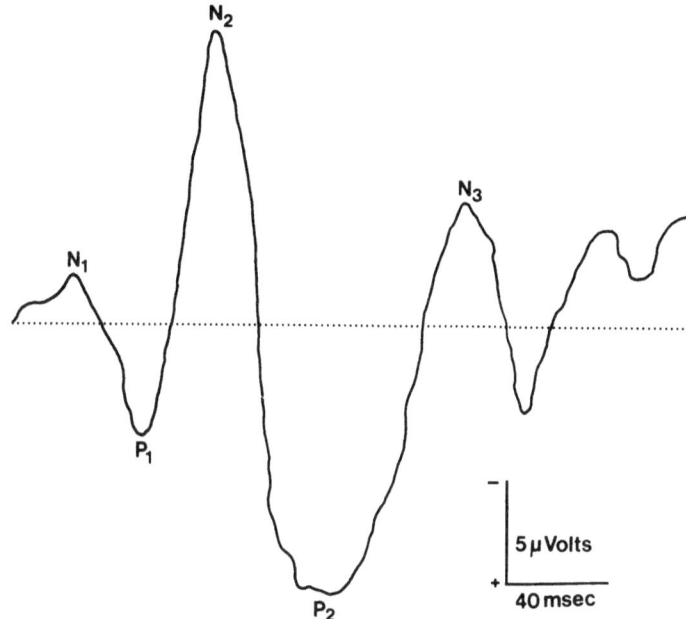

Fig. 1.   Typical VEP pattern recorded in normal subject.

and of latencies are reported in Table 1. Several repetitions of the VEP recording in these subjects on different days showed that pattern and latencies were constant while a slight variation of amplitudes can occur.

After that, 44 liver cirrhosis patients of mixed etiology and sex (age within 36-50 years) were examined. These patients were classified according to EEG[10] into 16 having encephalopathy degree 0 (HE_0), 8 degree 1 (HE_1), 6 degree 2 (HE_2), 6 degree 3 (HE_3) and 8 degree 4 (HE_4). Mean values of amplitudes and of latencies are reported in Table 1.

HE_1 differed from normal subjects by a progressive delay of latencies reaching statistical difference at the last wave N_3 ($P < 0.001$ vs control value). HE_2 showed the disappearance of N_1 wave. HE_3 had a pattern similar to HE_2 but with a further delay of N_3 wave ($P < 0.01$ vs HE_2). HE_4 showed a further simplification of VEP pattern with the disappearance of N_1 and P_1 waves.

VEPs recorded in the 16 patients without EEG evidences of HE showed two different patterns: one (HE_{0-I}) similar to those of controls, the other (HE_{0-II}) with a delayed N_3 latency ($P < 0.01$ vs controls) similar to that of HE_1 group. Attempting to identify the reasons for this discrepancy, we considered the biohumoral pattern of these patients. For biohumoral studies blood samples were

Table 1. Mean ± 1 SD of VEP parameters in all studied subjects

	N° cases	Amplitudes (μVolts)					Latencies (msec)				
		N_1	P_1	N_2	P_2	N_3	N_1	P_1	N_2	P_2	N_3
Controls	10	3.7+1.6	5.1+3.0	9.6+2.6	24.4+4.1	12.1+4.2	37+2	51+9	78+12	125+13	180+9
HE_{0-I}	6	4.2+1.5	5.7+1.7	7.2+1.6	22.3+8.2	10.5+5.2	28+9	64+10	81+10	134+25	173+8
HE_{0-II}	10	3.9+1.7	4.0+1.6	10.1+5.3	13.2+7.1	16.7+9.9	44+5	69+13	105+19	149+27	234+19•
HE_1	8	5.1+1.3	5.0+2.9	6.8+3.2	20.5+7.0	13.0+5.9	40+2	64+10	98+16	146+14	264+35••
HE_2	6	---	8.3+2.1	21.3+9.2	33.4+5.2	8.2+4.1	---	46+9	90+21	163+21	251+27
HE_3	6	---	10.0+7.5	29.0+11.5	39.3+18	16.3+8.4	---	45+15	108+16	195+28	383+53•••
HE_4	8	---	---	20.1+7.0	22.2+7.0	15.1+6.0	---	---	77+28	187+39	370+47

Student's t-test: •$p < 0.01$, ••$p < 0.001$ vs controls, •••$p < 0.01$ vs HE_2

collected simultaneously with EEG and VEP recordings. Amino acids in
the plasma were assayed with amino acid Analyzer Kontron, free tryptophan was separated by dialysis[11] and evaluated with chromatogra-
phic-fluorimetric method,[12] venous ammonia was assayed with Biochemia
Kit and octopamine with radioenzymatic method.[13] We could observe
(Figure 2) that group HE_{0-I} differed from controls only by a reduction
of the molar ratio of branched to aromatic amino acids. In agreement
with other reports[14,15] this phenomenon is compatible with the
cirrhotic status of the patients and independent of encephalopathy.

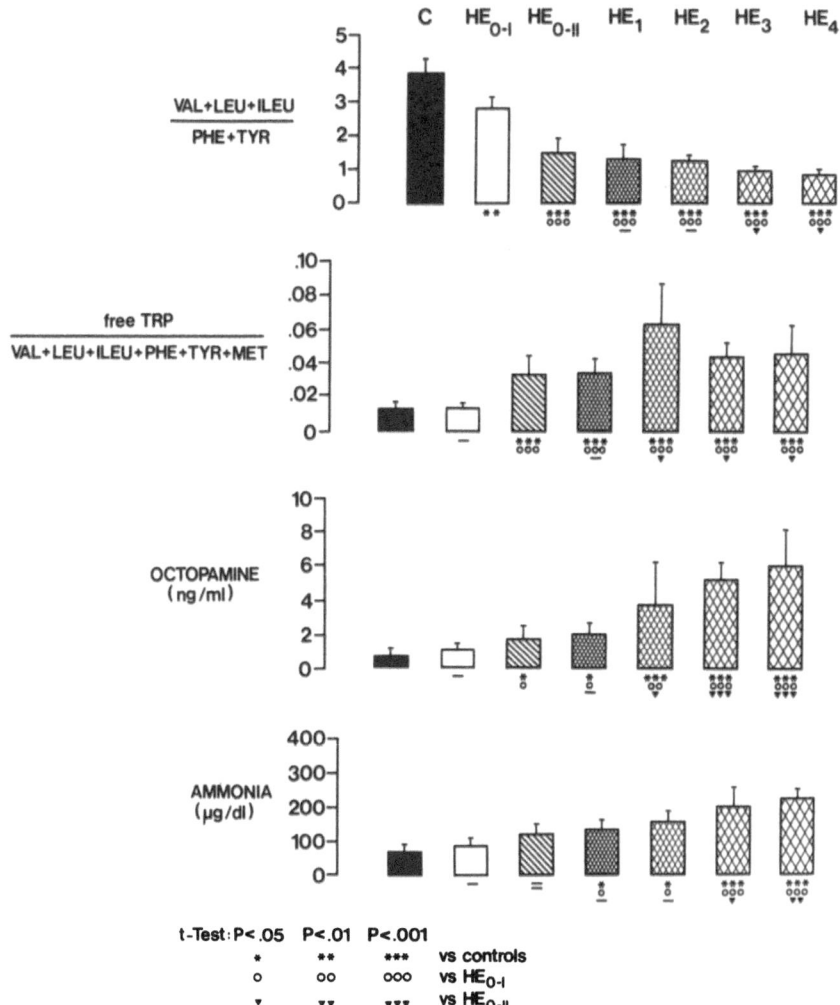

Fig. 2.   Biohumoral parameters recorded in all studied subjects and
          Student's t test of the most meaningful comparison. Values
          are reported as mean ± 1 SD. C means control subjects, va-
          line (Val), leucine (Leu), isoleucine (Ileu), phenylalanine
          (Phe), tyrosine (Tyr), tryptophan (Trp), methionine (Met).

Instead group HE_{0-II} revealed significant changes of the ratio of
free tryptophan to the sum of neutral amino acids, of ammonia and
of octopamine. While these observed parameters were significantly
different from controls and from values of HE_{0-I}, no differences
were detected when compared to HE_1 values. On the basis of these
similarities and on the appearance of manifested encephalopathy in
two of these patients after a short time we could consider HE_{0-II} as
patients in a preclinical stage of HE at the time of the study.
Incidentally, from these data we could infer, according with others,
[16] that the preclinical stage of HE is a frequent feature in liver
cirrhosis patients.

CONCLUSIONS

   This preliminary observation seems to indicate that VEP recording could satisfy the above-mentioned 4 points: 1) does not induce
tolerance, 2) performance and evaluation require only a few minutes,
3) evaluation is based on measurement of latency of N_3 and on the
pattern of waves so that every component of the staff can grade HE
in an objective way, 4) VEP seems sensitive enough in grading the
four degrees of coma and in evidentiating the preclinical stage of
coma using a unified criterion of evaluation.

REFERENCES

1. H. O. Conn and M. M. Lieberthal, Assessment of mental status,
    in: "The Hepatic Coma Syndromes and Lactulose," H. O. Conn
    and M. M. Lieberthal eds., Williams and Wilkins, Baltimore
    (1979).
2. P. Eggles, S. E. Christensen, L. Ranek, A. Theilgaard, and N.
    Tygstrup, Continuous reaction time in patients with hepatic
    encephalopathy. A quantitative measure of changes in con-
    sciousness, Scand. J. Gastroent. 16: 441 (1981).
3. K. H. Chiappa and A. H. Ropper, Evoked potentials in clinical
    medicine, (first of two parts), New Engl. J. Med. 306: 1140
    (1982).
4. C. Shagass and J. J. Straumanis, Drugs and human sensory
    evoked potentials, in: "Psycopharmacology. A Generation of
    progress," M. A. Lipton and K. F. Killam eds., Raven Press,
    New York (1978).
5. I. Bodis-Wollner and M. Onofry, System disease and visual
    evoked potential diagnosis in neurology: changes due to
    synaptic malfunction, Ann. N. Y. Acad. Sci. 388: 327 (1981).
6. M. L. Zeneroli, A. Penne, G. Parrinello, C. Cremonini, and E.
    Ventura, Comparative evaluation of visual evoked potentials
    in experimental hepatic encephalopathy and in pharmacologi-
    cally induced coma-like states in rat, Life Sci. 28: 1507
    (1981).
7. D. F. Schafer, L. E. Brody, and E. A. Jones, Visual evoked
    potentials: an objective measurement of hepatic encephalo-

pathy in the rabbit, Gastroenterology 77: 38A (1979).

8. M. L. Zeneroli, C. Cremonini, C. Gollini, G. Pinelli, A. Penne, E. Messori, and M. Baraldi, Effects of hyperammonemia and of hypoglycemia on visual evoked potentials in rat: comparison with hepatic encephalopathy, Riv. Fermacol. Terap. 13: 35 (1982).

9. M. L. Zeneroli, E. Ventura, M. Baraldi, A. Penne, E. Messori, and L. Zieve, Ammonia, mercaptans and short chain fatty acids as pathogenetic agents of hepatic encephalopathy: evaluation by visual evoked potentials, Hepatology 2: 532 (1982).

10. F. Rohmer and D. Kurtz, EEG et ammoniémie dans les troubles nerveux des affections hépatiques, in: Proceedings of the VII International Congress of Neurology, Rome (1961).

11. E. Stefanini and G. Biggio, A simple method for determination of free tryptophan in serum, Riv. Farmacol. Terap. 6: 49 (1975).

12. E. Costa, P. F. Spano, A. Groppetti, S. Algeri, and N. H. Neff, Simultaneous determination of tryptophan, tyrosine, catecholamines and serotonin specific activity in rat brain, Atti Accad. Med. Lomb. 23: 1100 (1968).

13. J. M. Saavedra, Enzymatic-isotopic method for octopamine at the picogram level, Anal. Biochem. 59: 628 (1974).

14. A. Cascino, C. Cangiano, V. Calcaterra, F. Rossi-Fanelli, and L. Capocaccia, Plasma amino acids imbalance in patients with liver disease, Am. J. Dig. Dis. 23: 591 (1978).

15. M. Morgan, J. P. Milson, and S. Sherlock, Plasma ratio of valine, leucine and isoleucine to phenylalanine and tyrosine in liver disease, Gut 10: 1068 (1978).

16. G. Marchesini, M. Zoli, C. Dondi, L. Cecchini, A. Angiolini, F. B. Bianchi, and E. Pisi, Prevalence of subclinical hepatic encephalopathy in cirrhotics and relationship to plasma amino acid imbalance, Dig. Dis. Sci. 25: 763 (1980).

SECTION 4

THERAPEUTIC ASPECTS OF HEPATIC ENCEPHALOPATHY

BROMOCRIPTINE IN THE TREATMENT OF CHRONIC HEPATIC ENCEPHALOPATHY

M. Y. Morgan

Department of Medicine, Royal Free Hospital School of
Medicine, Hampstead, London, NWE 2PF, Great Britain

Chronic hepatic encephalopathy (chronic porto-systemic encephalopathy) is a neuropsychiatric syndrome which occurs as a well-
recognised though rare complication of chronic liver disease.[1-5]
Patients show persistent clinical, psychometric and electroencephalographic evidence of encephalopathy and often present as neurological rather than hepatic problems. Profound changes in central
neurotransmitters, particularly of the adrenergic system have been
documented in these patients,[6,7] including decreased concentrations
of norepinephrine and dopamine and increased concentrations of the
week neurotransmitters octopamine and β-phenylethanolamine.[8-10]
Changes also occur in cerebral energy metabolism, namely a fall in
cerebral blood flow and cerebral oxygen consumption[11,12] together
with an abnormality of glucose handling.[13] Clinical improvement is
associated with an increase in oxygen utilization.[11,12,14]

Bromocriptine, 2 bromo- α-ergocryptine, is a semi-synthetic
ergot alkaloid, comprising a lysergic acid residue and a cyclic
tripeptide moiety. It is a specific dopamine receptor agonist with
a prolonged action,[15] and should on theoretical grounds benefit
chronic hepatic encephalopathy. A therapeutic trial of bromocriptine was undertaken in six male patients with cirrhosis and severe
hepatic encephalopathy.[16] Their mean age was 48.3 years (range 32-67).
Three of the patients had alcoholic cirrhosis although none had
abused alcohol for five or more years; two had cryptogenic cirrhosis
and one hepatitis B virus associated cirrhosis. The liver lesions in
five of the patients was biochemically and histologically inactive
and in the remaining patient the liver lesion showed only mild
activity.

In most patients the encephalopathy was of long-standing ran-

ging from six-months to eight years. In three patients the encephalopathy developed following portal-systemic shunt surgery performed
for the relief of portal hypertension three, eight and nine years
previously. In the remaining three patients there was evidence of
extensive spontaneous portal-systemic shunting of blood.

All patients suffered intermittent or persistent drowsiness,
inability to concentrate, poor memory, inversion of sleep pattern
and mood fluctuations. Speech was slurred; tremor and incoordination
were prominent features. Four patients had difficulty in walking,
three because of ataxis and one because of a spastic paraparesis.
Thus clinically they showed a mixed picture of cortical, extra-pyramidal and cerebellar dysfunction with one patient in addition showing
evidence of involvement of the cortico-spinal tracts. None had
worked for two or more years.

All patients showed consistently abnormal electro-encephalo-
grams (EEGs) and significant reductions in their cerebral blood flow
and cerebral oxygen and glucose consumption. All showed impairment
of both motor and cognitive function on psychometric testing.

None of the patients had sustained improvement with a low
protein diet and lactulose in doses up to 120 ml daily. Throughout
the trial patients remained on a protein restricted diet and were
prescribed lactulose 40 ml daily to avoid constipation.

Patients were admitted to hospital for an initial two-week
assessment period during which their clinical state and EEG were
assessed daily. Towards the end of the period computer-based psychometric testing[13] was undertaken and cerebral blood flow and metabolism[18,19] were measured. The assessments made during this period
gave a good indication of the patient's performance under controlled
conditions.

At the end of the assessment period, bromocriptine was introduced in a dose of 2.5 mg daily with food and increased in increments of 2.5 mg daily every third day to a maximum of 15 mg daily.
Once established on the maximum maintenance dose of bromocriptine
patients were discharged from hospital to be followed for eight to
12 weeks as outpatients. Throughout this period they were monitored
weekly by two clinicians working independently, by serial EEGs and
by computer based psychometric testing. Patients were then read-
mitted to hospitals for a further assessment period during which
measurements of cerebral blood flow and metabolism were repeated.
Performance during this second assessment period was thought to
fairly represent the effects of eight to 12 weeks of treatment with
bromocriptine.

The trial then continued on a double-blind randomized cross-
over basis during which patients were maintained on either bromo-

criptine or placebo (lactose) for two further eight-week periods. All six patients completed the first phase of the trial but one was excluded from the cross-over section of the trial because of severe monitoring difficulties. Two patients therefore crossed to placebo after eight to 12 weeks on bromocriptine while the remaining three patients were crossed-over after 16 to 20 weeks on bromocriptine (Figure 1). Monitoring during the cross-over trial continued on a weekly basis; cerebral blood flow and metabolism were measured again after each arm of the cross-over.

As a result of treatment with bromocriptine all six patients showed remarkable clinical improvement obvious within 48 to 72 hours. Most patients reported greatest improvement in their powers of concentration and memory. Speech, tremor and incoordination improved and gait became normal in two of the three patients with ataxia.

In all six patients there was definite overall clinical improvement so much so that eventually three patients were able to return to gainful full-time and one to part-time employment.

When patients were crossed-over to placebo clinical deterioration occurred. This was obvious within three days in patients who had received bromocriptine for only eight to 12 weeks, but was not detectable for at least seven days in patients who had received bromocriptine for longer before cross-over to placebo.

Before bromocriptine all patients showed mild to moderate abnormalities on EEG with slowing of the mean cycle frequency to 7.6+0.5 (1SE) cycles per second (cps). The mean cycle frequency in normal alert adults is greater than 8.9 cps. On bromocriptine the mean cycle frequency increased significantly to 8.1+0.6 cps (p < 0.05). In three patients the EEG became normal. Cross-over to placebo resulted in significant deterioration in the EEG in all patients with return to the previously slower recordings. This deterioration occurred more quickly in patients who had crossed to placebo after eight to 12 weeks on bromocriptine than in those who had received active treatment for longer before placebo.

While taking bromocriptine all six patients showed overall improvement on psychometric testing. All six showed improvement in cognitive function and four showed improvements in motor function. In general, the greatest improvements were seen in those complicated tasks that require higher mental function. Cross-over to placebo resulted in a deterioration in psychometric performance to pre-treatment levels. This deterioration occurred more quickly in patients who received placebo following a shorter period on bromocriptine.

Before bromocriptine the mean cerebral blood flow in the six patients was 32.7 $\pm$ 2.4 ml compared with a mean value of 50.0 $\pm$ 2.0 ml/100 g brain/min in 30 control subjects (P < 0.001). During treat-

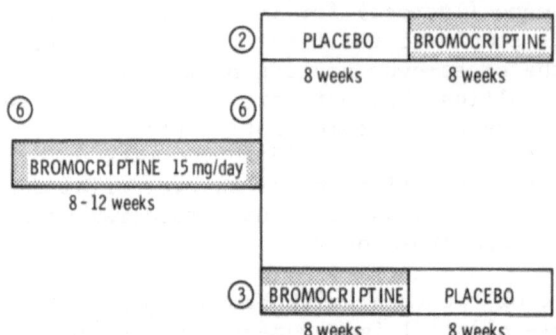

Fig. 1. Design of the bromocriptine trials. During the first eight
to 12 weeks all six patients received the drug in a single
-blind trial. Five patients were then randomised to the
double-blind cross-over phase of bromocriptine versus placebo.

ment with bromocriptine the mean cerebral blood flow in the six
patients increased significantly to 40.5 ± 1.5 ml/100 g/min (P <0.05)
(Figure 2).

The response to cross-over to placebo again varied with the
time previously spent on active treatment. Thus in the two patients
who crossed to placebo after eight to 12 weeks on bromocriptine the
cerebral blood reduced while on placebo and subsequently improved
when active treatment was restarted (Figure 3). These changes were
paralleled by changes in the clinical condition, the EEG and psychometric testing. In the three patients who crossed to placebo following a longer period on bromocriptine significant improvements in
cerebral blood flow were seen during treatment but little change
occurred when placebo was substituted (Figure 4). These changes in
cerebral blood flow were paralleled by much less marked changes in
clinical condition, EEG and psychometric performance than in the
short treatment group.

Before bromocriptine the mean cerebral oxygen consumption in
the six patients was 2.2 ± 0.4 ml compared with a mean value of
3.3 ± 0.1 ml/100 g brain/min in 30 control subjects (P < 0.02).
During treatment with bromocriptine the mean cerebral oxygen consumption in the six patients increased significantly to 3.3 ± 0.4 ml/
100 g brain/min (P < 0.02) (Figure 5).

Similarly, before bromocriptine the mean cerebral glucose consumption in the six patients was significantly reduced, 2.1 ± 0.6
mg compared with the mean value in control subjects, 4.8 ± 0.2 mg

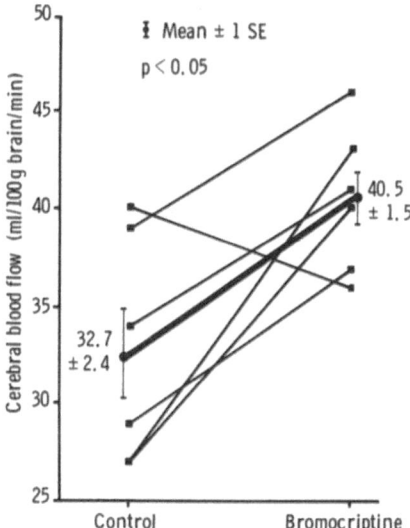

Fig. 2. Changes occurring in cerebral blood flow in six patients
with chronic hepatic encephalopathy during treatment with
bromocriptine.

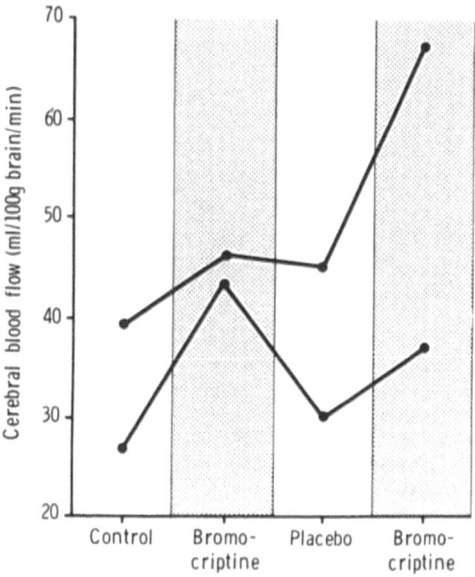

Fig. 3. Changes occurring in cerebral blood flow in two patients
with chronic hepatic encephalopathy during cross-over to
placebo after eight to 12 weeks treatment with bromocriptine and subsequent re-introduction of active treatment.

(P < 0.05), but improved significantly during treatment with bromocriptine to 6.6 ± 1.6 mg/100 g brain/min (P < 0.02) (Figure 6).

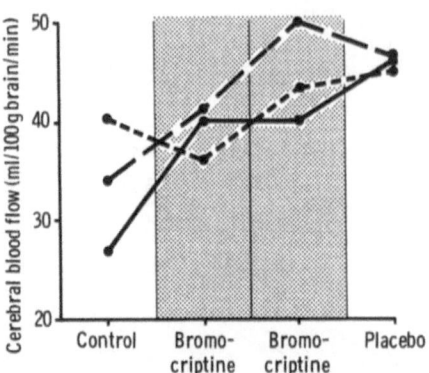

Fig. 4.   Changes occurring in cerebral blood flow in three patients
          with chronic hepatic encephalopathy during cross-over to
          placebo following 16 to 20 weeks treatment with bromocrip-
          tine.

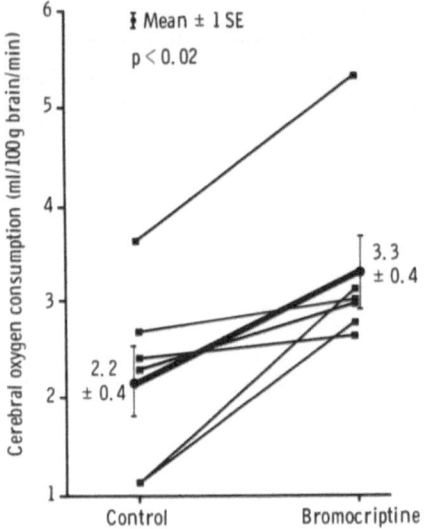

Fig. 5.   Changes occurring in cerebral oxygen consumption in six
          patients with chronic hepatic encephalopathy during treat-
          ment with bromocriptine.

     The changes in cerebral oxygen and glucose metabolism during
the cross-over phase of the trial paralleled those seen in cerebral
blood flow.

     One patient experienced a transient attack of hypomania in the
first few weeks of treatment. Bromocriptine was continued as the
patient failed to report the event and the symptoms abated in approximately one week. No other early side-effects were noted and no

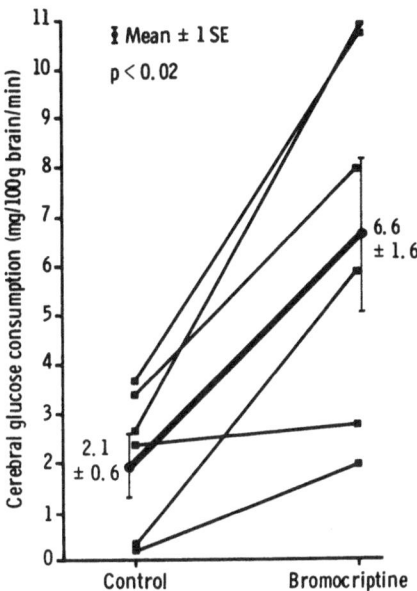

Fig. 6.   Changes occurring in cerebral glucose consumption in six
patients with chronic hepatic encephalopathy during treatment with bromocriptine.

haematological, biochemical or electrocardiographic changes occurred.
The drug was well-tolerated in a dose of 15 mg daily.

Thus in this group of six patients with severe chronic hepatic
encephalopathy treatment with bromocriptine resulted in significant
improvements in clinical condition, EEG, psychometric performance
and cerebral blood flow and metabolism.

Four years after the original trial two patients have died from
incidental causes while the remaining four patients are alive
and well on maintenance bromocriptine. After two years on bromocriptine 15 mg daily the patient who had experienced hypomania in
the early trial period complained of hearing loss and audiograms
suggested a drug-related ototoxicity (Figure 7a). As the patients'
only other medications were lactulose and spironolactone it was
suggested that the patient stop bromocriptine. This he preferred
not to do although he agreed to reduce the dose under close super-
vision. Over the next six months his hearing gradually improved and
the audiograms returned to near normal while the patient continued
to take bromocriptine 10 mg daily (Figure 7b). Repeat audiograms
over the past eighteen months have shown no further changes on this
dose of the drug. The remaining five patients although asymptomatic,
were screened for evidence of ototoxicity. In two patients the au-

diograms showed suggestive abnormalities, though one had taken considerable quantities of neomycin in the past. Bromocriptine was reduced in both patients with improvement occurring in the patient who had not received neomycin. The mechanism of the ototoxicity is unknown but might be related to changes occurring in fluid balance in the middle ear. Reduction of the bromocriptine dosage resulted in no loss of efficacy.

Since the original trial six further patients with severe stable hepatic encephalopathy, but well-compensated liver disease, have been treated with bromocriptine with equal success. One further patient with hepatic encephalopathy but poor liver function was treated with this drug but developed profound hyponatraemia possibly the result of inappropriate secretion or response to anti-diuretic hormone.[20] The hyponatraemia resolved when bromocriptine was discontinued.

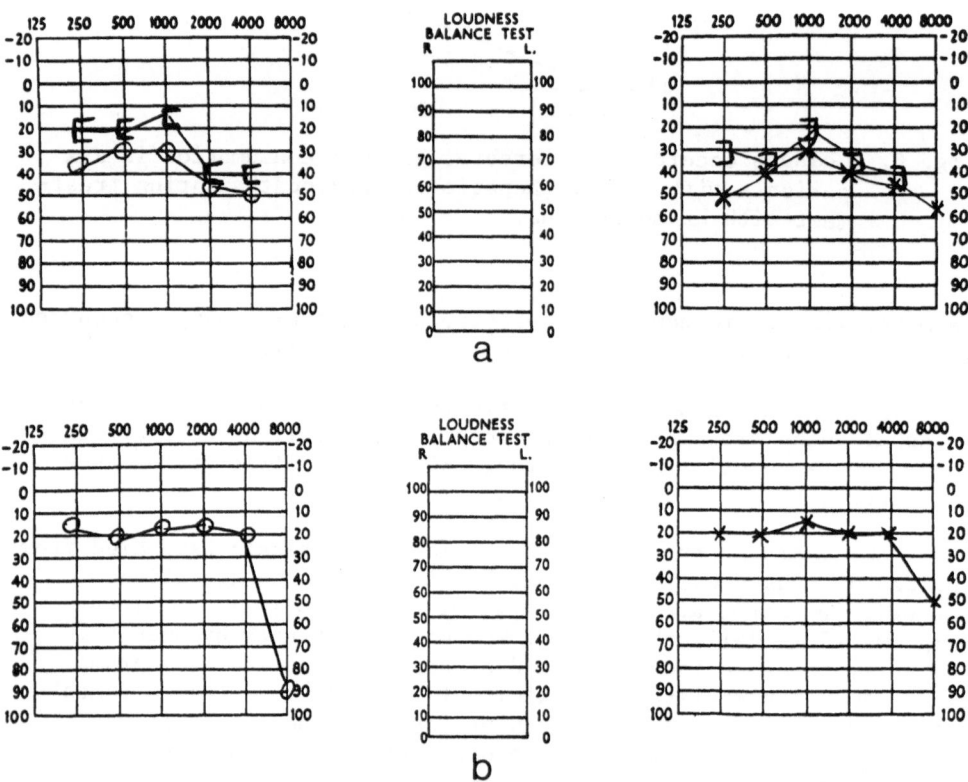

Fig. 7.   Audiogram in a patient with chronic hepatic encephalopathy (a) treated for two years with bromocriptine 15 mg daily showing reduction in both air and bone conduction in both ears, and (b) treated with bromocriptine six months after reduction of drug dosage to 10 mg daily. Right ear: 0 air, ⊏ bone; left ear: X air, ⊐ bone.

The mechanism of the effect of bromocriptine in this condition is speculative. Experimental work in baboons has shown that stimulation of dopaminergic receptors can result in marked increases in cerebral blood and metabolism.[21] The increase in cerebral blood flow has been attributed variously to either a direct vascular action of the dopaminergic agent causing vasodilation or to an inhibition of the vasoconstrictory noradrenergic tone mediated by prejunctional dopamine receptors.[23] However it is unlikely that the changes observed in clinical condition, EEG and psychometric function in these patients could result simply from the changes occurring in cerebral blood flow. The drug may however produce its beneficial effects as a result of peripheral rather than central dopaminergic effects as has been suggested for L-dopa.[24]

Prolonged treatment with bromocriptine was followed by a persistent beneficial effect when the drug was stopped. This is similar to the effect seen with various antihypertensive drugs where discontinuation of treatment is followed by a continued therapeutic effect for some time. In the case of bromocriptine, this effect may represent changes in dopaminergic receptor responsiveness or in the blood-brain barrier permeability, which may be self-perpetuating.

Bromocriptine is recommended as a safe, well-tolerated and highly-effective treatment for chronic hepatic encephalopathy in patients with well-preserved liver function who have failed to sustain improvement with conventional medical measures. It should always be used as an adjunct to these measures and never as an alternative. Thus these patients must still restrict their dietary protein intake and rigorously avoid constipation by use of lactulose. Patients should be stabilized initially on 15 mg bromocriptine daily for three or four months and then the dosage gradually reduced to 10 mg daily for long-term maintenance. Audiograms should be assessed before the drug is introduced and periodically throughout treatment.

No claim can be made for benefit from bromocriptine therapy in acute hepatic encephalopathy or in the prevention or treatment of recurrent hepatic encephalopathy in patients with less stable chronic liver disease.[25]

REFERENCES

1. S. Sherlock, W. H. J. Summerskill, L. P. White and E. A. Phear, Portal systemic encephalopathy. Neurological complications of liver disease, Lancet 2:453 (1954).
2. W. V. McDermott, Jr. and R. D. Adams, Episodic stupor associated with an Eck fistula in the human with particular reference to the metabolism of ammonia, J. Clin. Invest. 33: 1 (1954).
3. W. H. J. Summerskill, E. A. Davidson, S. Sherlock, and R. E. Steiner, The neuropsychiatric syndrome associated with hepatic cirrhosis and an extensive portal collateral circulation, Q.

J. Med. 25: 245 (1956).

4. M. Victor, R. D. Adams, and M. Cole, The acquired (non-Wilsonian) type of chronic hepato-cerebral degeneration, Medicine 44: 345 (1965).

5. A. E. Read, S. Sherlock, J. Laidlow, and J. G. Walker, The neuropsychiatric syndrome associated with chronic liver disease and an extensive portal-systemic collateral circulation, Q. J. Med. 36: 135 (1967).

6. R. J. Baldessarini and J.E. Fischer, Serotonin metabolism in rat brain after surgical diversion of the portal venous circulation, Nature New Biol. 254: 25 (1973).

7. J. M. Dodsworth, J. H. James, M. C. Commungs, and J. E. Fischer, Depletion of brain norepinephrine in acute hepatic coma, Surgery 75: 811 (1974).

8. J. E. Fischer and R. J. Baldessarini, False neurotransmitters and hepatic failure, Lancet 2: 75 (1971).

9. K. C. Lam, A. R. Tall, G. B. Goldstein, and S. F. Mistilis, The role of a false neurochemical transmitter, octopamine, in the pathogenesis of hepatic and renal encephalopathy, Scand. J. Gastroenterol. 8: 465 (1973).

10. K. K. Manghani, M. R. Lunzer, B. H. Billing, and S. Sherlock, Urinary and serum octopamine in patients with porto-systemic encephalopathy, Lancet 2: 943 (1975).

11. J. F. Fazekas, H. E. Ticktin, W. R. Ehrmantraut, and R. W. Altman, Cerebral metabolism in hepatic insufficiency, Am. J. Med. 21: 843 (1956).

12. J. B. Posner and F. Plum, The toxic effects of carbon dioxide and acetazolamide in hepatic encephalopathy, J.Clin. Invest. 39: 1246 (1960).

13. I. M. James, S. Nashat, D. Sampson, H. S. Williams, and M. Garassini, Effect of induced metabolic alkalosis in hepatic encephalopathy, Lancet 2: 1106 (1969).

14. E. Polli, G. Bianchi Porro, and A. T. Maiolo, Cerebral metabolism after portocaval shunt, Lancet 1: 1341 (1969).

15. T. Hökfelt and K. Fuxe, Effects of prolactin and ergot alkaloids on the tubero-infundibular dopamine (DA) neurons, Neuroendocrinology 9: 100 (1972).

16. M. Y. Morgan, A. W. Jakabovits, I. M. James, and S. Sherlock, Successful use of bromocriptine in the treatment of chronic hepatic encephalopathy, Gastroenterology 78: 663 (1980).

17. D. Jones and J. Weinman, Computer based psychological testing, in: "Human and Artificial Intelligence", D. Jones and A. Elithorn, eds., Elsevier, Amsterdam (1973).

18. D. J. Wyper, G. A. Lennox, and J. O. Rowan, Two minute slope inhalation technique for cerebral blood flow measurement in man 1. Method, J. Neurol. Neurosurg. Psychiatry 39: 141 (1976).

19. D. J. Wyper and J. O. Rowan, The construction and use of nomograms for cerebral blood flow calculations using a ^{133}Xe inhalation technique, Phys.Med.Biol. 21: 406 (1976).

20. A. W. Marshall, A. W. Jacobovits, and M. Y. Morgan, Bromocriptine-associated hyponatraemia in cirrhosis, Br. Med. J. in press (1982).

21. J. McCulloch and A. M. Harper, Dopaminergic systems and the cerebral circulation, Acta Neurol. Scand. (Suppl.) 56: (64) 100 (1977).

22. L. Edvinsson, J. E. Hardebo, A. M. Harper, J. McCulloch, and Ch. Owman, Action of dopamine agonist on brain vessels in vitro and after in vivo micropuncture, Acta Neurol. Scand. (Suppl.) 56 (64): 350 (1977).

23. A. G. Boulu, M. Plotkine, and C. Gueniau, Effects of dopaminergic agonists upon oxygen availability for cerebral cortex, Acta Neurol. Scand. (Suppl.) 56 (64): 352 (1977).

24. L. Zieve, W. M. Doizaki, and R. F. Derr, Reversal of ammonia coma by L-dopa: a peripheral effect, Gut 20:28 (1979).

25. M. Uribe, A. Farca, M. A. Marquez, G. Garcia-Romos, L. Guevara, A. Briones, and S. Gils, Treatment of chronic portal systemic encephalopathy with bromocriptine, Gastroenterology 76: 1342 (1979).

BROMOCRIPTINE TO TREAT PORTAL SYSTEMIC ENCEPHALOPATHY

M. Uribe

Instituto Nacional de la Nutriciòn Salvador Zubiràn

Liver Unit, Vasco de Quiroga No. 15 14000 Mexico, D.F.

Clinical Forms of Portal Systemic Encephalopathy

The clinical spectrum of portal systemic encephalopathy (PSE) is very wide. It may occur as a subclinical form, sometimes only detected by the electroencephalogram, frequently occurs as acute or chronic recurrent syndrome (spontaneous or induced by gastro-intestinal bleeding, diuretics, sepsis, etc.), and as a rare form in which neurological rather than hepatic signs are predominant, these groups of patients represent chronic hepatocerebral degeneration.[1]

In the majority of the PSE patients, hyperammonemia is part of the features and therefore the treatment of these cases has been directed towards either the direct removal of ammonia from the gut or the elimination of sources of ammonia production.

False neurotransmitters hypothesis

The provocative hypothesis postulated by Fischer and Baldes-sarini to explain PSE, has promoted a series of studies with L-dopa and dopa agonists. These authors suggested that accumulation of false neurotransmitters in the brain may replace dopamine and norepine-phrine, the true neurotransmitters. This hypothesis suggests that PSE might be explained by a defect in dopaminergic neurotransmission. Therefore L-dopa and bromocriptine (a specific dopamine agonist) should have a beneficial effect on PSE.

To date there are few studies in regard to the use of dopami-nergic agents in hepatic encephalopathy. The first of these drugs used to treat patients with PSE was L-dopa.

L-DOPA

In the first controlled study Lunzer et al.[2] administered L-dopa to six patients, with chronic PSE. Only three of the six tolerated the medication, and only one showed a significant beneficial response. Despite these unimpressive results the authors concluded that L-dopa "may provide a safe and more effective method of treatment of intractable chronic hepatic encephalopathy."

In a more recent prospective trial Michel et al.[3] studied 75 cirrhotic patients randomized to receive L-dopa plus a dopa decarboxylase inhibitor (37 cases) or placebo (38 patients). In this study only twelve of the 37 patients with L-dopa improved. This figure was similar in the placebo group in which 14 out of 38 patients demonstrated some degree of improvement. It is clear from this study that in controlled fashion L-dopa has little beneficial effect in PSE.

BROMOCRIPTINE

Bromocriptine, 2-bromo α ergocritine is a semi-synthetic ergot alkaloid, comprising a lysergic acid residue and a cycle trypeptide moiety. It is a specific dopamine receptor agonist.

In an uncontrolled study performed in one patient with PSE, bromocriptine 15 mg/day improved the clinical condition of a previous "intractable" patient,[4] this report motivated several groups of investigators to evaluate in controlled studies the efficacy of bromocriptine in various types of PSE.

A) Bromocriptine in Spontaneous Chronic PSE.

There are two controlled trials. In our study[5] we included 7 patients with chronic PSE. Two of the patients had a portocaval shunt. Patients were stable at the entry of the study and they had responded to the standard therapy of neomycin and milk of magnesia.

The study was carried out in a double blind fashion to compare bromocriptine (15 mg/day) versus placebo. The study included four periods. In control period I, patients were stabilized by the ingestion of neomycin 3 g/day and milk of magnesia as cathartic. After this 10 day period bromocriptine or placebo was administered during two weeks (treatment period A). Control period II followed and was identical to control period I, finally the other medication pair (bromocriptine or placebo) was given for 2 weeks. Cathartics and neomycin were discontinued during placebo and bromocriptine periods.

All patients responded adequately to neomycin plus milk of magnesia. Consequently they were all awake, and showed no remarkable clinical signs of PSE during control periods I and II.

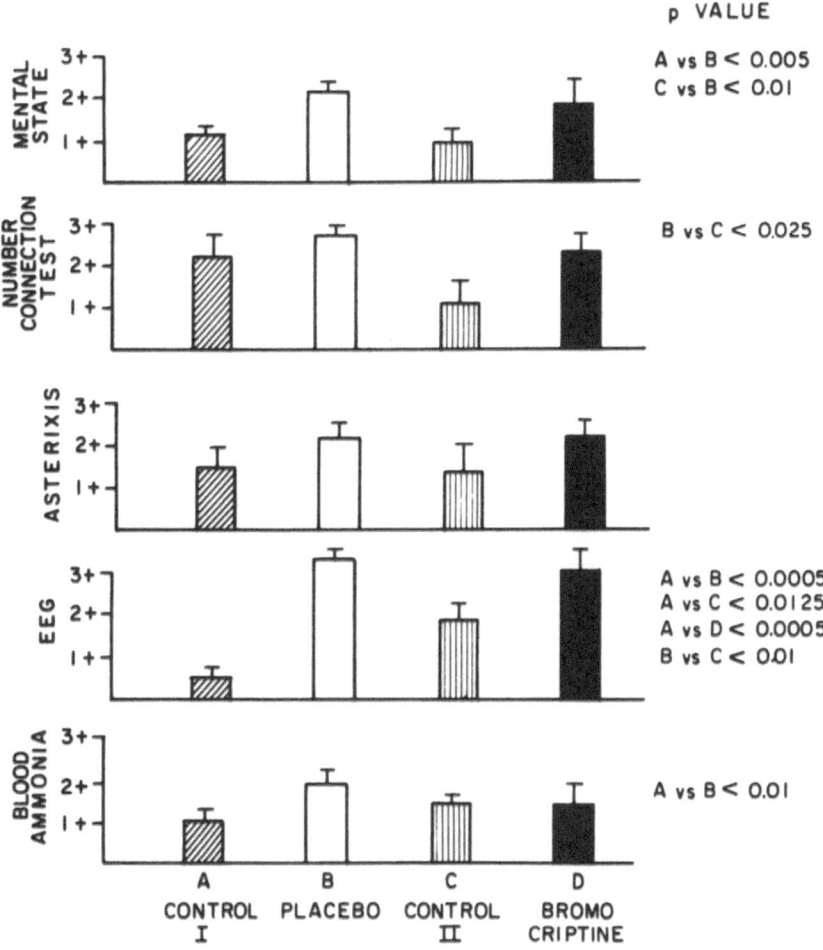

Fig. 1. Comparison of neomycin and milk of magnesia (control periods
         I and II), placebo, and bromocriptine. In the majority of
         the PSE parameters, bromocriptine was comparable to placebo.
         Placebo was significantly inferior than control periods I
         or II regarding mental state. NCT, EEGs, and blood ammonia.
         Bromocriptine was significantly inferior than neomycin and
         cathartics regarding EEGs. The height of the bars depicts
         mean ± SD.

Three patients developed signs of precoma when ingesting both placebo
and bromocriptine. Two patients developed precoma only while receiving placebo, one patient only while receiving bromocriptine. Another
patient remained awake throughout the study. In summary, 5 of 7 patients developed precoma signs when ingesting placebo (72%) and 4
of the 7 developed precoma when ingesting bromocriptine (57%), differences between placebo and bromocriptine were non significant.

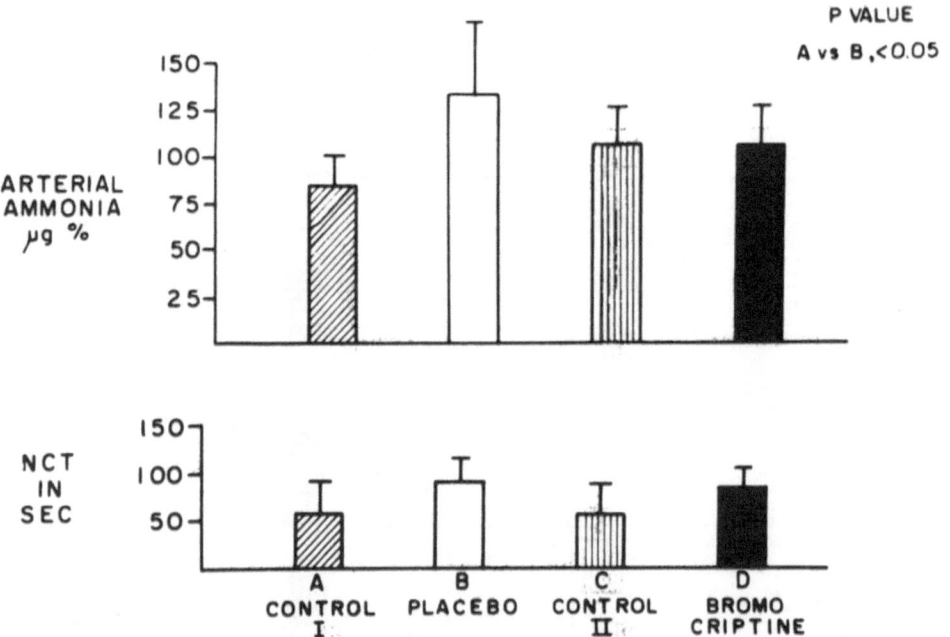

Fig. 2. Arterial ammonia concentration and NCT expressed in their
original units. Raw data show significant differences in
ammonia levels only between control period I and placebo.

Results regarding mental state, asterixis, EEG's, psychometric
tests and blood ammonia are shown (Figures 1 and 2). These parameters demonstrated that bromocriptine was not superior to placebo and
was always inferior to neomycin cathartics. PSE index (Figure 3)
showed very similar values for control periods I and II (0.32+0.1
and 0.31+0.1) and for placebo and bromocriptine periods 0.56+0.4
and 0.50+0.1.

In a more recent study in 11 patients with chronic PSE, Messner
et al.[6] compared bromocriptine (20 mg/day) plus sorbital (80 ml/day)
versus placebo tablets plus lactulose adjusted to produce 2-3 bowel
movements/day. Two of the eleven patients had a portocaval shunt.
The study was performed in a cross-over fashion. During the first
course of treatment with bromocriptine sorbitol (6 cases) two patients improved, two remained stable and two deteriorated. During
lactulose-placebo (5 cases) 3 cases improved and two remained stable.

SCPSE (spontaneous chronic portal systemic encephalopathy) some
improved with lactulose and deteriorated with bromocriptine. These
investigators found no differences in plasma aminoacids after either
treatment. It can be concluded from these two studies that bromo-

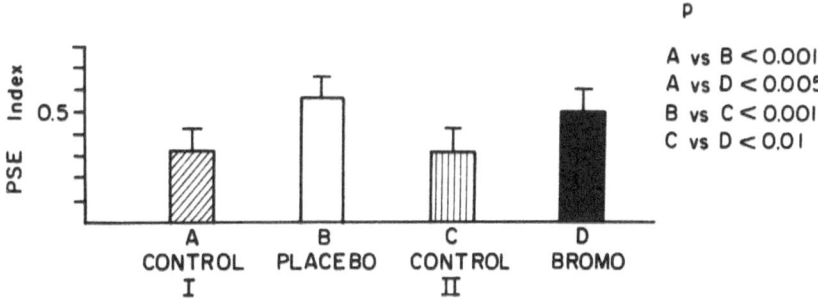

Fig. 3. Effect of bromocriptine, placebo, neomycin, and milk of
magnesia (control periods I and II) on PSE index. The PSE
index (mean $\pm$ SD) improved significantly during neomycin
and milk of magnesia administration when compared to placebo and bromocriptine. Control periods I and II were comparable. There were no significant differences between
placebo and bromocriptine.

criptine alone or combined with cathartics is not a useful treatment
in this type of PSE. Therefore, this drug should not be recommended
for chronic PSE patients who are adequately controlled with standard
therapy.

PSE After Portocaval Shunt

A single blind study of bromocriptine versus placebo was carried
out in 6 patients with portocaval shunt by Ubiria et al.[7] In this
study two patients presented serious side effects and bromocriptine
was discontinued. Two other patients developed PSE signs, both with
the dopamine agonist and placebo and one patient developed deep
coma during bromocriptine therapy. These authors concluded that in
the treatment of chronic recurrent PSE induced by portocaval shunt
bromocriptine is similar to the administration of placebo.

Acute PSE

Recently we studied 4 patients with severe mental state deterioration (grade 2-3 + of mental state) who were not adequately controlled by standard therapy.[8] These patients were included in a
single blind cross-over study using 15 and 30 mg of bromocriptine
versus neomycin 4 g/day plus tap water enemas (to avoid constipation). In each patient bromocriptine 15 mg or 30 mg/day resulted
inferior to standard therapy.

In a controlled study Granier et al.[9] administered bromocrip-

Table 1. Response to bromocriptine in PSE patients

Author	No. of patients	Predominant type of PSE	Bromocriptine mg/day	Concomitant Medication	Response	Deterioration	Same
Morgan	1	Hepatocerebral degeneration	15	Lactulose	1	0	0
Morgan*	5	Hepatocerebral degeneration	15	Lactulose	5	0	0
Uribe*	7	Chronic spontaneous	15		0	4	3
Messner*	6	Chronic spontaneous	20	Sorbital	2	2	2
Ubiria*	6	After portocaval	15		0	5	1
Granier	12	Acute PSE	20	L-Dopa Lactulose	3	9	0
Uribe*	4	Acute PSE	15-30	Enemas	0	4	0
TOTAL	41				11 (27%)	24 (59%)	6 (15%)

*Controlled studies.

tine to 13 patients with acute PSE. Only 3 of the 13 patients showed some degree of improvement.

Bromocriptine for Chronic Hepatocerebral Degeneration

The Royal Free Hospital group has found striking clinical response in six patients with chronic Parkinson-like encephalopathy treated with bromocriptine plus lactulose.[10] They will discuss their findings.

SUMMARY

At present, there are evidences that dopaminergic or dopamine agonist drugs (Table 1) in controlled trials have fail to demonstrate beneficial effect in patients with chronic spontaneous PSE, acute PSE and porto caval shunt induced PSE. Furthermore in a double blind fashion the dopamine antagonist metochlopramide was unable to induce changes in PSE parameters when administered during two weeks to 4 cirrhotic patients.[11] These findings and the clinical results with dopaminergic drugs provide with additional argument against the false neurotransmitters hypothesis to fully explain PSE.

There is a single report which suggests benefit of bromocriptine in the rare group of patients with Parkinson-like PSE. In the majority of the studies nausea, vomiting, and neurological side effects appeared.

Patients who are adequately controlled with neomycin or disaccharides should not be placed on L-dopa or bromocriptine. Bromocriptine is perhaps useful for the relatively rare disorder of hepatocerebral degeneration in which parkinsonism features are predominant.

REFERENCES

1. A. M. Hoyumpa, P.V, Desmond, and G. R. Avanti, Hepatic encephalopathy, Gastroenterology 76: 184 (1979).
2. M. Lunzer, I. M. James, and R. Weinman, Treatment of chronic hepatic encephalopathy with levodopa, Gut 15: 555 (1974).
3. H. Michel, H. Solere, and P. Gravier, Treatment of cirrhotic hepatic encephalopathy with L-dopa. A controlled trial, Gastroenterology 79: 207 (1980).
4. Y. M. Morgan, A. Jocobovitz, and A. Ellithorn, Successful use of bromocriptine in the treatment of a patient with chronic portal systemic encephalopathy, N. Engl. J. Med. 296: 793 (1977).
5. M. Uribe, A. Farca, and M. A. Marquez, Treatment of chornic portal systemic encephalopathy with bromocriptine. A double blind controlled trial, Gastroenterology 76: 1347 (1979).
6. M. Messner, P. Brissot, and P. Toulouse, Comparison of bromo-

criptine and lactulose in the treatment of spontaneous chronic portal systemic encephalopathy, Hepatology, in press (1983).

7. J. Ubiria, M. Morales, and M. Vila, Tratamiento de la encefalopatia crónica portosistémica con bromocriptina, Rev. Esp. Enf. Ap. Digest. 58: 21 (1980).

8. M. Uribe, M. A. Márquez, and L. Guevara, Bromocriptine for severe chronic portal systemic encephalopathy, Gastroenterology 82: 1201 (1982).

9. P. Granier, G. Cauvet, and G. Guilleret, A propos du traitment de l'encephalopathie hepatique par la bromocriptine, Gastroenterologie Clin. Biol. 3: 210 (1979).

10. M. Y. Morgan, A. W. Jacobovitz, and I. M. James, Successful use of bromocriptine in the treatment of chronic hepatic encephalopathy, Gastroenterology 78: 667 (1980).

11. M. Uribe, A. Ballesteros, and J. Rosales, Do dopamine antagonist drugs induce hepatic encephalopathy? Hepatology 2: 746 (Abst. #/ 293) (1982).

LACTITOL, A POTENTIAL SECOND GENERATION DISACCHARIDE DRUG

FOR THE TREATMENT OF PORTAL-SYSTEMIC ENCEPHALOPATHY

M. Bührer and J. Bircher

Department of Clinical Pharmacology, University of Berne

Berne, Switzerland

INTRODUCTION

In 1966 the first report of the beneficial effects of lactulose in the treatment of chronic portal systemic encephalopathy was published.[1] In the meantime, this drug has become accepted as drug of choice for this condition,[2] but also some disadvantages of lactulose - available only as syrup with a very sweet taste and contamination by other sugars - have now been recognized. Unfortunately these features may lead to aversion against the drug, to nausea related to the hyperosmolarity of the syrup and consequently to suboptimal treatment. In view of these difficulties it is surprising that no analogs with more favorable physiochemical properties have as yet been investigated.

Recently the chemical and nutritional properties of lactitol have been described.[3] It appears that this disaccharide can easily be produced in a chemically pure crystalline form and may be formulated into nonhygroscopic powders or tablets which are easy to handle. Lactitol is much less sweet than lactulose, but otherwise it seems to be similar in that it is not absorbed by the small intestine, but metabolized extensively by the colonic bacterial flora. It therefore might be the ideal successor of lactulose. In view of these facts pilot studies on the clinical effects of lactitol were initiated.[4]

Case Report

Pertinent clinical details of the two cases are summarized in Table 1. Case 1 was hospitalized and examined at the end of several one-week treatment periods. A complete report has been published elsewhere[4] and 2 relevant treatment results are given in Table 2.

275

Table 1. Clinical and laboratory data in the examined
          patients

	Case 1	Case 2[a]
Age, sex	62 male	60 male
History		
alcohol intake (g/day)	> 100	> 40
duration (years)	40	40
end-to-side portocaval anastomosis	1980	1980
Physical examination		
body weight (kg)	62	76
height (cm)	149	174
hepatomegaly	++	+
spider angiomata	+	+
ankle edema	+	−
Laboratory tests		
total bilirubin (mg/dl)	3.0	0.9
fasting conjugated bile acids (µmol/1)	63	96
serum albumin (g/dl)	3.5	4.0
galactose elimination capacity (mg/min/kg)	4.0[b]	3.5[b]
initial BSP-elimination (min^{-1})	0.031[c]	−
serum potassium (meq/1)	3.5	3.8
blood urea nitrogen (mg/dl)	9.3	12.6

[a] Insulin dependent diabetes since 1980
[b] Normal value 7.5 $\pm$ SD 1.0/mg/min/kg
[c] Normal value 0.125 $\pm$ 0.015 min^{-1}

DISCUSSION

The difficulties to handle a sticky syrup, the very sweet taste
and the nausea presumably caused by an excessive osmotic load are
minor disadvantages of lactulose. Nevertheless, they may lead to
suboptimal treatment because they may compromise the incentives for
patient compliance in a group of patients who a priori have difficulties to follow a strict treatment regimen. On the basis of the
two observed cases it appears that lactitol is superior to lactulose
in this respect since both patients clearly preferred lactitol. Two
additional patients who currently are under observation also confirm

Table 2. Clinical evaluation during therapy with lactitol and lactulose

Drug	Case 1		Case 2	
	lactitol[a]	lactulose[b]	lactitol[a]	lactulose[b]
Dosage (g/day)	75	100	54	50
Protein intake (g/day)	40	40	approx 60	approx 60
Coma grade (0-V)[c]	I-II	I-II	I	I
Trail test (sec)[d]	120	102	30	35
EEG-grade (0-V)[c]	II	II	II	II
Arterial NH_3 (µg/dl)	120	158	135	274

[a] Lactitol was given as 3 g tablets.

[b] given as commercial syrup (Duphalac[R]). An amount of 100 g corresponds to 150 ml, which was given in 3 divided doses. The 150 ml also include 16.5 g of galactose and 9 g of lactose. Case 2 received half the dose.

[c] 0 - V according to Parsons-Smith et al.[5]

[d] according to Zeegen et al.[6]

this observation. The drug, therefore warrants exploration of its true therapeutic potential in controlled studies.

It should be noted that lactitol like lactulose may produce bloating and flatulescence. Usually these symptoms improve upon continued treatment, presumably because gas forming clostridia do not survive when colonic contents are consistently acidified. Diarrhea resulting from overdosage can occur equally with lactitol as with lactulose. These latter adverse effects are probably related to mode of action of these disaccharides and therefore are unlikely to be improved by other sugars. If further studies confirm the efficacy of lactitol in the treatment of portal-systemic encephalopathy and its reduced rate of adverse effects this sugar may truly become a second generation disaccharide drug for the treatment of portal systemic encephalopathy.

REFERENCES

1. J. Bircher, J. Müller, p. Guggenheim, and U. P, Hämmerli, Treatment of chronic portal-systemic encephalopathy with lactulose, Lancet 1: 890 (1966).
2. H. O. Conn and M. M. Lieberthal,"The hepatic coma syndromes and lactulose," The Williams and Wilkins Co., Baltimore (1979).
3. J. A. van Velthuijsen, Food additives derived from lactulose; lactitol and lactitol palmitate, J. Agricult. Food Chem. 27: 680 (1979).
4. J. Bircher, M. Bührer, K. Franz, and J. A. van Velthuijsen, Erstmalige Anwendung von Lactitol in der Behandlung der portosystemischen Encephalopathie, Schweiz. Med. Wschr. 112: 1306 (1982).
5. B. G. Parsons-Smith, W. Summerskill, A. M. Dawson, and S. Sherlock, The electroencephalograph in liver disease, Lancet II: 867 (1957).
6. R. Zeegen, J. E. Drinkwater, and A. M. Dawson, Methods for measuring cerebral dysfunction in patients with liver disease, Brit. Med. J. II: 633 (1970).

LACTOSE TO TREAT ACUTE AND CHRONIC PORTAL SYSTEMIC ENCEPHALOPATHY

M. Uribe

Liver Unit, Instituto Nacional de la Nutritiõn
Salvador Zubiràn, Vasco de Quiroga No. 15, 14000 Mexico
D.F.

INTRODUCTION

The therapeutic effect of the semi-synthetic disaccharide lactulose, in the management of patients with acute and chronic portal
systemic encephalopathy (PSE) has been demonstrated in controlled
trials.[1,2] However, in developing countries the high cost and unavailability of lactulose constitute a serious drawback. In the
majority of developing countries there is a high prevalence of
primary lactase malabsorption. Lactose malabsorption ranges from 6%
in predominant Caucasian populations to 90-95% in countries with
predominantly oriental or black population.[3] In Mexico 74% of the
people is lactase deficient.

For this lactase deficient population, nature has provided the
possibility of an inexpensive manner of treatment. In lactase deficient individuals, lactose exerts the same effects than lactulose
does in general population, in whom there is no lactulase to degrade
the disaccharide (since lactulose is a semi-synthetic sugar). By
analogy lactase deficient patients with PSE can be theoretically
treated with lactose.

In vitro studies

Indeed, in vitro studies have demonstrated similar behavior of
lactulose and lactose in fecal incubation.[4] Both sugars were similarly degraded by fecal flora and their acidic metabolites lowered
the medium pH as compared to control incubation or compared to those
with the addition of neomycin (Figure 1). Simultaneous measurement
of ammonia in the culture demonstrated a reduction of fecal ammonia
generation after disaccharide addition and it was also noted a mild

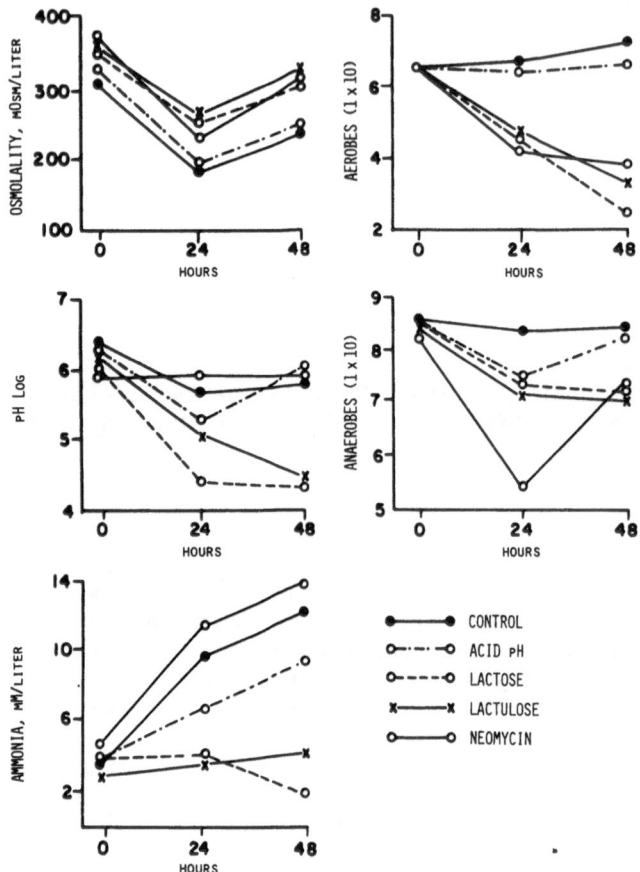

Fig. 1. In vitro fecal stool incubation demonstrated pH acidifica-
         tion, lowered bacterial counts and decrease in vitro ammonia
         generation after both lactose and lactulose (n=8).

reduction of aerobes and anaerobes fecal counts. If the same occurs
in vivo, the stool acidification may lower ammonia generation, bacterial growth and induce acidic diarrhea. This and other studies are
in agreement with the concept that colonic acidification may play an
important role in regard to disaccharide therapeutic effects.

CLINICAL USE OF LACTOSE

A) Chronic Portal Systemic Encephalopathy

     Because of the similar in vitro effects of lactose and lactulose
we decided to evaluate in a controlled trial the efficacy of lactulose p.o. in patients with cirrhosis, PSE and primary adult type
lactase deficiency.

Ten patients with chronic PSE were included.[5] The study was carried out in a cross over fashion to compare lactose versus neomycin plus milk of magnesia.

All patients were clinically and biochemically stable at entry and in all lactose malabsorption was demonstrated by a standard lactose tolerance test. The study was designed to compare lactose (50 mg twice p.o.) versus neomycin (3 g/day) plus milk of magnesia (70 mg/day) in a cross-over pattern in which each patient serves as his own control. To have better control patients were crossed over twice. Each period lasted two weeks and protein diet was kept at 40 g/day throughout the study.

Seriam semiquantitative-quantitative assessments were done including: mental state, asterixis, number connection tests, electroencephalograms and blood ammonia.

A significant improvement of mental state, asterixis, number connection tests, and electroencephalogram was evident during lactose therapy as compared with neomycin (Figure 2). None of the patients developed acute PSE and all remained awake during lactose treatment. Apart from mild diarrhea and bloating no serious side effects were noticeable during lactase treatment. The lactose dose of 50 g bid was enough to induce 3-4 bowel movements/day. Although this dose is mainly recommended for lactose intolerant patients, actually in terms of adult population every one has a relative lactase deficiency. Therefore, if a large dose of lactose is given to "lactose absorbers" the amount of lactase available can be overhelmed and the excess undegraded disaccharide can be taken by the intestinal bacteria (lower part of small intestine and colon) and degraded to beneficial, acidifying products. Therefore larger doses of lactose in lactase tolerant patients can be used.

B) Lactose Enemas to Treat Acute PSE

Patients with acute PSE (mental state grade 3-4, precoma or deep coma) are unable to ingest medications, the same occurs in patients with ilei in whom the oral administration of lactose or lactulose is not feasible. In these cases rectal disaccharides can be administered. Using the rectal route it is not mandatory that patients be lactose intolerant since the sugar can be deposited into the colon, where the fecal germs can easily metabolize the disaccharide.

The disaccharides given directly into the colon can be rapidly metabolized. Bond and Levitt[6] infused lactulose into the cecum and have noted the appearance of hydrogen gas in expired air within 4 or 5 minutes. These observations may explain the rapid clinical response obtained with lactose and lactulose enemas.

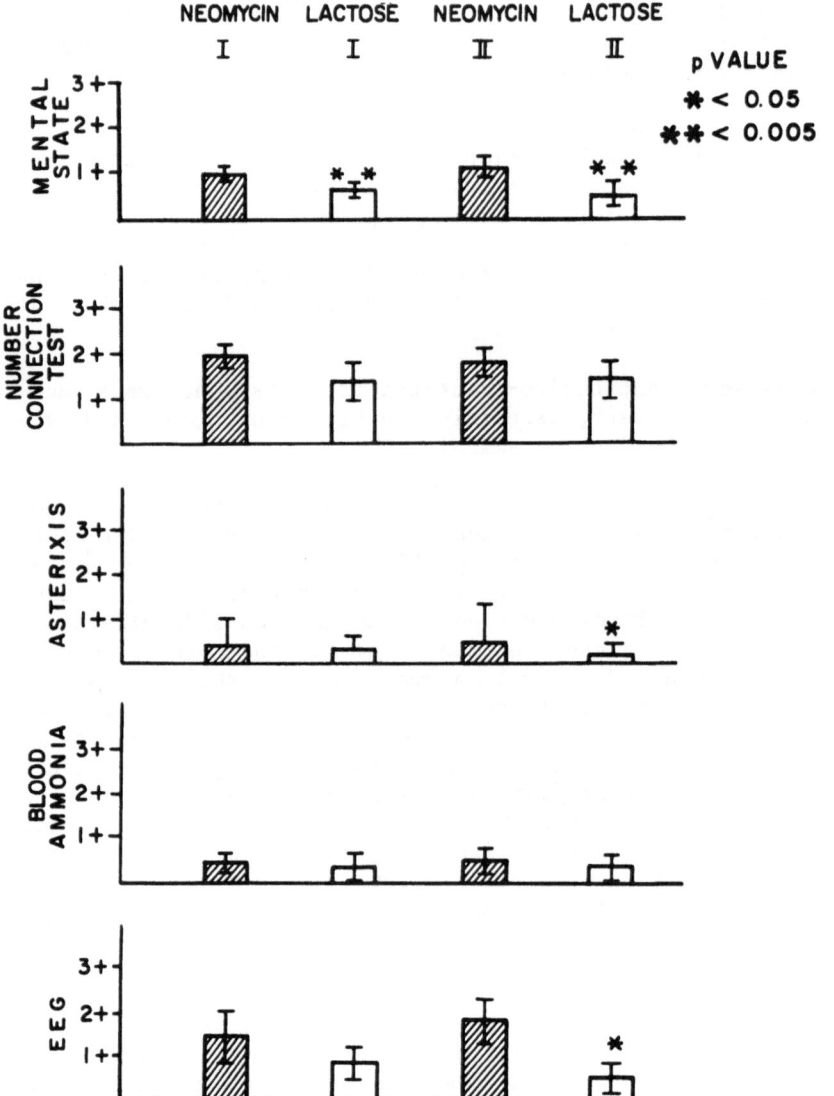

Fig. 2.   Effect of neomycin plus cathartics (neomycin I and II) and
          lactose (I and II) on PSE parameters. (Semiquantitative
          scale.)

Controlled Studies With Lactose Enemas

        In a randomized double blind study[7] we compared lactose enemas
plus placebo tablets versus neomycin tablets plus starch enemas in
a group of 18 patients with acute PSE. Ten patients were randomized
to receive starch enemas (10%; 1000 ml tid) plus neomycin tablets

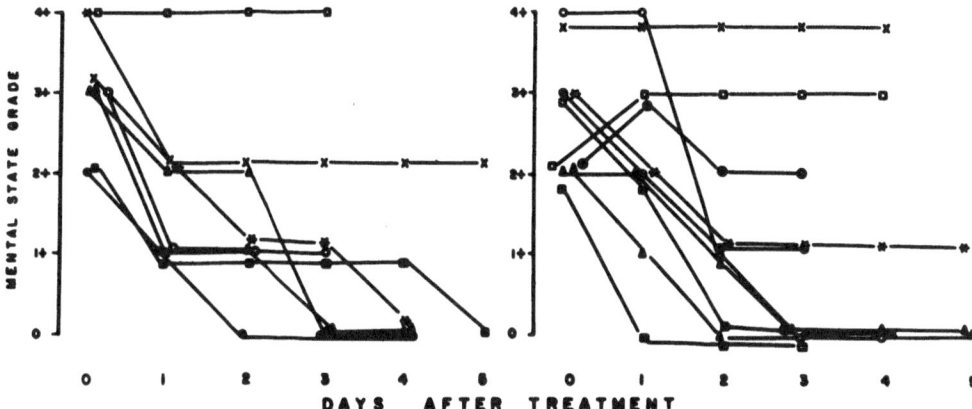

Fig. 3.   Changes in mental state as blindly evaulated after starch
enemas-neomycin (right) and lactose enemas (left). Each
symbol represents 1 patient.

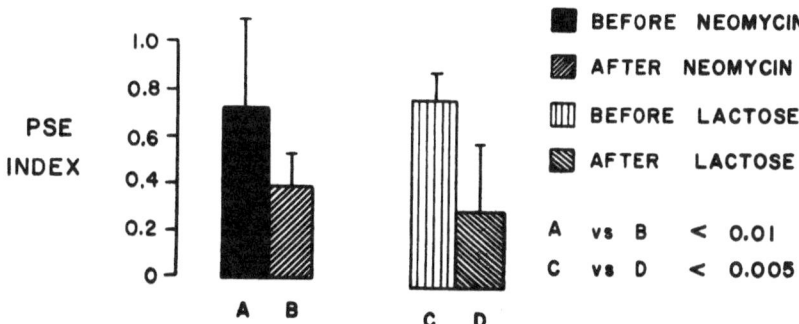

Fig. 4.   Effect of starch enemas-neomycin and lactose enemas-placebo
tablets on PSE Index.

(3 g/day) and 8 patients received lactose enemas (20%; 1000 ml tid)
plus placebo tablets.

Clinical improvement was observed in 7 of 8 patients treated
with lactose enemas (87%) and mental state significantly improved
from 2.8+0.8 to 0.8+1.4 (p < 0.025). A similar response was obtained

with starch enemas plus neomycin (Figure 3). Five patients of each
group were discharged with normal mental state (grade I). In all
patients who responded to lactose enemas, one grade of mental state
improvement was noticeable within the first 25 h.

After both treatments mental state, EEGs, asterixis, number
connection tests and blood ammonia significantly improved. The combination of PSE parameters as determined by the PSE index, significantly improved from $0.72 + 0.38$ ($p < 0.01$) after neomycin and from
$0.8 + 0.1$ to 0.32 ($p < 0.005$) after lactose enemas (Figure 4). Stool
pH decreased from $6.0 + 0.8$ to $4.8 + 1.0$ after lactose enemas.
Changes in stool pH after starch-neomycin therapy were non significant (Figure 5).

This study demonstrated the possibility of using lactose enemas
in acute PSE in patients with lactose tolerance. In this study, 50%
of patients were lactose intolerant and 50% were lactose tolerant.

COMMENTS

As occurs with lactulose, lactose may exert its beneficial
effect by lowering intestinal pH, reducing the absorption of unionized
ammonia and favoring the growth of weak ammonia producing bacteria.
The sugar may serve as a substrate in increasing bacterial assimi-
lation of ammonia. The sugar may reduce deamination of nitrogenous
compounds and also, by incuding osmotic diarrhea it may decrease
the transit time available both for production and absorption of
ammonia.

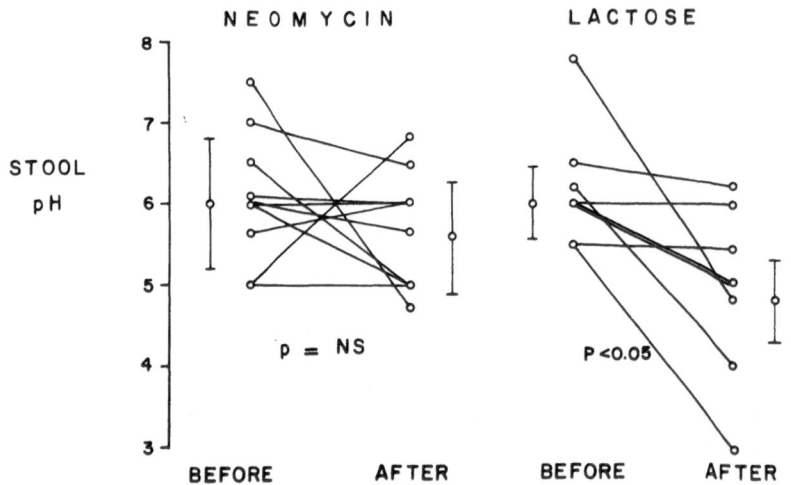

Fig. 5. Changes in stool pH after treatment with starch enemas
         neomycin and lactose enemas-placebo.

Caution With Simultaneous Disaccharides Antacid Administration

In a controlled study the administration of commonly used antacids diminished the intensity of both lactose and lactulose induced effects and in some patients prevented stool acidification which is the base of sugars' therapeutic effect.[8]

REFERENCES

1. C. E. Atterbury, W. C. Maddrey, and H. O. Conn, Neomycin-sorbitol and lactulose in the treatment of acute portal systemic encephalopathy, Am. J. Dig. Dis. 23: 398 (1978).
2. H. O. Conn, C. M. Leevy, and Z. R. Vlahczevic, Comparison of lactulose and neomycin in the treatment of chronic portal systemic encephalopathy, Gastroenterology 72: 573 (1977).
3. T. Gilat, Lactase deficiency: the world pattern today, Israel J. Med. Sci. 15: 369 (1979).
4. H. Lewis, S. Rojas, and M. Uribe, Similar effect of lactose and lactulose on in vitro fecal ammonia generation and bacterial flora. (Abstr.) Gastroenterology 78: 1206 (1980).
5. M. Uribe, M. A. Marquez, and R. G. Garcìa, Treatment of chronic portal systemic encephalopathy with lactose in lactase deficient patients, Dig. Dis. Sci. 25: 924 (1980).
6. J. M. Bond and M. D. Levitt, Investigation of small transite time utilizing pulmonary hydrogen (H_2) measurements, J. Lab. Clin. Med. 85: 546 (1979).
7. M. Uribe, J. Moreno-Berthier, and H. Lewis, Lactose enemas plus placebo tablets versus neomycin tablets plus starch enemas in acute portal systemic encephalopathy, Gastroenterology 81: 101 (1981).
8. M. Uribe and H. O. Conn, Effect of antacids on intestinal response and stool acidification induced by lactose and lactulose in lactose intolerant subjects, Gastroenterology 82: 1248 (1982).

DO BRANCHED-CHAIN AMINO ACIDS HAVE A ROLE IN THE TREATMENT OF

HEPATIC ENCEPHALOPATHY?

L. S. Eriksson and J. Wahren

Departments of Medicine and Clinical Physiology,
Huddinge University Hospital, S-141 86 Stockholm, Sweden

INTRODUCTION

The last decade has witnessed a dramatic growth of interest in
the administration of branched-chain amino acids as a possible therapy
in patients with liver cirrhosis and hepatic encephalopathy. These
patients show elevated levels of the aromatic amino acids (tyrosine,
phenylalanine and tryptophan) as well as methionine, while the concentrations of the branched-chain amino acids (BCAA) leucine, isoleucine and valine are decreased.[1,2,3] The aromatic amino acids are
of particular interest since they serve as precursors for the physiological neurotransmitters norepinephrine, dopamine and serotonin.
Moreover, they compete with the BCAA for transport across the blood-
brain barrier via the same transport system, the L-system.[4] As a
result of the increased availability of aromatic amino acids, the
reduced levels of BCAA and probably also an augmented permeability
of the blood-brain barrier,[5] the brain uptake of aromatic amino
acids may increase. This in turn has been suggested to result in the
formation of "false" neurotransmitters such as octopamine and phenylethanolamine.[6] These amines are less biologically active than the
physiological neurotransmitters and are thought to accumulate and
displace the latter, thereby causing cerebral dysfunction.

Influence of BCAA Administration on Amino Acid Metabolism

In accordance with the "false" neurotransmitter hypothesis it
has been suggested that normalization of the amino acid pattern in
patients with liver cirrhosis and encephalopathy may exert a beneficial effect by reducing the brain influx of aromatic amino acids.
In this context, administration of amino acid mixtures enriched in
BCAA has been proposed.[7,8] These mixtures have contained not only

287

the BCAA but also small amounts of other amino acids, among these
methionine and phenylalanine. Since these two amino acids are both
increased in plasma in cirrhotic patients and it is desirable to
lower their levels, it could be an advantage to use a solution containing just the BCAA.

A recent study demonstrated that intravenous administration of
leucine alone, resulting in a six-fold rise in its arterial concentration, was accompanied by a pronounced decrease in the blood
levels of the aromatic amino acids and methionine in healthy
subjects.[9] In contrast, valine infusion resulted in only a slight
decrease in tyrosine concentration, and isoleucine administration
gave no significant changes in amino acid concentrations.[10] (Figure
1). Thus, of the three BCAA, leucine was by far the most effective
in influencing the amino acid pattern in blood. However, during
leucine infusion, lowered concentrations were seen not only for
tyrosine, phenylalanine and methionine but also for valine and
isoleucine. As mentioned in the introduction, the latter two amino
acids are already low in the cirrhotic patients. Therefore, it was
suggested that a mixture consisting mainly of leucine (70%) but also
small amounts of valine and isoleucine (20% and 10%, respectively)
might be employed in patients with hepatic encephalopathy.[10]

The metabolic effects of a mixed BCAA solution - composed as
described above - were studied in patients with documented liver
cirrhosis but without clinical signs of encephalopathy and the
results were compared to those obtained in a group of healthy volunteers.[11] The BCAA solution was given as an intravenous infusion
(300 μmol/min) for 150 min. In the basal state the patients demonstrated the characteristic changes in amino acid pattern; the concentrations of the three BCAA were 20-30% lower than in the healthy
controls, while the levels of tyrosine (+115%), phenylalanine (+30%)
and methionine (+50%) were increased (Figure 2). Interestingly, the
whole blood determinations used in this study revealed a marked
reduction (-75%) in the concentration of aspartic acid as compared
to the healthy controls (Figure 2). Together with the increased
plasma levels of aspartate previously reported[3] this suggests a
partial depletion of aspartate from the intracellular space in cirrhotic patients. Since aspartate serves as a nitrogen donor in the
urea cycle, an intracellular aspartate depletion might be limiting
for the ammonia detoxification. Furthermore, since aspartate is an
excitatory brain neurotransmitter,[12] its low blood concentration
could have a direct implication for the etiology of hepatic coma.

The brain exchange of amino acids was also examined in the basal
state and during BCAA infusion. Catheters were introduced percuta-
neously into an artery and a jugular vein in both patients and controls. The brain uptake of amino acids could be estimated on the
basis of the arterio-venous concentration differences. In the basal
state, both groups showed an uptake of all three BCAA, glutamine,

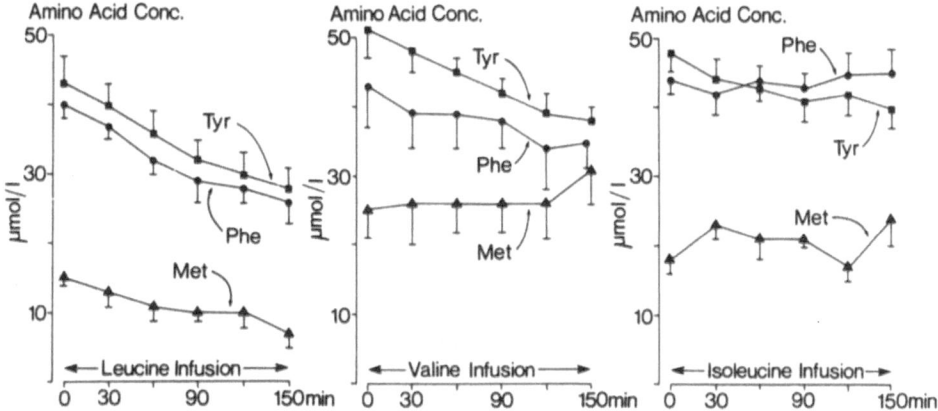

Fig. 1. Changes in concentrations of individual amino acids in
response to intravenous infusion of leucine (300 μmol/min),
valine (600 μmol/min) and isoleucine (150 μmol/min),
respectively, in healthy subjects. Mean ± SE are indicated.

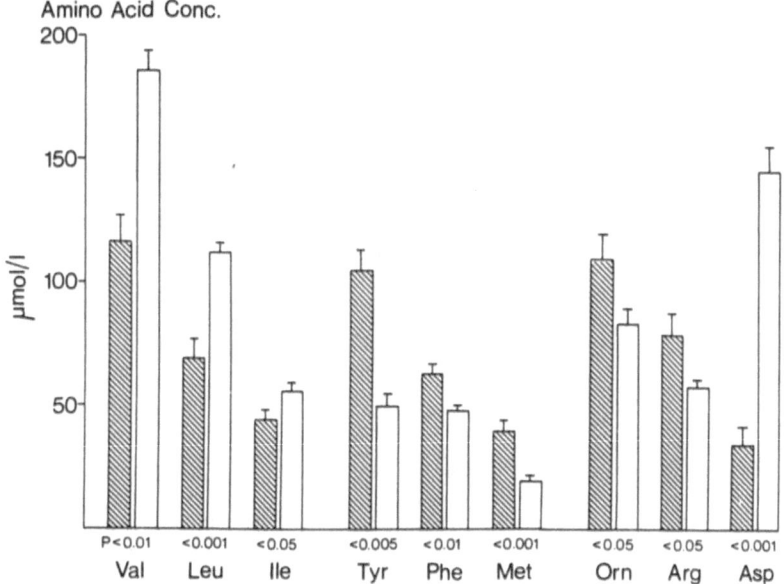

Fig. 2. Arterial whole-blood amino acid concentrations in the basal
state in patients with liver cirrhosis (hatched bars) and
in controls (open bars). Mean ± SE are shown.

serine and lysine, while an uptake of tyrosine and phenylalanine
was found in the patients only. It is noteworthy that the uptake of
the BCAA was similar in both groups; the lower arterial concentra-

tions in the patients was compensated by an increased brain fractio-
nal extraction for BCAA, suggesting an increased blood-brain barrier
permeability in the patients, as previously demonstrated in portacaval shunted animals.[5] Moreover, it is of interest that the patients
showed a net brain uptake of glutamine rather than a release, as
previously suggested on the basis of animal experiments.[13] During
the BCAA infusion the arterial levels of aromatic amino acids decreased (Figure 3) and the BCAA concentrations increased in parallel
with those of the controls. The brain uptake of leucine increased
two- to three-fold in both groups and was significantly higher (50%,
$P < 0.05$) in the patients than the controls. The basal uptake of
tyrosine seen in the patients was abolished during BCAA infusion
(Figure 4) and the controls displayed a similar tendency. This was
also the case for phenylalanine and methionine. In addition, histidine uptake in the patients was inhibited during the BCAA infusion.

These findings thus demonstrate that in patients with liver
cirrhosis an increase in the blood concentration of aromatic amino
acids is accompanied by an augmented brain uptake of these amino
acids. Moreover, the observations show that an elevation of the BCAA
concentrations results in a diminished brain uptake of aromatic amino
acids, primarily of tyrosine. Thus, with respect to amino acid
transport kinetics, the above findings go along with the theory of
"false" neurotransmitters. In addition, the results suggest that
administration of the BCAA solution employed in this study may possibly be of therapeutic value in patients with liver cirrhosis and
encephalopathy.

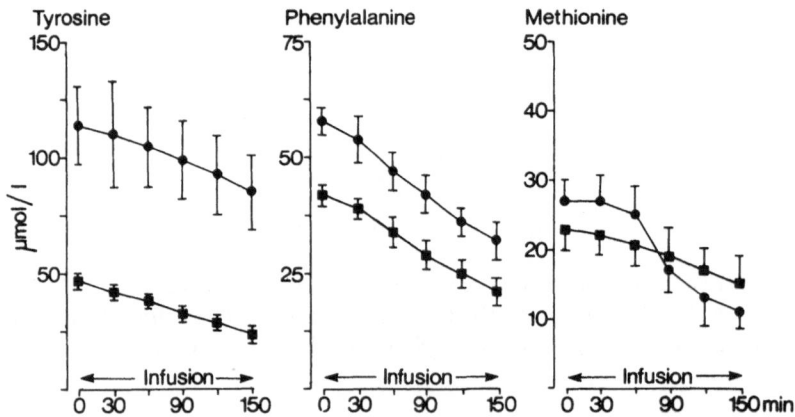

Fig. 3.   Decrease in tyrosine, phenylalanine and methionine concen-
          trations in cirrhotic patients (●) and in healthy controls
          (■) during BCAA infusion. Mean ± SE are indicated.

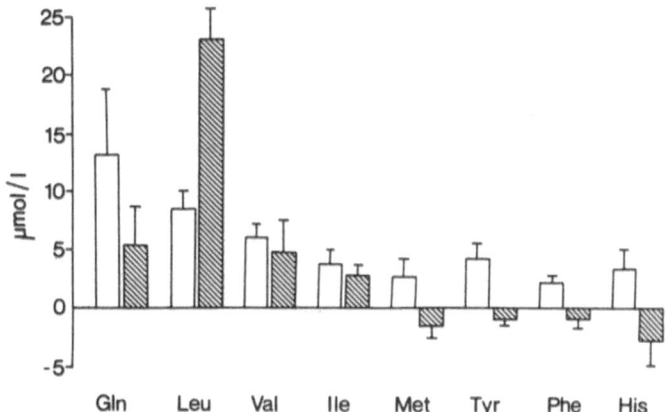

Fig. 4. Brain exchange of amino acids in patients with liver cirrhosis in the basal state (open columns) and during BCAA
infusion (hatched columns). Column height represents
arterial-jugular venous concentration difference.

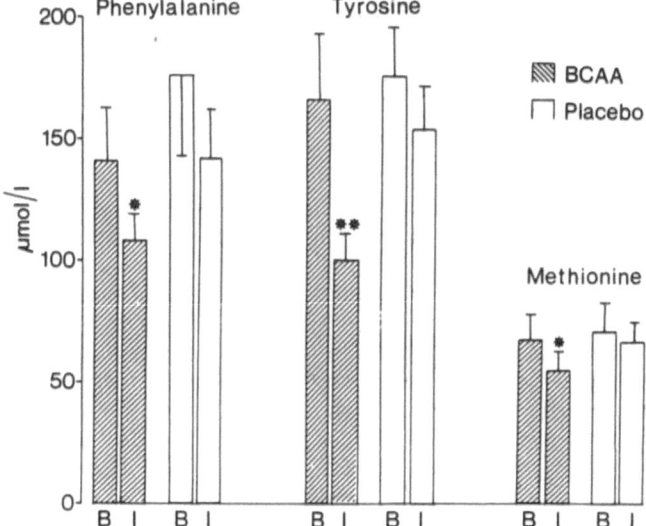

Fig. 5. Amino acid concentrations in patients with hepatic encephalopathy receiving BCAA (hatched columns) or placebo (open
columns) before (B) and during treatment (I). Asterisks
denote the probability that differences are caused by
random factors.

BCAA Administration in Acute Hepatic Coma

The possible beneficial effect of the mixed BCAA solution in patients with liver cirrhosis and acute hepatic coma has been investigated in a multicenter study involving four medical centers in France – Paris, Lille, Montpellier and Marseille – and one in Sweden, Huddinge.[14]

In this study a double blind, randomized design was used. BCAA (70% leucine, 20% valine and 10% isoleucine; 20 g/l in 5.5% glucose) or placebo (5.5% glucose) was given i.v. for 20 hours a day. Nutritional support was provided with equal proportions of carbohydrate and fat (Intralipid). Patients were accepted to the study if they had a history of liver cirrhosis and acute encephalopathy grade II or more, as disclosed at two consecutive neurological examinations with at least a 6-hour interval. Patients with massive gastrointestinal bleeding (requiring more than two units of blood), uremia, sepsis or respiratory insufficiency were excluded from the study. The treatment was continued for a maximum of five days or until the patient woke up.

A total of 52 patients were included in the study; 31 were in grade IV encephalopathy, 19 in grade III and 2 in grade II. When the treatment code was broken it turned out that 27 patients, 13 females and 14 males, had received placebo. The BCAA group was somewhat older than the placebo group (60 $\pm$ 2 and 52 $\pm$ 2 years, respectively; P <0.05) but otherwise no differences were seen between the two groups with regard to the etiology of the cirrhosis, laboratory findings, the grading of encephalopathy, precipitating factors or number of patients with ascites.

Samples for determination of plasma amino acid concentrations were taken before the trial and in the morning of each day during the study. Figure 5 illustrates the effect of the BCAA administration on plasma levels of phenylalanine, tyrosine and methionine. Before the trial these amino acids were elevated in both groups. In the group receiving BCAA infusion the concentrations of all three amino acids decreased significantly, while no similar decline was seen in the group receiving placebo. With regard to the BCAA levels, only minor changes were noted after the BCAA infusion. This seemingly surprising finding is most likely explained by the fact that the samples for amino acid analysis were taken 4 hours after the end of infusions. Previous studies have demonstrated that the concentrations of the three BCAA decline rapidly after the end of a BCAA infusion (Figure 6), although the reductions in levels of aromatic amino acids and methionine persisted for several hours.[10] It is therefore probable that the BCAA levels were in fact elevated during the 20 hours of BCAA infusion and that this rise caused the observed fall in the concentrations of aromatic amino acids.

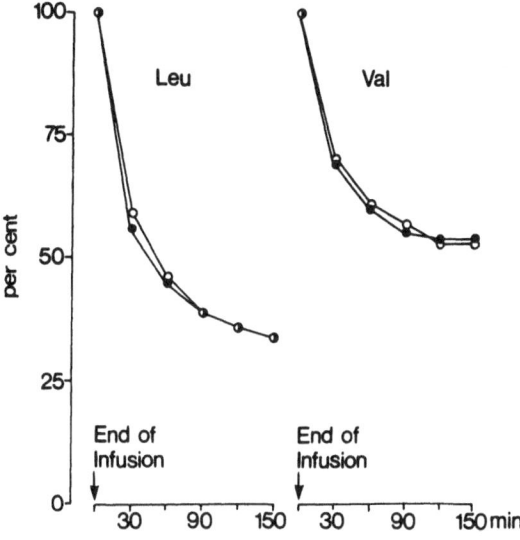

Fig. 6. Disappearance rates for leucine and valine in patients with
         liver cirrhosis (●) and in healthy controls (o) after the
         end of BCAA infusion.

In spite of the observed amino acid changes, the results for
clinical grading and EEG did not differ between the BCAA-treated
group and the placebo group. Thus, 14 of 27 patients in the BCAA
group and 12 of 25 in the placebo group improved during the treatment
(n.s.). Moreover, the number of patients who died during the course
of the trial was significantly greater in the BCAA group - 13 of 27
as compared to 5 of 25 in the placebo group (P < 0.05). The immediate
cause of death varied (gastrointestinal bleeding, infection, etc.).
However, when factors other than encephalopathy were excluded, a
higher mortality rate still remained in the BCAA-treated patients.
Clearly, these results from a controlled clinical trial contrast
those previously obtained under less rigorously controlled circumstances[8,15,16,17] and render no support for the notion that administration of BCAA to patients with liver coma may be beneficial.

Oral Administration of BCAA to Patients with Chronic Encephalopathy

In a recent report of a single case, it was suggested that
ingestion of a diet enriched in BCAA may improve cerebral function
in patients with chronic encephalopathy.[18] In order to evaluate the
possible effect of oral BCAA administration in patients with chronic
encephalopathy in a more systematic manner, a randomized, double-
blind, crossover study was designed.[19] Seven patients with hepatic
encephalopathy of grade I or II were treated with a mixture of either
BCAA or placebo (maltodextrine) for 14 days each. The crystalline

BCAA mixture (70% leucine, 20% valine, 10% isoleucine) was dispensed
in sachets (7.5 g BCAA) and taken orally as powder dissolved in
orange juice four times daily, 30 g/day. Before and after each treatment period the patients cerebral function was examined by clinical
evaluation, EEG recording and psychometric testing.

     Five patients showed improvement clinically as well as in their
psychometric test results during the first treatment period. The
improvement occurred regardless of whether the patients received
BCAA or placebo and was probably an effect of hospitalization and
increased clinical attention. For the psychometric tests, part of
the improvement may be related to learning or recognition of the
test situation, although different tests were used on each occasion.
However, a comparison of the results from the psychometric tests and
EEG as well as the clinical status for the BCAA and placebo periods
respectively, failed to indicate significant differences (Table 1),
suggesting no beneficial effect of BCAA over placebo. Likewise, in
four patients treated with BCAA for an additional period of three to
five months after the double-blind period, clinical evaluation and
psychometric tests continued to show no further improvement in cerebral function.

     The plasma amino acid levels were determined in the fasting
state before and once or twice weekly during the trial. In the basal
state a characteristic pattern of low BCAA and increased phenylalanine, tyrosine and methionine concentrations was observed. However,
no consistent changes were noted during either of the two treatment
periods. The BCAA levels were as low during BCAA administration as
during the placebo period. In order to verify an adequate uptake of
BCAA from the gastrointestinal tract, the plasma amino acid and
ammonia concentrations were studied in five patients before and for
three hours after oral intake of 7.5 g of BCAA. After 60 min the
BCAA concentrations had increased 200-800%; one to two hours later
they had returned to the basal levels. Tyrosine, phenylalanine and
methionine levels fell progressively during the 3 hours of observation (Figure 7). This pattern thus resembles that seen during intravenous BCAA infusion[19] and the results imply that the effect of oral
intake on amino acid levels is similar to that of intravenous BCAA
administration. The ammonia levels were unchanged throughout the
three hours of observation.

     The rapid decline in BCAA levels after oral intake is intriguing,
since it could mean that a possible effect of oral BCAA was so brief
that it may not give rise to a consistent lowering of the aromatic
amino acid levels. Therefore one of the patients was studied before
and during four days of continuous i.v. BCAA infusion (30 g/day).
The plasma concentrations of valine, isoleucine, methionine and phenylalanine normalized during the infusion, while leucine levels were
three times higher than in normal controls. In spite of this, no
improvement was seen in the patient's clinical status, EEG or psycho-

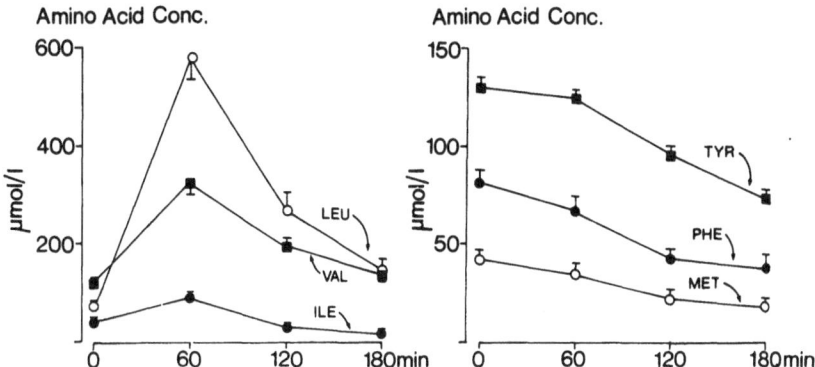

Fig. 7.   Venous plasma amino acid concentrations following the in-
          gestion of 7.5 g of BCAA. Data are given as mean + SE.

metric test results.

      It should be noted that despite an extra amino nitrogen load
of 30 g daily, the patients with chronic encephalopathy did not
deteriorate during the BCAA intake. Although no comparable increase
in mixed protein ingestion was given during the placebo period it
is possible that BCAA were in fact less toxic than an isonitroge-
nous load of protein. These considerations together with the unal-
tered ammonia concentration during the absorption studies, indicate
that BCAA may constitute a means of increasing nitrogen intake in
cirrhotic patients without causing a deterioration in encephalopathy.
This is in agreement with recent results comparing a BCAA-enriched
diet with dietary protein in cirrhotic patients. On the other hand,
the present data clearly indicate that the BCAA regimen fails to
improve cerebral function in the present group of patients with
chronic encephalopathy.

Biochemical Alterations vs Clinical Findings after BCAA Administration

      The present studies demonstrate that intravenous and oral admi-
nistration of BCAA are both accompanied by reduced blood levels of
aromatic amino acids and, most likely, also by a decreased brain
uptake of these amino acids in patients with acute and chronic encephalopathy. Yet, in neither patient-group can an improved cerebral
function be detected. Similar results were reported in another
controlled trial employing a BCAA-enriched amino acid solution in
hepatic coma patients. Moreover, in patients with chronic encephalopathy, crossover studies with either oral or intravenous administration of BCAA enriched solutions (F080) have proven equally

Table 1.   Psychometric Test Results in Patients with
           Chronic PSE

Test	Before treatment	After BCAA	After Placebo
Trail making A (Sec)	90 + 9	59 + 9**	53 + 12*
Trail making B (Sec)	142 + 8	127 +15	126 + 15
Colour Test (Sec)	76 +16	58 +16	54 + 16
Digit Symbol (No. correct)	49 +14	62 +14*	65 + 13**

*P < 0.05, **P < 0.01 as compared with the corresponding
measurement before treatment.

negative with regard to amelioration of the cerebral symptoms.[22,23]
These findings are at variance with the notion that the altered
amino acid metabolism seen in the encephalopatic patients bears a
simple relationship to the pathogenesis of hepatic encephalopathy
as suggested by the "false" neurotransmitter hypothesis. In fact,
recent measurements of brain concentrations of norepinephrine and
octopamine showed no differences between patients with hepatic encephalopathy and controls.[24] Consequently, other already established
or as yet undiscovered metabolic alterations may be of greater importance in the etiology of the disturbed brain function in this disorder.

     It might be argued that the absence of any beneficial effect of
BCAA administration in the hepatic coma patients could have to do
with the fact that they received a fat emulsion as part of their
nutritional support.[25] Theoretically, this could raise the concentration of free fatty acids and cause a displacement of tryptophan
from their common binding sites on albumin. This in turn would augment
the free tryptophan levels in plasma resulting in an increased brain
uptake with a possible deleterious effect on brain neurotransmitter
synthesis and brain function. However, this is unlikely to be of importance since in the present as well as the previously reported
study both the BCAA and the placebo-treated patients received the
fat emulsion.[21] In addition, direct measurements of tryptophan in
plasma of 15 patients with acute hepatic encephalopathy did not show
any significant change in either free tryptophan levels or in the free
to total tryptophan ratio before and during infusion of fat emulsion.

Acknowledgements

     This study was supported by grants from the Swedish Medical
Research Council (No. 3108), the Petrus and Augusta Hedlund Founda-
tion and the Karolinska Institute. The amino acid mixtures were generously supplied by KabiVitrum AB, Stockholm, Sweden.

REFERENCES

1. F. L. Iber, H. Rosen, S. M. Levenson, and T. C. Chalmers, The
    plasma amino acids in patients with liver failure, J. Lab.
    Clin. Med. 50: 417 (1957).
2. V. Iob, W. W. Coon, and M. Sloan, Free amino acids in liver,
    plasma, and muscle of patients with cirrhosis of the liver,
    J. Surg. Res. 7: 41 (1967).
3. J. E. Fischer, N. Yoshimura, A. Aguirre, J. H. James, M. G.
    Cummings, R. M. Abel, and F. Deindoerfer, Plasma amino acids
    in patients with hepatic encephalopathy. Effect of amino
    acid infusions, Am. J. Surg.127: 40 (1974).
4. D. L. Oxender and H. N. Christiansen, Distinct mediating systems
    for the transport of neutral amino acids by the Ehrlich cell,
    J. Biol. Chem. 238: 3686 (1963).
5. J. H. James, J. Escourrou, and J. E. Fischer, Blood-brain neutral
    amino acid transport activity is increased after portacaval
    anastomosis, Science 200: 1395 (1978).
6. J. E. Fischer and R. J. Baldessarini, False neurotransmitters
    and hepatic failure, Lancet ii: 75 (1971).
7. J. E. Fischer and R. J. Baldessarini, Pathogenesis and therapy
    of hepatic coma, in: "Progress in Liver Diseases," Popper
    and Schaffner, eds., Grune & Stratton, New York (1976).
8. J. E. Fischer, H. M. Rosen, A. M. Ebeid, J. H. James, J. M.
    Keane,and P. B. Soeters, The effect of normalization of plasma
    amino acids on hepatic encephalopathy in man, Surgery 80: 77
    (1976).
9. L. Hagenfeldt, S. Eriksson, and J. Wahren, Influence of leucine
    on arterial concentrations and regional exchange of amino
    acids in healthy subjects, Clin. Sci. 59: 173 (1980).
10. S. Eriksson, L. Hagenfeldt, and J. Wahren, Intravenous infusion
    of α-ketoisocaproate - influence on amino acid and nitrogen
    metabolism in patients with liver cirrhosis, Clin. Sci. 62:
    285 (1981).
11. Y. Sato, S. Eriksson, L. Hagenfeldt, and J. Wahren, Influence
    of branched-chain amino acid infusion on arterial concentra-
    tions and brain exchange of amino acids in patients with
    hepatic cirrhosis, Clin. Physiol. 1: 151 (1981).
12. K. Krnjević, Chemical nature of synaptic transmission in verte-
    brates, Physiol. Rev. 54: 418 (1974).
13. J. H. James, V. Ziparo, B. Jeppsson, and J. E. Fischer, Hype-
    rammonaemia, plasma amino acid imbalance, and blood-brain

aminoacid transport: a unified theory of portal-systemic encephalopathy, Lancet ii: 772 (1979).

14.   J. Wahren, P. Denis, P. Desurmont, L. S. Eriksson, J.-M. Escoffier, A. P. Gauthier, L. Hagenfeldt, H. Michel, P. Opolon, J. C. Paris, and M. Veyrac, Is intravenous administration of branched chain amino acids effective in the treatment of hepatic encephalopathy? Hepatology, submitted (1983).

15.   E. Holm, J. P. Striebel, E. Meisinger, P. Haux, W. Langhans, and H. D. Becker, Aminosäurengemische zur parenteralen Ernährung bei Leberinsuffiziens, Infusionstherapie 5: 274 (1978).

16.   T. C. F. Aguilar and J. L. M. Picouto, Nutriciòn parenteral en 29 enfermos afectos de encefalopatia hepàtica tratodos con F.080, Rev. Clin. Esp. 155: 355 (1979).

17.   H. Freund, J. Dienstag, J. Lehrich, N. Yoshimura, R. R. Bradford, R. Rosen, S. Atamian, E. Slemmer, J. Holroyde, and J. E. Fischer, Infusion of branched-chain enriched amino acid solution in patients with hepatic encephalopathy, Ann. Surg. 196: 209 (1982).

18.   H. Freund, N. Yoshimura, and J. E. Fischer, Chronic hepatic encephalopathy. Long-term therapy with a branched-chain amino-acid-enriched elemental diet, JAMA 242: 347 (1979).

19.   L. S. Eriksson, A. Persson, and J. Wahren, Branched-chain amino acids in the treatment of chronic encephalopathy, Gut 23: 801 (1982).

20.   D. Horst, N. Grace, H. O. Conn, E. Schiff, S. Schenker, A. Viteri, D. Law, and C. E. Atterbury, A double-blind randomized comparison of dietary protein and an oral branched chain amino acid (BCAA) supplement in cirrhotic patients with chronic portal-systemic encephalopathy. Annual Meeting of the American Association for the Study of Liver Diseases, Abstract 288 (1981).

21.   H. Michel, G. Pomier-Layrargues, O. Duhamel, B. Lacombe, G. Cuilleret, and H. Bellet, Intravenous infusion of ordinary and modified amino acid solutions in the management of hepatic encephalopathy (controlled study, 30 patients). Abstract, Gastroenterol. 79: 1038 (1980).

22.   W. J. Millikan, J. M. Henderson, W. D. Warren, S. P. Riepe, M. H. Kutner, L. Wright, J. Ziffer, and R. B. Parks, Total parenteral nutrition with F080 in cirrhotics with subclinical encephalopathy, Ann. Surg.(1982) in press.

23.   A. McGhee, J. M. Henderson, W. J. Millikan, J. C. Bleier, M. Kassouny, R. Vogel, and D. Rudman, Comparison of the effects of hepatic-aid and a casein modular diet on encephalopathy, plasma amino acids, and nitrogen balance in cirrhotic patients, Ann. Surg, in press (1982).

24.   G. Cuilleret, G. Pomier-Layrargues, F. Pons, J. Cadilhac, and H.

Michel, Changes in brain catecholamine levels in human cirrhotic hepatic encephalopathy, J. Brit. Soc. Gastroent. 21: 565 (1980).

25. J. E. Fischer, Amino acids in hepatic coma, Dig. Dis. Sci 27: 97 (1982).

TREATMENT OF HEPATIC ENCEPHALOPATHY BY INFUSION OF A MODIFIED AMINO

ACID SOLUTION: RESULTS OF A CONTROLLED STUDY IN 47 CIRRHOTIC PATIENTS

H. Michel, G. Pomier-Layrargues, J. P. Aubin, P. Bories,
D. Mirouze, H. Bellet-Hermann

Clinique des Maladies de l'Appareil Digestif and Laboratoire de Biochimie B, Hôpital Saint-Eloi, Montpellier
France

INTRODUCTION

The mechanism of hepatic encephalopathy (HE) is still unknown.
A characteristic amino acid pattern in HE has been described: an
increased level of plasma free tryptophan, a fall in plasma branched
chain amino acids (BCAA) valine, leucine and isoleucine and a rise
in plasma aromatic amino acids (AAA) phenylalanine and tyrosine.[1]
The brain uptake of AAA would increase; the ensuing depletion of
brain dopamine and norepinephrine and increase of brain octopamine,
which is considered as a false neurotransmitter, would result in
perturbation of cerebral neurotransmission.[2]

Infusion of modified amino acid solutions, with high levels of
BCAA and low levels of AAA can normalize the deranged plasma amino
acid pattern found in HE, especially the $\frac{BCAA}{AAA}$ molar ratio.

Such solutions are thought to be of value in the treatment of
HE as shown by several reports.[3-10] But, to our knowledge, there
are no published controlled clinical trials that demonstrate convincingly the efficacy of this treatment. The purpose of our study
will be to investigate the validity of such a therapeutic approach.

MATERIALS AND METHODS

Patients

47 patients with liver cirrhosis were admitted in the trial.
Cirrhotic patients with HE and uncontrolled gastrointestinal bleeding or HE and renal failure with anuria were excluded from the

301

study. Diagnosis of cirrhosis was confirmed by peritoneoscopy with
or without liver biopsy, or post mortem examination. The aetiology
of the cirrhosis was chronic alcoholism in 39 patients, chronic
infection with B virus in 4 patients, chronic biliary tract obstruc-
tion in 1 patient. In 3 patients, cirrhosis was thought to be cryptogenic. All the patients had acute HE as assessed by clinical examination and EEG. HE was secondary to gastro-intestinal bleeding (8
patients), diuretic abuse (7 patients), pneumonia, urinary tract
infection or spontaneous bacterial peritonitis (10 patients). In 22
patients, there were no obvious precipitating factors.

Evaluation of HE

    Clinical signs. The stage of HE was determined twice daily in
the morning and in the afternoon, by the same two physicians (G. P.,
J. P. A.), one day prior to and during the 5 days of treatment. HE
was graded in 3 stages according to the following criteria: stage I
(impending coma), asterixis, abnormal sleeping cycle, occasional
drowsiness, euphoria or depression and ability to maintain sphincter
control; stage II (stupor), asterixis, asleep most of the time but
can be awakened, marked confusion and disorientation; stage III,
asleep all of the time with or without response to painful stimuli.

    EEG evaluation. Each patient received a standard EEG on day 1,
3 and 5 of the treatment: stage I, primarily distinct slow alpha
waves activity with synchronized bilateral theta waves in the frontal leads; stage II, no detectable alpha rhythm, synchronized bilateral theta waves with some monomorphous or polymorphous delta waves
and occasional di-or triphasic spikes, and stage III, numerous di-or
triphasic waves interspersed with bilateral rhythmic fronto-temporal
delta waves.

    Overall assessment of HE evolution was made by the clinical
and EEG staging and classified as follows: improved, unchanged or
deteriorated. The final comparison was made using day 1 and day 5.

Laboratory study

    The following biochemical tests were performed on the first
and fifth day : serum glucose, BUN, electrolytes, bilirubin, ASAT,
alkaline phosphatases, prothrombin level, albumin, globulin, hemoglobin, creatinine. Arterial ammonia was measured by the Berthelot
method.[11] Plasma amino acids were determined with a 121 M Beckman
autoanalyser as previously described.[12] Samples were taken at 8 a.m.,
after the amino acid infusion had been stopped for 30 minutes. After
centrifugation, plasma was quickly frozen until analysis.

Treatment

    Therapy was started 48 hours after admission or within 48 hours of onset of HE when arising during hospitalisation. We felt this 48-hour delay was necessary for two reasons 1) to make the diagnosis of HE, 2) to exclude the least sick patients who spontaneously wake up or the very sick patients who die within 48 hours. All patients received parenteral nutrition consisting of 500 ml of 30% hypertonic dextrose solution, 500 ml of 20% lipid emulsion and one of two amino acid solutions. A total of 1600 calories was administered daily. Patients were randomly assigned into two groups (Table 1). Group I received a commercially available preparation while group II received a modified amino acid solution. The infusions for this second group had the BCAA and glycine concentrations increased by 80% and 50%, while the phenylalanine, methionine and arginine were decreased by 37%, 71% and 50% respectively; tyrosine was absent. This solution was prepared from the appropriate crystallized amino acids, solubilized in sterile distilled water, at the concentrations shown in Table 2. Sterility was assessed by repeated bacteriologic analysis. In both groups, 6.25 g of nitrogen were infused on the first day, 9.12 g on the second and third days, 12.50 g on the fourth and fifth days. The patients received electrolytes as needed: 75 mEq of KCl, 4.9 mEq/l of Ca, 8.2 mEq of Mg 50_4. As the total duration of treatment was short, no vitamins or mineral were deemed necessary. Additional treatment of HE such as neomycin and lactulose was intentionally omitted.

The trial was approved by the Human Experimental Committee in 1978. Informed consent was obtained from the patient or a responsible relative prior to the study.

Statistical analysis

To compare the clinical and EEG staging of the patients before the treatment and at the end of the amino acid infusions, the corrected Chi square test was used. The changes in biochemical values were tested by the Student's t test for within group differences and by the paired t test for between-group differences.[13]

Table 1. Comparison of the groups: clinical characteristics at randomization

	Group I (n = 24)		Group II (n = 23)	
Age (Yrs)	59.9 + 2.4		59.9 + 2.4	
(range)	(32 - 84)		(34 - 78)	
Sex	19 M	5 F	18 M	5 F
Jaundice	15		15	
Ascites	18		18	
G.I. bleeding	3		5	
Infection	5		5	

RESULTS

The 24 patients of group I received a commercially available amino acid solution and the 23 patients of group II received a modified amino acid solution. The 2 groups were identical, with respect to age, sex, previous episodes of HE associated complications and baseline laboratory data except in group II, in which the albumin was significantly lower (Table 3). Clinically, there were no significant differences between the 2 groups neither in the delay between onset of HE and treatment nor the stage of HE at the beginning of the infusions nor the precipitating factors (Table 4).

Clinical efficiency

Concerning the clinical efficiency in the patients of group I (Figure 1) 6 improved, 11 patients experienced no change, in 7 the clinical condition deteriorated. By the end of the study 6 patients were dead: on the third day 1 of these patients had stage I and 1 had stage III HE; death was due to gastrointestinal bleeding. On the fourth day 2 patients had stage III and 1 had stage II HE; death was due to gastrointestinal bleeding,[1] hepatocellular carcinoma[1] and spontaneous bacterial peritonitis.[1] On the fifth day 1 patient had stage III HE and death was due to septicemia. In group II (Figure 2) treated with the modified amino acid solution, 8 patients improved, 8 did not change and 7 deteriorated. By the end of the study 7 patients were dead; on the third day 3 of these had stage III HE and death was due to massive gastrointestinal bleeding in all 3 cases. On the fourth day 1 patient had stage I and 1 had stage III HE and death was due to massive gastrointestinal haemorrhage in one and mesenteric infarction in the other. By the fifth day 1 patient had stage I and 1 had stage III HE and the death was due to gastrointestinal bleeding in one and hepatocellular carcinoma in the other. There was no significant difference between the 2 groups.

Evolution of EEG in the 2 groups did not differ significantly. 13 patients in group I and 12 in group II had no EEG performed on the fifth day, due to mortality or technical unavailability.

Laboratory data

When comparing the biochemical tests at the beginning and at the end of the treatment, there were no significant differences except for the plasma amino acids.

Arterial ammonia. On day 1, arterial ammonia concentration (normal value < 25 µmol/l) was elevated in the 2 groups: 85.6 ± 13.3 µmol/l (mean $\pm$ SEM) in group I, and 75.6 ± 3.1 µmol/l in group II. Infusions of amino acids did not modify these values on day 5:

Table 2. Composition of the two amino acid solutions BCAA: branched chain amino acids; AAA: aromatic amino acids

	Group I (Commercial solution) g/l	Group II (Modified solution) g/l
Essential AA		
L isoleucine	2.55	9
L leucine	6.95	11
L lysine	9.75	7.6
L methionine	4.70	1
L phenylalanine	6.25	1
L threonine	2.50	4.5
L tryptophan	1.30	0.76
L valine	6.25	8.4
Non essential AA		
L alanine	4.75	7.5
L arginine	12.5	6
L histidine	2.5	2.4
L proline	4	8
L serine	0.65	5
L tyrosine	0.12	0
L glycine	4.5	9
L cysteine	0.75	0.4
Total nitrogen	12.50	12.50
BCAA/AAA ratio	2.42	28.4

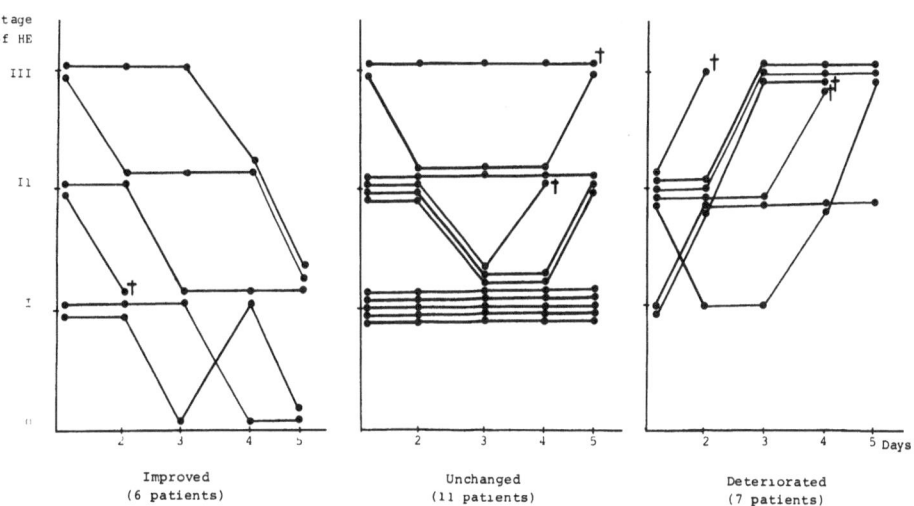

Fig. 1. Clinical efficiency of non modified amino acid solution in HE (group I).

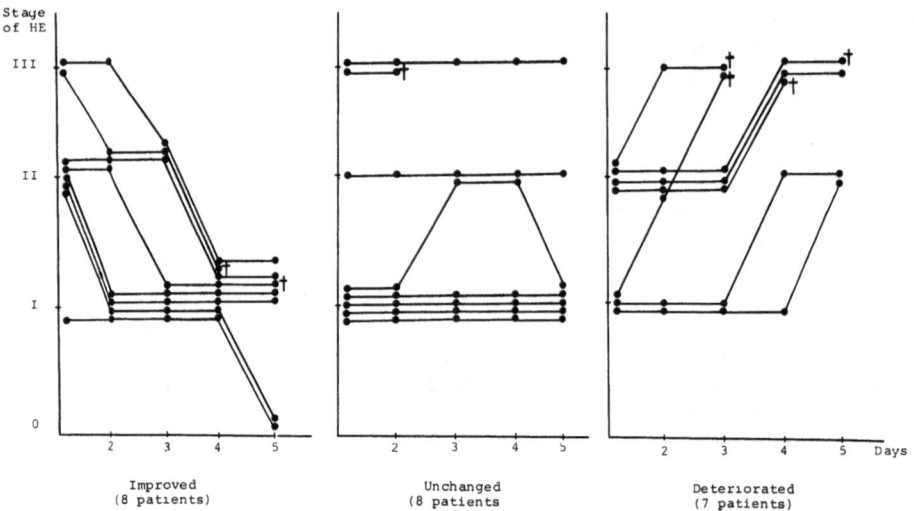

Fig. 2.   Clinical efficiency of modified amino acid solution in HE
          (group II).

Table 3.   Comparison of the groups: laboratory data at rando-
           mization (results are expressed as mean ± SEM)
           *(P < 0.02 (Student's t test).

	Group I (n=24)	Group II (n=23)
Bilirubin (μmoles/1)	73 ± 15	87 ± 15
ASAT (IU)	44.3 ± 4.3	68.6 ± 20
ALAT (IU)	30.4 ± 3.5	43.7 ± 9.3
Albumin*(μmoles/1)	420 ± 116	377 ± 116
Prothrombin (%)	43 ± 4	47 ± 4.6
Hemoglobin (n moles/1)	68.8 ± 2.5	67 ± 3.1
Creatinine (μmoles/1)	150.6 ± 26.5	151.6 ± 17.7
Urea (m moles/1)	10.7 ± 1.5	14 ± 2
Natremia (m moles/1)	130 ± 8	131 ± 6
NH_3 (μmoles/1)	85.6 ± 13.3	75.6 ± 3.1
Nitrogen balance (gN/day)	-12.7 ± 2.3	-10 ± 2.3

82.3 ± 17.8 μmol/1 in group I and 79.8 ± 17.2 μmol/1 in group II.

    Plasma amino acids (Table 5). Before treatment, the plasma
amino acid pattern was identical as those previously described in
cirrhotic patients with HE. BCAA (leucine, valine and isoleucine)
were decreased, AAA (tyrosine and phenylalanine) were increased.

Table 4. Initial clinical pattern of HE

		Group I (n=24)	Group II (n=23)
Stage	I	9	9
	II	11	10
	III	4	4
Precipitating factors	Infection	5	5
	Diuretic	4	3
	G.I. bleeding (moderate)	3	5
	Spontaneous	12	10
Previous episodes			
	0	15	13
	1	5	5
	2	1	1
	unknown	3	4
Delay between onset and treatment (days)*		2.8 ± 0.6	2.7 ± 0.7

*mean $\pm$ SEM.

The molar ratio BCAA/AAA was low. The 2 groups were not significantly different. On the fifth day, patients in group I had a significant increase of valine and phenylalanine. Isoleucine, leucine, tyrosine and the molar ratio BCAA/AAA remained unchanged. Of the patients in group II, valine, leucine and isoleucine were increased significantly. Tyrosine and phenylalanine remained unchanged. Thus, the molar ratio BCAA/AAA increased significantly and was even reversed.

DISCUSSION

HE is a neuropsychiatric disorder resulting from acute or chronic liver failure. To date, the exact mechanism of this syndrome remains unknown.[14] Many authors have reported, in cirrhotic HE, a fall in plasma BCAA and a rise in plasma AAA. These abnormalities would result in a perturbation of the synaptic neurotransmission (false neurotransmitters theory). Several authors have suggested the infusion of modified amino acid solutions with high levels of BCAA and low levels of AAA; this could normalize the plasma amino acid unbalance in HE and result in improvement of the mental state.

Our study clearly demonstrates that such infusions have no beneficial effects on the clinical course of HE in cirrhotic patients, when compared to commercially available solutions. However, modified solutions have induced a rise in plasma BCAA, and a highly significant increase in the BCAA/AAA molar ratio.

Table 5. Plasma amino acid (μmoles/l) before and after therapy values are mean values ± SEM. *Significance of differences between values at randomization and after therapy (paired t test).

	Group I			Group II		
	At randomization	After therapy	P*	At randomization	After therapy	P*
Valine	182 ± 39	344 ± 74	0.05	135 ± 14	586 ± 119	0.001
Leucine	111 ± 23	188 ± 54	NS	85 ± 11	346 ± 78	0.01
Isoleucine	48 ± 6	82 ± 19	NS	50 ± 8	293 ± 83	0.01
Phenylalanine	129 ± 24	232 ± 51	0.05	124 ± 17	112 ± 19	NS
Tyrosine	120 ± 11	126 ± 13	NS	126 ± 16	105 ± 30	NS
Molar ratio BCAA/AAA	1.29 ± 0.12	1.56 ± 0.11	NS	1.15 ± 0.10	6.65 ± 1.72	0.01

In comparison, our results differed from those of previous reports in which improvements of HE occurred with the same modified
amino acid solutions; variability in results might be due to the
project design an approach, to uncontrolled studies, to different
type and small number of patients in some series, to addition of
neomycin and lactulose in the treatment which might account for the
clinical improvements.

CONCLUSION

Infusion of modified amino acid solutions, with high levels of
BCAA and low levels of AAA can normalize and even reverse the deranged plasma amino acids abnormalities but have no beneficial effects
on the clinical course of cirrhotic HE.

REFERENCES

1. H. M. Rosen, N. Yoshimura, J. M. Hodgman, and J. E. Fischer,
   Plasma amino acid patterns in hepatic encephalopathy of differing etiology, Gastroenterology 72: 483 (1977).
2. J. E. Fischer and R. J. Baldessarini, False neurotransmitters
   and hepatic failure, Lancet 2: 75 (1971).
3. J. E. Fischer, H. M. Rosen, A. M. Ebeid, H. J. James, J. M.
   Keane, and P. B. Soeters, The effects of normalization of
   plasma amino acids on hepatic encephalopathy in man, Surgery
   80: 77 (1976).
4. A. Watanabe, A. Takesue, T. Higashi, and N. Nagashima, Serum
   amino acids in hepatic encephalopathy. Effects of branched
   chain amino acid infusion on serum aminogram, Acta Hepato-
   Gastroenterol. 26: 346 (1979).
5. A. Sieg, U. Gartner, J. P. Striebel, G. Lanzinger-Rossnagel,
   B. Kommerell, and P. Czygan, Parenterale amino saürenbehan-
   dlung bei patient en mit leberzirrhose, Inn. Med. 6: 209
   (1979).
6. T. Caparros Fernandez De Aguilar, J. Lopez Martinez, and F. Perez
   Picuoto, Nutricion parenteral en 29 enfermos afectos de
   encefalopatia hepatica tratados con F080, Rev. Clin. Esp.
   155: 355 (1979).
7. G. Kleinberger, R. Kotzaurek, H. Pall, M. Pichler, and S. Sze-
   less, Parenterale erährung bei coma hepaticum, Leber. Mogen.
   Darim. 6: 340 (1976).
8. P. Ferenci and F. Wewalka, Parenterale ernährung von patienten
   mit leberzirrhose mit hepatïsher enzephalopathie, Infusionsther Klin. Ernähr. 7: 72 (1980).
9. F. Fiaccadori, F. Ghinelli, G. Pelosi, D. Sacchini, G. L. Vaona,
   M. L. Zeneroli, E. Rocchi, V. Santunione, P. Gibertini, and
   E. Ventura, Selective amino acid solutions in hepatic encephalopathy treatment. (A preliminary report), La Ricerca
   Clin. Lab. 10: 411 (1980).

10. H. J. Reiter and J. C. Bode, Parenteral application of a special amino acid solution in the treatment of severe hepatic encephalopathy, Z. Gastroenterol. 16: 457 (1978).

11. G. Dropsy and J. Boy, Determination de l'ammoniémie (méthode automatique par dialyse), An. Biol. Clin. 19: 313 (1961).

12. D. H. Spackman, W. H. Stein, and R. Moore, Automatic recording apparatus for use in the chromatography of amino acids, Anal. Chem. 30: 1190 (1958).

13. G. W. Snedecor and W. G. Cochran, "Statistical Methods" sixth edition, Ames, Iowa, State University Press (1967).

14. L. Zieve, Hepatic encephalopathy: Summary of present knowledge with an elaboration on recent developments, in: "Progress in Liver Diseases," Vol. V, Grune and Stratton, New York, pp. 327-339 (1979).

EFFICACY OF BRANCHED-CHAIN AMINO ACIDS

IN THE TREATMENT OF HEPATIC ENCEPHALOPATHY

J. E. Fischer

Department of Surgery, University of Cincinnati

Medical Center, Cincinnati, Ohio

INTRODUCTION

A. Rationale

All therapy in patients with liver disease is a play for time,
until the well-known regenerative capacity of the liver can occur.
The regenerative capacity of the liver is an extremely complicated
process, involving a series of permissive and stimulatory factors,
such as steroids, triiodothyronine, insulin and glucagon and other
factors, such as the ileal factor, which remain unknown. Of all the
factors that are currently known which influence liver regeneration,
nutrition is the easiest one for the physician to manipulate.
Nutrition in the therapy of patients with liver disease has long been
important in hepatology.

In the surgical setting, the ability to provide nutrition is
complicated, since many of these patients are sick, septic, and
undergo extensive abdominal procedures, the complications of which
may prevent oral nutrition for a prolonged period of time. Under
such circumstances, we have utilized the techniques of hyperalimen-
tation by which amino acid-hypertonic dextrose solutions, with or
without some modicum or fat as a source of essential amino acid or
calories, for nutritional support. In patients with pre-existing
liver disease, it has been our experience in the surgical setting,
that approximately 50%-60% of such patients, even those with grade I
encephalopathy, will tolerate up to 60-80 g of a standard amino acid
mixture. In these patients, nitrogen equilibrium can be achieved, as
well as nutritional support, and there is no necessity for providing
a solution with a specialized amino acid configuration. In patients,
however, with a grade II-IV encephalopathy, or in patients in which

311

standard amino acid solutions are not tolerated, we have utilized a single amino acid configuration, now commercially available as HepatAmine, or previously known as F080(1). This solution is an amino acid solution in which 35% of the amino acids are available as a branched-chain amino acid, valine, leucine or isoleucine, as opposed to the normal 14%-25% in commercially available mixtures. In addition there are decreased amounts of phenylalanine and methionine, as well as increased amounts of arginine and alanine[1].

B. The Role of Branched-Chain Amino Acids in Normal Physiology

Under normal circumstances, the branched-chain amino acids are the only group of amino acids that is largely cleared by the liver following a meal. It has been estimated that between 60%-100% of the splanchnic clearance of amino acids through the liver is in the form of the branched-chain amino acids. Similarly, in a patient in nitrogen equilibrium, it is likely that between 60%-100% of the peripheral exchange of nitrogen is in the form of the branched-chain amino acids, which are utilized either for energy, directly by oxidation, by skeletal muscle and heart, or with energy for protein synthesis.[2] Under normal circumstances, the control of efflux of other amino acids through skeletal muscle is under the influence of exercise,[3] insulin,[4] and other factors, such as glucose,[5] with the plasma concentration of the branched-chain amino acids playing a relatively minor role.[6]

Under circumstances, however, of insulin resistance or catabolism, as in liver disease, it is possible that the branched-chain amino acids which normally make up 6%-7% of the total energy requirements, may have a much more potent role in the efflux of other amino acids through the myocyte membrane.

C. Theoretically Beneficial Effects of the Branched-Chain Amino Acids

There are approximately seven individual, theoretically beneficial, effects of the branched-chain amino acids:

1. As an energy source. Particularly under circumstances when glucose production and ketogenesis are decreased, the branched-chain amino acids which normally make up between 6%-7% of the energy requirements of the skeletal muscle, heart and brain, may theoretically constitute up to 30% of the energy requirement.

2. Under abnormal circumstances, especially when the influence of insulin is decreased, the branched-chain amino acids may regulate the flux of other amino acids across the myocyte membrane.[6]

3. In man, leucine is associated with increased protein synthesis

and decreased breakdown of muscle.[7] In rats, valine appears to be more potent.[8]

4. When given with an energy source, hepatic protein synthesis is increased by all branched-chain amino acids.[8,9]

5. Administration of the branched-chain amino acids decrease aromatic amino acids in plasma by decreased proteolysis, as well as increased protein synthesis. The latter effect requires an energy source, preferably glucose, for the utilization of the branched-chain amino acids.[10]

6. Branched-chain amino acids form the bulk of competition for transport by system-L across the blood brain barrier by competing with the other neutral amino acids, of which toxic aromatic amino acids are a part.

7. It has been demonstrated in hepatectomized animals that administration of the branched-chain amino acids will increase norepinephrine synthesis, specifically in certain brain regions.[11]

8. On a theoretical basis, it is possible that the branched-chain amino acids improve catecholamine synthesis in the periphery.

THE UTILIZATION OF BRANCHED-CHAIN AMINO ACIDS IN PATIENTS WITH LIVER DISEASE

A. Anecdotal Series

Numerous anecdotal series have been published since 1975,[12,13,14,15] in which branched-chain enriched amino acid solutions, usually given with hypertonic dextrose, have been utilized in patients with liver disease or who are intolerant to standard solutions and in hepatic coma. Several conclusions can be drawn from these studies, although conclusions of efficacy are not possible in a disease as variable as hepatic encephalopathy. The conclusions are:

1. In patients who are intolerant to standard solutions, infusions of up to 125 g of a branched-chain enriched amino acid solution for 24 h are well tolerated.

2. In many instances, awakening from hepatic encephalopathy accompanies the infusion of such amino acid solutions.

3. There are two forms of liver disease: fulminant hepatitis with a generalized hyperaminoacidemia, except for the branched-chain amino acids, which are normal. The hyperaminoacidemia, which may be due to release of amino acids from the dying liver, is so severe that infusion techniques alone, although lowering amino acids some-

what, are not sufficient to normalize the plasma amino acid pattern.[12] Perfusion techniques, such as polyacrylonitrile membrane,[16] charcoal, [17] or hemodialysis, are necessary as well.

4. In patients with cirrhosis and chronic exacerbation of encephalopathy due to intercurrent illness, infusion of 80 g/24 h of 35% enriched branched-chain amino acid mixture, such as HepatAmine, is associated with awakening from hepatic encephalopathy, and nitrogen equilibrium, as well as normalization of the plasma amino acid pattern.[15]

However, in a disease as variable as hepatic encephalopathy, only a properly done, randomized, prospective trial will be accepted as showing efficacy. A number of these are now available.

B. Randomized Prospective Trials in the Treatment of Hepatic Encephalopathy with Branched-Chain Amino Acids: Randomization Suspect

A number of such trials have now been reported; all appear to show efficacy for a branched-chain enriched amino acid solution, as compared to standard solutions.[18,19,20] However, the numbers in the various groups make the randomization suspect and suggest that some selection was utilized in which patients went into which groups. Thus they cannot be accepted as properly randomized trials.

C. Prospective Randomized Trials in the Utilization of Branched-Chain Amino Acids in the Treatment of Hepatic Encephalopathy

At present writing, I know of six apparently properly done randomized prospective trials, in which patients were randomized for receiving a branched-chain amino acid solution as against a standard form of therapy. In four of these trials, branched-chain amino acid solutions were combined with a hypertonic dextrose caloric source, but in two, between 60%-70% of the calories were given as intravenous fat. This is the most striking difference between the various studies and their outcome. First, we will discuss the trials in which the branched-chain amino acids are seen to be positive.

A multi-center, randomized prospective trial was reported by Rossi-Fanelli and his coworkers and is repeated elsewhere in this volume.[21] In this group, 40 patients with "acute-on-chronic" hepatic encephalopathy, or chronic recurrence of encephalopathy, were randomized for either receiving isocaloric hypertonic dextrose and lactulose, and the other group 60 g of branched-chain amino acids in isocaloric hypertonic dextrose. Patients were entered within 6 hrs of onset of hepatic encephalopathy. Three patients did not complete the trial in either group. The results show no difference between lactulose and the branched-chain amino acids, although the trend is clearly in favor of the branched-chain amino acid group which, if one looks at the pre-entry criteria, appeared to be sicker patients.

Wake-up occurred in 70% of the patients receiving the branched-chain amino acid, while only in 49% of the lactulose group, a trend, but not significantly significant in the number of patients so studied. There was no difference in survival.

The other three groups utilized a more complete amino acid nutritional mixture, generally based on FO80, as described by Fischer et al.[12] In another Italian trial, reported by Fiaccadori in this volume,[22] three groups of patients, 16 patients in each, were described. The first group received lactulose alone, the second group received a branched-chain enriched amino acid complete nutritional mixture with hypertonic dextrose, and the third group received both the nutritional mixture and lactulose. Wake-up appeared better in both groups receiving the nutritional mixture, as compared with lactulose alone. Wake-up appeared somewhat better in the group receiving both forms of therapy, and there were no deaths in the group receiving lactulose and the branched-chain amino acids, while there was one death in the group receiving branched-chain amino acids alone, and five deaths in the group with lactulose. This report suggests that the branched-chain amino acid may be of survival value in the treatment of acute hepatic encephalopathy.

Increased survival was also reported in the United States randomized prospective trial, in which FO80, now HepatAmine, was randomized against neomycin and isocaloric hypertonic dextrose in a group of 80 patients, by far the largest group entered in a randomized prospective trial, in which eight centers contributed patients.[23] In this study, patients were entered into the trial if they were perceived as requiring nutritional support, and if they did not respond to conventional therapy of hepatic coma within 48 hrs. Thus a rather more severe group of patients was treated in this study. The trial had a crossover provision, and patients must have completed 72 hrs of therapy in order to have considered entering the trial. In this study, global assessment, that is, did patients improve, was significantly improved in the group receiving HepatAmine and hypertonic dextrose, as opposed to the group receiving neomycin and isocaloric hypertonic dextrose. Wake-up was significantly better, both as measured clinically and by EEG, read in blinded fashion by several neurologists. Most striking, however, was the increased survival in the group receiving nutritional support (85%), as opposed to neomycin (55%). It is interesting to point out that, in this sick group of patients, the improved survival followed the same pattern in two other studies of nutritional support in patients with severe illnesses, that is, no difference in the two groups for a week, but improved survival thereafter.[24,25] This pattern may be taken, in my experience, as an index of the effect of nutrition and nutritional support on survival in severe illness. It is of interest that in the multiple, randomized prospective trial in the United States, the patients who died, died of liver failure, and very few of GI bleeding or other causes.

No difference in survival was seen in the Brazilian study, although wake-up was faster in the group receiving HepatAmine and hypertonic dextrose than neomycin and isocaloric hypertonic dextrose. Only 16 episodes of hepatic encephalopathy were included in each group; however, two patients in each group died. It is not clear, at the present writing, how selection was done, and whether these patients had failed to respond to standard therapy for hepatic encephalopathy.[26]

It is striking that the two trials in which negative reports for efficacy of BCAA have been reported have both utilized intravenous fat as the major caloric source. In Michel's study, carried out at Montpelier, a conventional amino acid solution containing 20% branched-chain amino acids and a high concentration of arginine was randomized against a 35% branched-chain amino acid solution containing less arginine. Sixty-seven percent of the calories were given as fat.[27] There was no difference in the rate of awakening between the two groups. It is not clear when patients were entered into the trial, and how long they were symptomatic with hepatic encephalopathy. However, they received little or no treatment other than conventional branched-chain solutions, including cathartics, etc.

Wahren et al. reported a multicenter trial conducted in Sweden and France. In this trial it is not clear how long patients had to remain in hepatic coma before they were entered. Massive GI bleeding was excluded, but 22 patients with lesser degrees of GI bleeding were entered in either group, and deaths from GI bleeding were extensive.[28] Here again, 50% of the calories were recorded as fat. The control group received no amino acid supplementation, while the treatment group received branched-chain amino acids consisting of 70% leucine and smaller amounts of isoleucine and valine. The results here fail to confirm any efficacy for the branched-chain amino acid solutions, but this study was marred by extremely high mortality in both groups within the first month. If deaths from GI bleeding are excluded, which probably should be excluded from a trial on hepatic coma, there is no statistically significant difference between the deaths in the various groups.

The marked difference between these two trials raises the issue of caloric source as being primary. Various groups have implicated free tryptophan as important in the etiology of hepatic coma[29] and, indeed, although the penetration of tryptophan across the blood brain barrier is complicated, there is little question that free tryptophan is important. Our own infusion experiments in dogs suggest that both phenylalanine and tryptophan are required for the production of hepatic coma.[30] Capocaccia and his group have derived evidence that, when branched-chain amino acids are given with glucose, free tryptophan falls.[31] However, when branched-chain amino acid solutions are given with glucose and fat, free tryptophan fails to fall and may even increase slightly. Whether the differences between these studies

can be explained on this basis, or on the fact that Sherwin and his
group have shown that the branched-chain amino acid utilization is
improved with glucose,[10] is not clear at the present time.

Taken together, the results from the various intravenous trials,
unequivocally show that the use of branched-chain amino acids in
hepatic coma with hypertonic dextrose as a caloric source, is associated with the rate of wake-up which is at least equivalent to that
of lactulose or neomycin in especially resistant patients. When given
with fat as a major caloric source, efficacy has not been demonstrated. The reasons for these findings are not clear at present.

D. Oral Branched-Chain Amino Acid Supplementation in the Treatment
   of Chronic Encephalopathy

Here again, the treatment of chronic hepatic encephalopathy
with oral branched-chain amino acids has focused on just a small
group of patients in anecdotal fashion.[32] In a somewhat larger group
of patients known to be protein-intolerant, A662, the precursor of
Hepatic-aid , given with polycose, was randomized against incremental
protein in a clinical research setting.[33] Nitrogen balance and encephalopathy were carefully monitored. The results in this study showed
clear superiority for the branched-chain amino acid solution given
with a glucose base, as opposed to mixed protein. One patient deteriorated; five improved. In contrast, eight patients with mixed protein deteriorated. The results clearly show that the branched-chain
enriched amino acid nutritional supplements are superior to mixed
protein in the prevention of hepatic encephalopathy in susceptible
patients.

A similar finding was described by Egberts et al. in 22 patients
with latent portal systemic encephalopathy, very carefully studied.[34]
In this group, a mixed tablet containing roughly equimolar amounts
with the branched-chain amino acids were given with a dietary base
and the variety of psychometric parameters tested. Clear evidence
for improvement in this crossover design trial against placebo was
evident, and there was little question that, in addition to its
nutritional efficacy, that the branched-chain amino acids also
improved psychometric testings in these susceptible patients.

Eriksson and Wahren have interpreted their results on a very
small number of patients in a crossover trial as being negative for
improvement in encephalopathy.[35] As has been so well pointed out by
Schomerus,[36] the absence of positive results in three patients subject
to a crossover trial in each group does not constitute a negative
study. Moreover, when carefully examined, Eriksson's data does show
improvement in the group of patients treated with branched-chain
amino acids in digital symbol tests, although there was a trend
toward improvement in both groups in the Reitan trial test, which
might have been due to learning. While Eriksson and Wahren interpret

their results as negative, it is clear that, with a larger number
of patients, were the trend to continue the results should be positive. This study cannot be taken as indicating an unfavorable result
in the treatment of chronic hepatic encephalopathy. Indeed, if anything, interpretation of the data as it presently stands shows a
trend toward improvement with BCAA.

SUMMARY AND CONCLUSIONS

A number of trials are now available which clearly show efficacy for the branched-chain amino acids in hepatic encephalopathy.
In the intravenous group, those studies in which the caloric source
has been derived principally from glucose are clear in showing efficacy as against lactulose, neomycin and, in one case, to show
improved survival in a severe group of patients, presumably on a
nutritional basis. In those studies in which branched-chain amino
acids were given intravenously and fat was used as a primary caloric
source, no efficacy was demonstrated. The reasons for this may be
several, but require further study.

No study in which oral branched-chain amino acids have been
administered in sufficient dosage has failed to show efficacy in a
randomized blind crossover fashion. The single trial, which has been
interpreted as being negative, has trends toward efficacy for the
branched-chain amino acids which, if carried to a sufficient number
of patients, will probably confirm the other two trials currently
available, which show efficacy for BCAA in treatment of patients
with chronic hepatic encephalopathy.

REFERENCES
1. J. E. Fischer, J. M. Funovics, A. Aguirre, J. H. James, J. M.
   Keane, R. I. C. Wesdorp, N. Yoshimura,and T. Westman, The
   role of plasma amino acids in hepatic encephalopathy, Surgery
   78: 276 (1975).
2. J. Wahren, P. Felig, and L. Hagenfeldt, Effect of protein ingestion on splanchnic and leg metabolism in normal man and in
   patients with diabetes mellitus, J. Clin. Invest. 57: 987
   (1976).
3. A. L. Goldberg, Mechanism of growth and atrophy of skeletal
   muscle in "Muscle Biology", New York, Dekker, vol. I, pp.
   89-118 (1972).
4. T. Pozedsky, P. Felip, J. S. Soeldner, and G. F. Cahill, Jr.,
   Insulin blockage of amino acid release by human forearm
   tissues, Trans. Assoc. Am. Physicians 81: 258 (1968).
5. H. N. Munro, J.G. Black,and W. S. T. Thomson, The mode of action
   of dietary carbohydrate on protein metabolism, Brit. J. Nutr.
   13: 475 (1959).
6. R. Oddessey and A. L. Goldberg, Oxidation of leucine by rat
   skeletal muscle, Amer. J. Phys. 223: 1376 (1972).

7. R. S. Sherwin, Effect of starvation on the turnover and metabolic response to leucine, J. Clin. Invest. 21: 1471 (1978).
8. H. R. Freund, H. J. James, and J. E. Fischer, Nitrogen sparing mechanisms of singly administered branched-chain amino acids in the injured rat, Surgery 90: 237 (1981).
9. A. Sakamoto, L. L. Moldawer, A. Bothe, B. R. Bistrian, and G. L. Blackburn, Are the nitrogen sparing mechanisms of branched-chain amino acid administration really unique? Surg. Forum 31: 99 (1980).
10. R. A. Gelfaud, R. G. Hendler, and R. S. Sherwin, Dietary carbohydrate and metabolism of ingested protein, Lancet i: 65 (1979).
11. J. H. James, P. M. Herlin, L. Edwards, C. A. Nachbauer, and J. E. Fischer, Effect of infusion of branched-chain amino acids on concentrations of amino acids in plasma and brain and on brain catecholamines after total hepatectomy in the rat, Life Sciences 30: 1361 (1982).
12. J. E. Fischer and R. J. Baldessarini, Pathogenesis and therapy of hepatic coma, in: "Progress in Liver Disease" H. Popper and F. Schaffner, eds., Grune and Stratton, New York, pp. 363-397 (1976).
13. A. Okada, S. Kamata, C. W. Kim, and Y. Kawashima, Treatment of hepatic encephalopathy with BCAA-rich amino acid mixture, in: "Metabolism and Clinical Implications of Branched-Chain Amino and Ketoacids," M. Walser, R. Williamson, eds., Elsevier North Holland, New York, pp. 447-452 (1981).
14. L. Capocaccia, V. Calcaterra, C. Cangiano, A. Cascino, F. Fiaccadori, S. Gentile, F. Ghinelli, G. Pelosi, O. Riggio, F. Rossi-Fanelli, D. Sacchini, and G. Giunchi, Therapeutic effect of branched-chain amino acids in hepatic encephalopathy: A preliminary study, in: "Medical and Surgical Problems of Portal Hypertension," Orloff, M. J., Stipa, S., Ziparo, V. eds., Academic Press, London, New York, pp. 239-249 (1979).
15. H. Freund, J. Dienstag, F. Lehrich, N. Yoshimura, R. R. Bradford, H. Rosen, S. Atamian, E. Slemmer, J. Holroyde, and J. E. Fischer, Infusion of BCAA solution in patients with hepatic encephalopathy, Ann. Surg. 196: 209 (1982).
16. D. B. Silk, M. A. Hanid, and P. N. Trewby, Treatment of fulminant hepatic failure by polyacrylonitrile membrane haemodialysis, Lancet ii: 1 (1977).
17. B. G. Gazzard, M. J. Weston, I. M. Murray-Lyon, H. Flax, C. O. Record, R. Williams, B. Portmann, P. G. Langley, E. H. Dunlop, P. J. Mellon, and M. B. Ward, Charcoal hemoperfusion in the treatment of fulminant hepatic failure, Lancet i: 1301 (1974).
18. S. Rakette, M. Fischer, H. J. Reimann, and S. V. Sommoggy, Effects of a special amino acid solution in patients with liver cirrhosis and hepatic encephalopathy, in: "Metabolism and Clinical Implications of Branched-Chain Amino and Ketoacids" M. Walser, R. Williamson eds., Elsevier, North-Holland, New York, pp. 419-427 (1981).

19. T. Higashi, A. Watanabe, S. Hayashi, T. Obata, N. Tanei, and
     H. Nagashima, Effect of branched-chain amino acid infusion
     on alterations in CSF neutral amino acids and their transport
     across the blood brain barrier in hepatic encephalopathy, in:
     "Metabolism and Clinical Implications of Branched-Chain Amino
     and Ketoacids," M. Walser, R. Williamson eds., Elsevier,
     North-Holland, New York, pp. 465-470 (1981).

20. E. Holm, J. P. Streibel, P. Moller, and M. Hartman, Amino acid
     solutions for parenteral nutrition and for adjuvant treatment
     of encephalopathy in liver cirrhosis, studies concerning 120
     patients, in: "Metabolism and Clinical Implications of Bran-
     ched-Chain Amino and Ketoacids," M. Walser, R. Williamson eds.,
     Elsevier, North-Holland, New York, pp. 513-518 (1981).

21. F. Rossi Fanelli, O. Riggio, C. Cangiano, A. Cascino, D. De Con-
     ciliis, M. Merli, M. Stortoni, and G. Giunchi, Branched-chain
     amino acids vs lactulose in the treatment of hepatic coma: a
     controlled study, Dig. Dis. Sci. 27: 929 (1982).

22. F. Fiaccadori, F. Ghinelli, G. Pedretti, G. Pelosi, D. Sacchini,
     M. L. Zeneroli, E. Rossi, P. Gibertini, and E. Ventura, Bran-
     ched-chain amino acid enriched solutions in hepatic encepha-
     lopathy, a controlled trial (submitted for publication).

23. F. B. Cerra, N. K. Cheung, J. E. Fischer, N. Kaplowitz, E. R.
     Schiff, J. L. Deinstag, C. D. Mabry, C. M. Leevy, and T.
     Kiernan, A multicenter trial of branched-chain enriched amino
     acid infusion (FO80) in hepatic encephalopathy (HE), Hepatology
     2: (5) 699 (1982).

24. R. M. Abel, C. H. Beck, Jr., W. M. Abbott, J. A. Ryan, G. O.
     Barnett, and J. E. Fischer, Improved survival from acute renal
     failure after treatment with intravenous essential L-amino
     acids and glucose, N. Engl. J. Med. 288: 695 (1973).

25. J. W. Alexander, B. G. McMillan, J. D. Stinnett, C. K. Ogle, R.
     C. Bozian, J. E. Fischer, J. B. Oakes, M. J. Morris, and R.
     Krummel, Beneficial effects of aggressive protein feeding in
     severely burned children, Ann. Surg. 192: 505 (1980).

26. E. Strauss, W. R. Santos, and E. C. DaSilva, A randomized con-
     trolled clinical trial for the evaluation of the efficacy of
     balanced amino acid solution compared to neomycin in hepatic
     encephalopathy (submitted for publication).

27. G. Polier-Layrargues, O. Duhamel, G. Cuilleret, P. Bovics, H.
     Bellet-Hermann, and H. Michel, Treatment of hepatic encepha-
     lopathy by infusions of a modified amino acid solution.
     Results of a controlled study in 33 cirrhotic patients (sub-
     mitted for publication).

28. J. J. Wahren, J. Denis, P. Desurmont, L. S. Erikson, J. M. Escof-
     fier, A. P. Gauthier, L. Hagenfeldt, H. Michel, P. Opolon,
     J. Paris, and M. Veyrac, Is i.v. administration of branched-
     chain amino acids effective in the treatment of hepatic ence-
     phalopathy? A multicenter study, Europ. Soc. Parent. Enter.
     Nutr. FC47: 61 (1981).

29. A. Cascino, C. Cangiano, V. Calcaterra, F. Rossi-Fanelli, and
     L. Capocaccia, Plasma amino acid imbalance in patients with
     liver disease, Am. J. Dig. Dis. 23: 591 (1978).
30. F. Rossi-Fanelli, F. H. Freund, R. Krause, A. R. Smith, J. H.
     James, S. Castorina-Ziparo, and J. E. Fischer, Induction of
     coma in normal dogs by infusion of aromatic amino acids and
     prevention by addition of branched chain amino acids,
     Gastroenterology 83: 664 (1982).
31. C. Cangiano, F. Rossi-Fanelli, and L. Capocaccia, Personal com-
     munication.
32. H. Freund, N. Yoshimura, and J. E. Fischer, Chronic hepatic
     encephalopathy. Long-term therapy with a branched-chain-
     amino-acid-enriched elemental diet, JAMA 242: 347 (1979).
33. D. Horst, N. Grace, H. O. Conn, E. Schiff, S. Schenker, A. Vi-
     teri, D. Law, and C. E. Atterbury, A double-blind randomized
     comparison of dietary protein and an oral branched chain amino
     acid (BCAA) supplement in cirrhotic patients with chronic
     portal-systemic encephalopathy (PSE) (ABS), Hepatology 5:
     518 (1981).
34. E. M. Egberts, W. Hampter, and P. Jurgens, Effective treatment
     of latent portosystemic encephalopathy (PSE) with oral bran-
     ched chain amino acids (BCAA). Presented at AISF Conference
     on Hepatic Coma, Rome, November 19-20, 1982 (this volume).
35. L. S. Eriksson, A. Persson, and J. Wahren, Branched chain amino
     acids in the treatment of chronic hepatic encephalopathy,
     Gut 23: 801 (1982).
36. H. Schomerus, In discussion of paper 39, AISF Conference on
     Hepatic Coma, Rome, November 19-20, 1982 (this volume).

BRANCHED CHAIN AMINO ACID ENRICHED SOLUTIONS IN THE TREATMENT

OF HEPATIC ENCEPHALOPATHY: A CONTROLLED TRIAL

F. Fiaccadori,[a] F. Ghinelli,[a] G. Pedretti,[a] G. Pelosi,[a]
D. Sacchini,[a] M.L. Zeneroli,[aa] E. Rocchi,[aa] P. Gibertini,[aa]
and E. Ventura[aa]

[a]Cattedra di Malattie Infettive, Università di Parma,
Parma, Italy, [aa]Istituto di Clinica Medica, Università
di Modena, Modena, Italy

MATERIALS AND METHODS

Patients

The study was performed on 48 patients consecutively admitted
to our departments between Sept. 1977 and April 1980 and selected
according to the following criteria: (1) presence of liver cirrhosis
(diagnosed on clinical and laboratory data and confirmed in all cases
but one by liver biopsy) (2) presence of HE (assessed by two different observers through the evaluation of mental state, asterixis
and number connection test (Reitan A) using the score system proposed
by Conn;[13] EEG performed in 36 out of the 48 cases were graded
according to the classification of Kurtz et al.:[14] only patients in
grade 2-3-4 HE were included in the study); (3) no evidence of hepa-
to-renal syndrome (assessed according to the criteria proposed at
the symposium held in Sassari[15].)

Study design

The 48 patients were randomly assigned to one of the following
therapeutic protocols:

Group A (16 cases): administration of lactulose, by means of nasogastric tube or enema, at a dose ranging from 150 to 300 mg/day,
able to produce a cathartic effect. Hypertonic glucose (30%) solutions were administered through a catheter introduced in the subclavian vein at a rate of 1.35 ml/min for 24 hr. (Total amount =
2000 ml/24 h; caloric intake = 2500 Kcal/24 h).

Group B (16 cases): total parenteral nutrition (TPN), through the subclavian vein, with hypertonic glucose in an isocaloric amount and at the same rate as in group A, plus a special AA mixture rich in BCAA and poor in AAA (supplied by Boehringer-Biochemia-Robin under the trade name of BS 666). The composition is compared with that of a commercially available solution in Table 1.

BS 666 infusion lasted 12 h and the protein intake was $\sim$ 0.8-1 g/kg/ bw/day.

Group C (16 cases): TPN, as in group B, plus lactulose, as in group A. Patients included in each group received the assigned treatment for 7 consecutive days.

Informed consent was obtained for each patient from the next of kin.

None of the patients received plasma or blood transfusions. Four patients (1 in group A, 1 in group B, 2 in group C) with a complicating gram negative sepsis were given specific antibiotic treatment. Insulin, electrolytes and vitamins were given as needed.

No placebo group was included as it was considered unethical; therefore the efficacy of a BCAA enriched solution was compared with that of lactulose which is still considered the best form of treatment in HE.

Assay procedures

Fasting blood samples were drawn prior to and during treatment from an antecubital vein for the determination of SGOT, SGPT, serum albumin, serum globulin, conjugated and unconjugated bilirubin, prothrombin time, hemoglobin, blood glucose, BUN, creatinine, alkaline phosphatase.

Fasting blood samples for the determination of AA and ammonia were collected before treatment (basal values) and on the 3rd and 7th day of treatment; in groups B and C blood samples were collected at least 10 h after completing the AA infusion.

Plasma AA were determined by column chromatography with a Technicon sequential Multisample amino analyzer on the supernatant of plasma made protein-free by precipitation with 4% sulfosalycilic acid. Blood ammonia was determined by an enzymatic UV method (Biochemia Monotest); normal values in our laboratory range from 25 to 94 µg/dl in males and from 18 to 82 µg/dl in females.

EEG recordings (O.T.E. Biochemia EEG model E8e) were also obtained before treatment and on the 3rd and 7th day.

Statistical analysis

Basal data were compared to those obtained on the 3rd and 7th day of treatment using Student's t test for paired data by matching the three groups with respect to the following parameters: 1) BCAA/AAA molar ratio, 2) blood ammonia, 3) incidence of patient awakening, mental state and neurological tests (evaluated according to the score system proposed by Conn[13].)

RESULTS

With the exception of G.I. bleeding the 3 groups were comparable for age, sex, type of cirrhosis, routine blood tests and precipitating causes of HE (Table 2).

Biochemistry

Routine blood chemistry was quite similar in the three groups before the beginning of the study and did not show significant variations during any of the three therapeutic regimens.

1) BCAA/AAA molar ratio (Table 3)

Group A: comparison between basal values and those on the 3rd and 7th day of treatment failed to reveal any statistical difference.

Group B: with respect to basal values, the molar ratio showed a significant increase both on the 3rd and 7th day ($p < 0.001$).

Group C: a statistically significant rise was recorded only on the 7th day ($p < 0.005$).

2) Blood ammonia

Blood ammonia levels showed no significant change in group A, whereas a statistically significant decrease was observed both in Groups B and C on the 3rd ($p < 0.05$) and 7th day ($p < 0.001$) (Table 4).

3) Neurological symptoms and EEG findings (Figure 1)

The neurological evaluation showed that after 3 days of treatment 5 out of 16 patients in group A, 9 out of 16 in group B and 11 out of 16 in group C came out of the coma; a statistical difference between groups B and A ($p < 0.01$) and between groups C and A ($p < 0.001$) was observed. By the 7th day 10 out of 16 patients in group A, 15 out of 16 in group B and all patients in group C were awake, a statistically significant difference being observed between groups B and A ($p < 0.01$), and between groups C and A ($p < 0.01$).

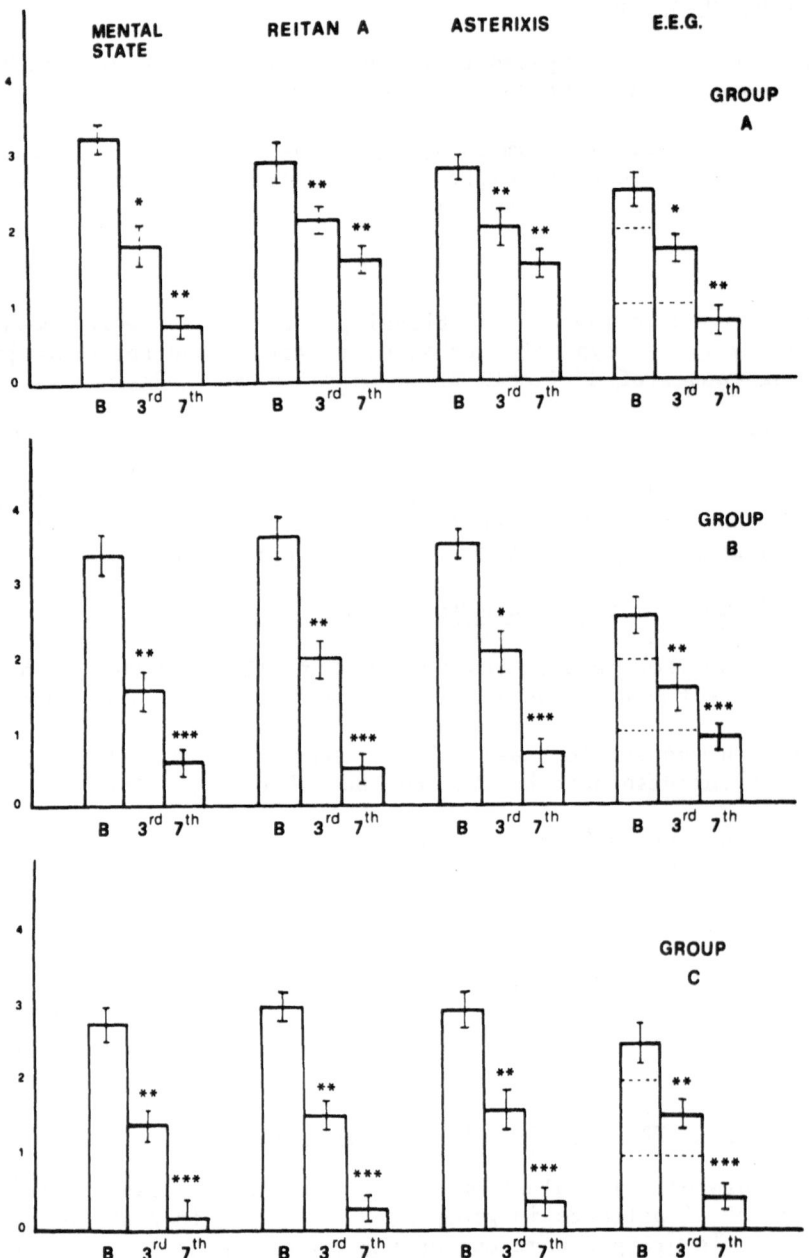

Fig. 1.   Statistical comparison of clinical, neurological, and
electroencephalographic parameters in groups A, B, C.
Mean + S.E. of the basal period vs third and seventh day
*p< 0.02, **p <0.05, ***p < 0.001).

Table 1. Comparison between a commercial amino acid mixture and the specially formulated solution (BS 666) used in this study.

Components	Commercial solution	BS 666
1 - L-Essentials	g/l	g/l
Isoleucine	2.95	4.50
Leucine	3.85	5.50
Valine	2.80	4.20
Methionine	2.25	0.50
Phenylalanine	2.40	0.50
Tryptophan	0.65	0.38
Threonine	1.70	2.25
Lysine - HCl	3.85	3.80
2 - L-Non Essentials		
Alanine	3.00	3.75
Arginine	1.55	3.00
Glycine	9.00	4.50
Histidine	1.20	1.20
Proline	4.75	4.00
Serine	2.50	2.50
Cysteine-HCl	0.02	0.25

Encephalopatic scores (mental state, asterixis, Reitan A) showed a significant decrease in each group of patients both at the third and seventh day. The statistical difference between basal values and those on the seventh day was greater ($p < 0.001$) in groups B and C than in group A ($p < 0.05$). Improvement in the EEG recordings was parallel to the recovery of mental activity.

DISCUSSION

On the basis of previous personal experience and in agreement with data reported by Fischer, we are of the opinion that the i.v. administration of conventional amino acid mixtures to patients with severe liver failure may precipitate or worsen HE, thus in the last few years all our patients with HE have been treated with specially formulated AA solutions designed to correct the altered plasma amino acid profile present in cirrhotics with HE. The encouraging results obtained led us to undertake the present study aimed at comparing

Table 2. Details of the 48 patients included in the study

Group	A	B	C
No. patients	16	16	16
Age (mean in yr)	52.37	51.90	48.00
Men	10	12	13
Women	6	4	3
Type of cirrhosis			
Cryptogenic	7	6	5
Postalcoholic	7	9	9
Postnecrotic	2	1	2
Precipitating causes			
Dehydration	4	3	4
G.I. Bleeding	1	6	1
Sepsis	1	1	3
Protein overload	1	1	2
Unknown	8	5	6
Clinical findings			
Previous episodes of HE	6	9	8
Ascites	12	10	13
Diabetes	2	2	2
Portasystemic anastomosis	2	4	3
Biochemical findings			
SGOT (UKW/dl)	38.12 ± 4.06	67.69 ± 12.95	70.31 ± 17.55
SGPT (UKW/dl)	34.5 ± 4.76	45.31 ± 10.38	48.75 ± 9.66
Serum albumin (g/dl)	2.54 ± 0.10	2.56 ± 0.13	2.49 ± 0.12
Serum globulin (g/dl)	2.49 ± 0.17	2.38 ± 0.10	2.42 ± 0.16
Conjugated bilirubin (mg/dl)	2.07 ± 0.6	1.95 ± 0.37	2.81 ± 1.44
Unconjugated bilirubin (mg/dl)	1.40 ± 0.18	1.50 ± 0.20	2.05 ± 0.6
Prothrombin activity (%)	62.25 ± 3.49	63.50 ± 6.20	59.25 ± 4.71
Hemoglobin (g/dl)	11.27 ± 0.51	11.72 ± 0.56	12.01 ± 0.76
Blood glucose (g/dl)	0.99 ± 0.08	1.15 ± 0.09	1.39 ± 0.23
BUN (g/l)	0.38 ± 0.04	0.38 ± 0.06	0.53 ± 0.07
Creatinine (mg/dl)	1.59 ± 0.63	0.99 ± 0.09	1.03 ± 0.07
Alkaline phosphatase (mU/ml)	151.13 ± 21.70	158.44 ± 13.56	159.56 ± 13.15

Table 3. Variations of BCAA/AAA molar ratio in the three groups of patients before, during and at the end of the treatments (Mean $\pm$ SE).

		Baseline values	3rd day	7th day
Group A	$\dfrac{BCAA}{AAA}$	1.25 ± 0.08	1.04 ± 0.08	1.17 ± 0.11
Group B	$\dfrac{BCAA}{AAA}$	1.04 ± 0.20 [**]	1.88 ± 0.20 [**]	1.75 ± 0.11 [**]
Group C	$\dfrac{BCAA}{AAA}$	1.09 ± 0.13	1.33 ± 0.13	1.92 ± 0.20 [*]

[*] $p < 0.005$, [**] $p < 0.001$

Table 4. Blood ammonia changes (μg/dl) before, during and after treatments in the three groups of patients (Mean $\pm$ SE).

	Baseline	3rd day	7th day
Group A	146.81 $+$ 9.73	132.56 $+$ 11.24	122.24 $+$ 11.20
Group B	184.93 $+$ 27.39	111.50 $+$ 10.56[*]	105.93 $+$ 7.58[**]
Group C	171.18 $+$ 18.70	144.25 $+$ 18.27[*]	103.27 $+$ 14.51[**]

[*]$p < 0.05$, [**]$p < 0.001$.

the efficacy of these special AA solutions with that of lactulose which is still considered the drug of choice in the treatment of HE.

The present study shows that the BCAA enriched solutions are extremely effective in reversing HE (93.7% of patients at the 7th day).

This efficacy is significantly higher than that of lactulose (62.3% of patients on the 7th day) which nonetheless is reconfirmed as an efficacious drug in reversing HE.

Similar conclusions, i.e., better efficacy of AA solutions vs lactulose, may be drawn from the changes in the neuroclinical and EEgraphic parameters, the statistical difference between basal findings and those at the 7th day being more significant in groups B (BS 666) and C (BS 666 + lactulose) than in group A (lactulose alone).

Since the best clinical results were obtained using a combination of lactulose and AA (group C, 100% of patients awake by the 7th day) a cumulative effect of lactulose is intestinal trapping of ammonia,[16] which, in excess may produce high levels of brain glutamine which, in turn, utilizing the same transport sites at the BBB as the neutral amino acids (NAA) would increase brain extraction of NAA ("Unified theory of HE").[17] Moreover, data have been reported[18] supporting the hypothesis that the plasma AA imbalance in cirrhosis may be partly due to ammonia induced changes in pancreatic hormones. The usefulness of NH_3 as a marker of HE was confirmed; improvement in clinical and neurological signs was constantly associated with a decrease in blood levels of NH_3 which failed to reach statistical significance only in group A.

The decrease in NH_3 in group B may be attributed to BCAA, and in group C to the combined action of BCAA and lactulose. It is tempting to suggest that BCAA reduces ammonia as a result of protein synthesis regulation and degradation as well as by stimulating glutamine synthesis in the muscle (the main route of ammonia clearance in liver cirrhosis).[19]

The BCAA/AAA ratio (significantly increased on the 3rd and 7th day in group B and on the 7th day in group C) appeared to be well correlated with the modifications in the metabolic and neurological parameters following treatment with BCAA enriched solutions.

Data emerging from the present trial suggest that, although the treatment of HE can not be necessarily identified with the treatment of hepatic failure, the use of BCAA rich solutions represents clear progress in the attempt to correct some metabolic alterations known to be pathogenetically and clinically related to hepatic encephalopathy.

Acknowledgement

The authors are grateful to Prof. Roberto Bernardi (Biochemia-Boehringer-Research Laboratories) for arranging the supply of amino acid mixtures.

REFERENCES

1. F. L. Iber, H. Rosen, and S. M.Levenson, The plasma amino acids in patients with liver failure, J. Lab. Clin. Med. 50: 417 (1957).

2. A. Cascino, C. Cangiano, V. Ca caterra, F. Rossi Fanelli, and L. Capocaccia, Plasma amino acid imbalance in patients with liver disease, Am. J. Dig. Dis. 23: 591 (1978).

3. J. E. Fischer, J. M. Funovics, A. Aguirre, J. H. James, J. M. Keane, R. I. C. Wesdorf, H. Yoshimura, and T. Westman, The role of plasma amino acids in hepatic encephalopathy, Surgery 78: 276 (1975).

4. H. M. Rosen, H. Yoshimura, J. M. Hodgman, and J. E. Fischer, Plasma amino acid patterns in hepatic encephalopathy of differing etiology, Gastroenterology 72: 483 (1977).

5. J. E. Fischer, H. M. Rosen, A. M. Ebeid, J. H. James, J. M. Keane, and P. B. Soeters, The effect of normalization of plasma amino acids on hepatic encephalopathy in man, Surgery 80: 77 (1976).

6. E. H. Egberts, W. Hamster, P. Jurgens, H. Schumacher, G. Fondalinski, U. Reinhard, and H. Schomerus, Effects of branched chain amino acid on latent portal systemic encephalopathy, in: "Metabolism and Clinical Implications of Branched Chain Amino and Ketoacids", M. Walser, J. R. Williamson eds., Elsevier North Holland, New York (1982).

7. T. Higashi, A. Watanabe, S. Shayashi, T. Obata, H. Takei, and H. Nagashima, Effects of branched chain amino acid infusion on alterations in CSF neutral amino acids and their transport across the blood brain barrier in hepatic encephalopathy, in: "Metabolism and Clinical Implications of Branched-Chain Amino and Ketoacids", M. Walser, J. R. Williamson eds., Elsevier North Holland, New York (1981).

8. E. Holm, J. P. Striebel, P. Moller, and M. Hartmen, Amino acid solutions for parenteral nutrition and for adjuvant treatment of encephalopathy in liver cirrhosis. Studies concerning 120 patients, in:"Metabolism and Clinical Implications of Branched-Chain Amino and Ketoacids", M. Walser, J. R. Williamson eds., Elsevier North Holland, New York (1981).

9. A. Okada, S. Kamata, C. W. Kim, and Y. Kawashima, Treatment of hepatic encephalopathy with BCAA rich amino acid mixture, in: "Metabolism and Clinical Implications of Branched Chain Amino and Ketoacids", M. Walser, J. R. Williamson eds., Elsevier, North Holland, New York (1981).

10. S. Rakette, M. Fischer, H. J. Reimann, and S. J. Sommogy, Effects
     of special amino acid solutions in patients with liver cirrho-
     sis and hepatic encephalopathy, in: "Metabolism and Clinical
     Implications of Branched Chain Amino and Ketoacids", M. Wal-
     ser, J. R. Williamson, eds., Elsevier North Holland, New York
     (1981).

11. G. Marchesini, M. Zoli, C. Dondi, G. Bianchi, M. Cirulli, and
     E. Pisi, Anticatabolic effect of branched-chain amino acid-
     enriched solutions in patients with liver cirrhosis, Hepato-
     logy 2: 420 (1982).

12. F. Fiaccadori, F. Ghinelli, G. Pelosi, D. Sacchini, G. L. Vaona,
     M. L. Zeneroli, E. Rocchi, V. Santunione, P. Gibertini, and
     E. Ventura, Selective amino acid solutions in hepatic ence-
     phalopathy treatment, Ric. Clin. Lab. 10: 377 (1980).

13. H. O. Conn, Assessment of mental state, in: "The Hepatic Coma
     Syndrome and Lactulose", Williams and Wilkins, Baltimore
     (1979).

14. D. Kurtz, J. P. Zenglein, M. Imler, M. Girardel, G. Grinspan,
     B. Peter, and F. Rohmer, Etude du summeil nocturne au cours
     de l'encephalopathie porto-cave, Electroencephalography and
     Clinical Neurophysiol. 33: 167 (1972).

15. L. E. Earley, Conclusive remarks and presentation of diagnostic
     criteria of the hepato-renal syndrome, in: "Hepato-Renal
     Syndrome" E. Bartoli, L. Chiandussi, eds., Medical Books
     Padova (1980).

16. H. O. Conn and M. M. Lieberthal, Lactulose in the management of
     chronic portal systemic encephalopathy, in "The Hepatic Coma
     Syndrome and Lactulose", Williams and Wilkins, Baltimore
     (1979).

17. J. H. James, B. Jeppson, V. Ziparo, and J. E. Fischer, Hyperam-
     monaemia plasma amino acid imbalance and blood-brain amino
     acid transport. A unified theory of portal-systemic ence-
     phalopathy, Lancet 2: 773 (1979).

18. G. Marchesini, M. Zoli, C. Dondi, A. Angiolini, A. Melli, and
     E. Pisi, Ammonia-induced changes in pancreatic hormones and
     plasma amino acids in patients with liver cirrhosis, Dig.
     Dis. Sci. 27: 406 (1982).

19. A. H. Lockwood, J. M. Donald, R. E. Reiman, A. S. Gelbard, S.
     J. Laughlin, T. E. Duffy, and F. Plum, The dynamics of am-
     monia metabolism in man, J. Clin. Invest. 63: 449 (1979).

BRANCHED-CHAIN AMINO ACIDS IN THE TREATMENT

OF SEVERE HEPATIC ENCEPHALOPATHY

F. Rossi Fanelli, C. Cangiano, A. Cascino, M. Merli, O.
Riggio, M. Stortoni, L. Capocaccia*

Clinica Medica III, University of Rome, Rome, Italy
*II^ Cattedra di Gastroenterologia, University of Rome
Rome, Italy

INTRODUCTION

The most characteristic feature of the plasma amino acid (AA)
profile in chronic liver failure is the rise in the three aromatic
AA (AAA), phenylalanine (PHE), tyrosine (TYR) and free tryptophan
(F. TRY) and the fall in the three branched-chain AA (BCAA), valine
(VAL) leucine (LEU) and isoleucine (ILEU).[1,2] These alterations of
plasma AA are in turn responsible for brain accumulation of AAA.
In fact, blood-brain entry of AAA is increased either because of a
decreased competition by BCAA which use the same transport system
across the blood-brain-barrier (BBB)[3] or because an increased activity of the transport system itself.[4,5] Brain accumulation of AAA
may profoundly alter the synthesis of neurotransmitters leading to
a depletion of putative neurotransmitters, norepinephrine and dopamine, and an accumulation of false neurotransmitters (such as octopamine and phenylethanolamine)[6,7,8] or inhibitory neurotransmitters
(such as serotonin).[9] The false neurotransmitters hypothesis offers
an appealing explanation for the neurologic disorders and coma that
complicate chronic liver failure.[6]

Normalization of plasma AA by intravenous administration of an
AA mixture enriched in BCAA and containing only minimal amounts of
PHE and TRY, (may) result in an improvement of hepatic encephalopathy (HE) both in experimental animals[10] and man.[11] In a preliminary, uncontrolled study[12] we found that a solution containing
exclusively BCAA was estremely effective in reversing severe HE. In
fact, all the 21 cirrhotic patients in grade 3-4 HE regained consciousness within 48 h (mean ± SE = 20.5+3.5 h) (Figure 1). As shown
in the Figure, the time of arousal was clearly influenced by the

335

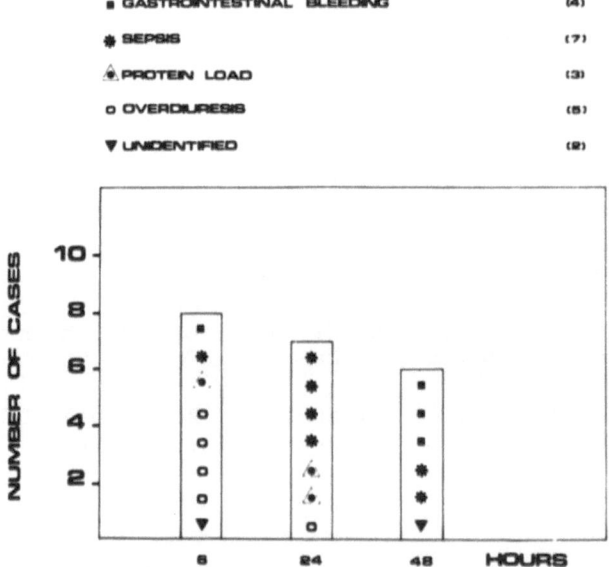

Fig. 1.   Time of arousal in the 21 patients in grade 3-4 HE treated
with BCAA infusions.

severity of the precipitating events, the G. I. bleeding requiring
the longest time while overdiuresis the shortest.

To confirm these extremely promising results, we carried out
a prospective, randomized, controlled study, in which the efficacy
of BCAA was compared to that of lactulose in reversing severe HE.[13]
Lactulose is very effective, and is considered the drug of choice
in the treatment of HE.[14] We considered it unethical to use a placebo control. Forty consecutive patients were randomly assigned to
receive either BCAA (treatment A - Group A) or lactulose (treatment
B - Group B). All patients had a clinically, biochemically and histologically proven liver cirrhosis and were in grade 3-4 HE as assessed
by two independent neurologists according to the Adams and Foley
classification[15] as reported by Fischer [11] (Table 1). Only patients
with hepatorenal syndrome, assessed according to Sassari's criteria,[16] were excluded from the study. Six patients, three in each
group, dropped out from the study either because they were sent to
surgery because of uncontrollable bleeding or because the consent
from their next of kin was withdrawn. Therefore, two groups of 17
patients each were actually compared. The two groups were well
matched for sex, age, type of cirrhosis and precipitating events
(Table 2). Also the routine blood chemistry and the liver function

Table 1. Criteria used to assess HE

Grade 1:   fluctuant mild confusion with euphoria and/or
           depression slowed speech, disorder of sleep
           rhythm.

Grade 2:   (impending coma) accentuation of grade 1 with
           drowsiness inappropriate behavior and inabi-
           lity to maintain sphincter control.

Grade 3:   (stupor) sleeps most of the time but arousable,
           marked confusion is present with lack of know-
           ledge of surroundings.

Grade 4:   (coma) physical response to painful stimuli may
           or may not be present.

Table 2. Comparison between the two groups of patients
          included in the study

	Treatment A	Treatment B
No. of patients	17	17
Age (mean in yr)	57	61
Men	10	11
Women	7	6
Type of cirrhosis:		
Cryptogenic	11	8
Postalcoholic	3	8
Postnecrotic	3	1
Precipitating events of hepatic coma		
Infections	6	6
Bleeding varices	3	4
Constipation	1	–
Protein overload	1	2
Paracentesis	1	–
Overdiuresis	1	1
Alcohol abuse	1	–
Surgery	1	1
Unknown	2	3

---

tests were quite similar in the two groups with the exception of
the protrombin time which was significantly lower in the group

treated with the BCAA (Table 3). As shown in Table 4, the clinical picture was somewhat worse in patients receiving BCAA than in those given lactulose.

Table 5 shows the details of the two treatments. Treatment A consisted in a solution of leucine g 1.1%, isoleucine 0.9% and valine 0.8% in 20% dextrose in water administered through a catheter inserted in a subclavian vein. The flow rate was set at 60 ml/h (1500 ml/day) for the first 24 h and at 80 ml/h (2000 ml/day) thereafter by means of a peristaltic pump. Patients in group B received lactulose either via a nasogastric tube (30-40 g every 4 h until catharsis occurred, then the dose was tapered to ensure two bowel movements per day) or by intermittent enemas (200-300 g/day) in those patients who were preferred not to receive lactulose orally (bleeding, etc.). 23% dextrose in water was administered with the same modalities as in the BCAA group. The events which precipitated the episodes of coma received a prompt treatment, however no other specific treatment for HE was given. It was decided not to give cathartics to patients receiving BCAA in order to have a more clear-cut evaluation of their therapeutic effect.

During the study, the patient's neurological status was assessed twice a day by two independent and experienced neurologists who did not know which treatment was being given. The study was planned as follows: if patients receiving either treatment A or B, regained consciousness (grade 0-1 HE) within 48 h, either treatment was continued for further 48 h. If no response occurred, the two treatments were combined (treatment C). After the given treatment (A or B) was

Table 3. Biochemical findings

	Treatment A	Treatment B
	BCAA + glucose	Lactulose + glucose
GTP(mμ/ml)	36.60+47.30	37.20+47.60
Serum albumin (g/dl)	2.78+0.37	2.94+0.68
Serum globuline (g/dl)	2.69+0.83	2.26+0.63
Total bilirubine (mg/dl)	8.20+6.88	8.13+7.02
Protrombin time (in %)	49.70+14.90	66.70+19.70
Ammonia (γ/dl)	179.30+86.30	165.50+64.90
Hemoglobin (g/dl)	11.50+1.90	11.50+1.20
Blood glucose (mg/dl)	158.80+94.90	120.50+46.00
Creatinine (mg/dl)	1.30+0.67	1.88+1.16

Table 4.   Clinical picture of the two groups of patients

	Treatment A	Treatment B
Previous episodes of hepatic encephalopathy	8	2
Ascites	12	7
Severe jaundice (direct bilirubin 5 mg/100 ml)	9	5
Severe renal insufficiency (creatinine 3 mg/100 ml)	1	2
Diabetes	7	3
Porto-systemic anastomosis	3	2

discontinued all patients were put on a protein restricted diet (0.5 g/kg BW/day) and oral lactulose in an amount to ensure a cathartic effect. The study was considered concluded ten days after commencement of therapy. Routine blood chemistry was monitored daily throughout the study. Blood samples for ammonia and amino acid determinations were collected before starting therapy (baseline, Sample 1), when patients regained consciousness (Sample 2), six h after the treatment was stopped (Sample 3) and at the tenth day (Sample 4).

The clinical results are reported in Table 6. Of the seventeen patients treated with BCAA, twelve regained consciousness within 48 h (70.5%), whilst eight out of seventeen patients responded to lactulose (47.1%). The mean ($\pm$ SE) time of arousal (in h) during treatment A or B was $27.6+6.48$ and $31.5+4.4$ respectively. Either the rate or the time of recovery (as assessed by the x^2 test or the Student's t test for unpaired data) did not differ significantly between the two groups. It must be considered, however, that patients in the control group did not receive a placebo, if this were the case, the difference between the two groups would have certainly become significant. The aim of this study, however, was not to prove the superiority of BCAA over lactulose, a well established active drug in the treatment of HE, but just to confirm their efficacy. The recovery rate in group C as well as the death rate in the three groups are listed in the Table.

The modifications of plasma amino acids and ammonia observed during both treatments are of particular interest. The baseline values of all the AA were similar in the two groups showing the characteristic profile with high AAA and low BCAA (Figure 2). Normal values of plasma AA are reported in Table 7 . As it could be expected, in patients receiving BCAA, plasma valine, leucine and isoleucine rose significantly ($p < 0.001$), upon mental recovery (Figure 2). Concomi-

Table 5. Details of the two treatments

Treatment A

Valine	0.84	g %
Leucine	1.1	g %
Isoleucine	0.9	g %
Glucose	20	g %

2000 ml/24 h

Treatment B

Lactulose per os or enemas

| Glucose | 23 | g % |

(2000 ml/24 h)

Table 6. Clinical results in the 34 patients included
in the study

	Treatment A BCAA + Glucose	Treatment B Lactulose + Glucose	Treatment C BCAA + Lactulose + Glucose	
			A+B	B+A
No. of Pts	17	17	5	2
Responsive	12 (70,5%)	8 (47.1%)	2 (40%)	1
Unresponsive	5 (29.5%)	9 (52.9%)	3 (60%)	1

tantly, PHE, TYR and F. TRY decreased considerably, though only F. TRY significantly ($P < 0.05$). The reduction of plasma AAA during i.v. infusion confirms our previous reports[2,12] and should be attributed to the regulatory effect of BCAA on muscular protein turnover.[17,18] In fact the increased degradation of muscle protein is mostly responsible for plasma AAA accumulation in chronic liver failure.[19] When BCAA infusion was stopped either BCAA or AAA plasma levels tended steadily to return to their baseline values with the exception of F. TRY which remained within the values expected in cirrhotics without HE (Table 7). We were not surprised that, except for F. TRY, the plasma AA profile when the patients were fully alert (i.e. at the 10th day) was quite similar to that observed when patients were in deep coma. This is in keeping with our previous observations, in which we failed to demonstrate a significant corre-

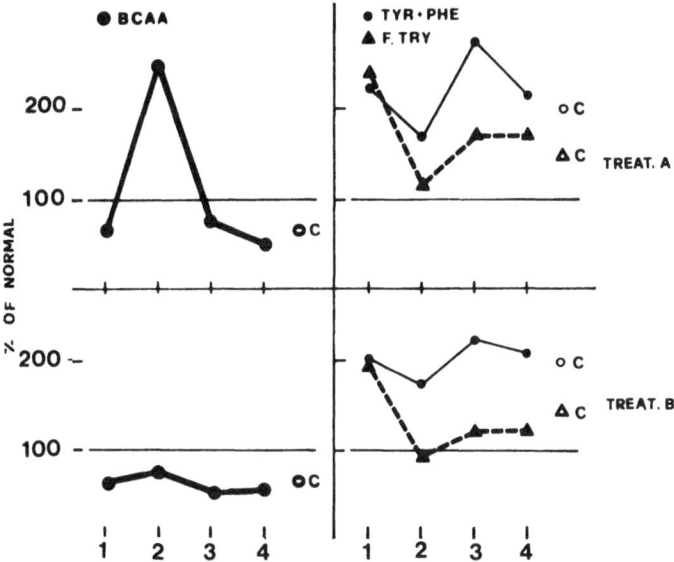

Fig. 2.   Plasma amino acid modifications observed during the two
          different forms of treatment.

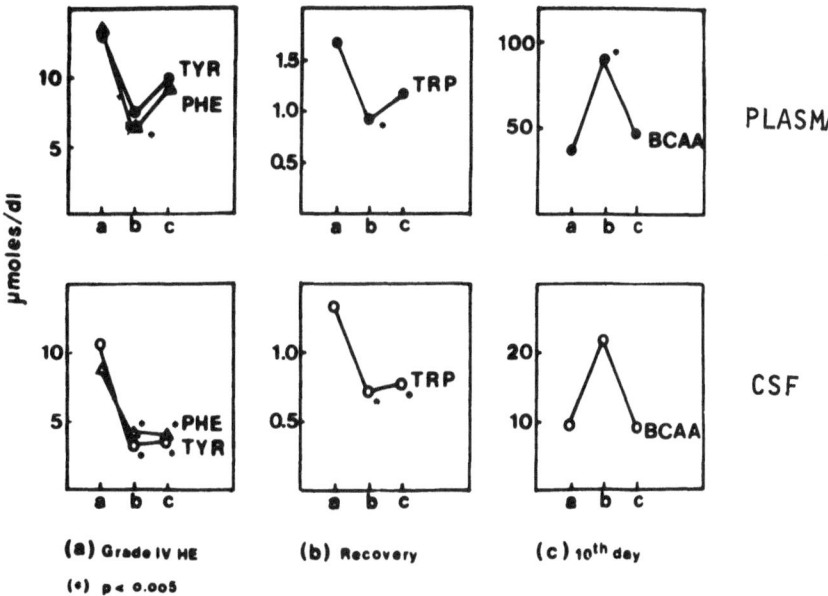

Fig. 3.   Plasma and CSF amino acid changes observed in 10 patients
          in grade 3-4 HE treated with BCAA infusions. Reproduced
          with permission of S. Karger AG, Basel (7/12/83).

lation between HE and plasma AA patterns.[2,12] Although data from our [2,20,21] and other laboratories[22,23] support the role played by F. TRY in HE, we are reluctant to accept that only F. TRY is involved in HE. Indeed, very recent data indicate that also PHE and TYR play a major role in the pathogenesis of HE.[24]

It is conceivable that AA modifications in plasma did not parallel those in the CNS. Data from dogs[25] and monkeys[26] with portocava shunt have shown that plasma and CSF AA profiles were quite different when the animals became comatose. In a group of ten patients in grade 3-4 HE receiving BCAA with the same modalities as those in group A of the controlled study we have contemporaneously investigated the AA modifications occurring in plasma and in CSF. As shown in Figure 3 BCAA and AAA behavior in plasma was quite similar to that already observed in the previous study. Conversely, the AA patterns in the CSF was quite different: the BCAA rose and the AAA fell significantly upon mental recovery, but, unlikely in plasma, they remained low throughout the study.

The plasma AA changes in the group of patients receiving lactulose and glucose were irrelevant with the exception of F. TRY, which decreased significantly ($P < 0.05$) upon mental recovery and remained at low levels thereafter. Rather than to lactulose, TRY behavior in group B should be mostly attributed to the insulin-induced fall in NEFA exerted by glucose and to the consequent increased number of albumin binding sites for F. TRY.

Interestingly, plasma ammonia decreased significantly under both treatments paralleling the clinical evolution. While the "intestinal trapping" of ammonia is a well established effect of lactulose[13] much less is known of the mechanism(s) through which BCAA reduce blood ammonia. However, at least two modalities may be involved: (1) as already mentioned ammonia is released by muscles under catabolic conditions[27] and BCAA may reduce muscular protein degradation;[17] (2) BCAA may act by stimulating muscular glutamine synthesis which has been reported as the major route of ammonia clearance in chronic liver failure.[27] An exciting hypothesis has been recently proposed linking ammonia to brain glutamine, increased blood-brain AA transport, plasma and brain AA patterns and false neurotransmitters synthesis.[28]

From what has been discussed, it must be concluded that BCAA are extremely effective in reversing severe HE. They likely act by decreasing plasma levels of AAA and ammonia as well as by directly competing with AAA for the transport system through the BBB. This latter mechanism probably accounts for the greater, (more evident) efficacy of BCAA with respect to lactulose whose major effect on HE is exerted only through a reduction of plasma ammonia levels.

REFERENCES

1. J. E. Fischer, J. M. Funovics, J. H. James, J. M. Keane, R. J. C.
    Wesdrop, N. Yoshimura, and T. Westman, The role of plasma
    amino acids in hepatic encephalopathy, Surgery 78: 276 (1975).
2. A. Cascino, C. Cangiano, V. Calcaterra, F. Rossi Fanelli, and
    L. Capocaccia, Plasma amino acids imbalance in patients with
    liver disease, Am. J. Dig. Dis. 23: 591 (1978).
3. W. M. Pardridge, Regulation of aminoacid availability to the
    brain, in: "Nutrition and the Brain." Vol. I, R. J. Wurtman
    J. J. Wurtman Ed., Raven Press, New York (1977).
4. H. J. James, J. Escorrou, and J. E. Fischer, Blood-brain neutral
    amino acids transport activity is increased after portacaval
    anastomosis, Science 200: 1395 (1978).
5. P. Cardelli-Cangiano, C. Cangiano, J. H. James, V. Jeppsson, W.
    Brenner, and J. E. Fischer, Uptake of amino acids by brain
    microvessels isolated from rats after portocaval anastomosis,
    J. Neurochem. 36: 627 (1981).
6. J. E. Fischer and R. J. Baldessarini, Pathogenesis and therapy
    of hepatic coma, in: "Progress in Liver Diseases," Vol. 5,
    H. Popper, F. Schaffner, eds., Grune and Stratton, New York,
    pp. 367-397 (1976).
7. F. Rossi Fanelli, C. Cangiano, A. Attili, M. Angelico, A. Ca-
    scino, L. Capocaccia, R. Strom, and C. Crifò, Octopamine plas-
    ma levels and hepatic encephalopathy: a re-appraisal of the
    problem, Clin. Chim. Acta 67: 255 (1976).
8. C. Cangiano, F. Rossi Fanelli, A. Bozzi, V. Calcaterra, A. Ca-
    scino, and L. Capocaccia, Plasma phenylethanolamine in hepatic
    encephalopathy, Eur. J. Clin. Invest. 8: 183 (1978).
9. A. J. Knell, A. R. Davidson, R. Williams, B. D. Kantamaneni, and
    G. Curzon, Dopamine and serotonin metabolism in hepatic en-
    cephalopathy, Br. Med. J. 1: 549 (1974).
10. J. E. Fischer, J. M. Funovics, A. Aguirre, J. H. James, J. M.
    Keane, R. I. C. Wesdorp, N. Yoshimura, and T. Westman, The
    role of plasma amino acids in hepatic encephalopathy, Surgery
    78: 276 (1975).
11. J. E. Fischer, H.M. Rosen, A.M. Ebeid, J. H. James, J. Keane, and
    P. B. Soeters, The effect of normalization of plasma amino
    acids on hepatic encephalopathy in man, Surgery 80: 77 (1976).
12. L. Capocaccia, V. Calcaterra, C. Cangiano, A. Cascino, F. Fiac-
    cadori, S. Gentile, F. Ghinelli, G. Pelosi, O. Riggio, F.
    Rossi Fanelli, D. Sacchini, and G. Giunchi, Therapeutic effect
    of branched-chain amino acids in hepatic encephalopathy: a
    preliminary study, in: "Medical and Surgical Problems of
    Portal Hypertension." M. J. Orloff, S. Stipa, V. Ziparo eds.,
    Academic Press, London, pp. 239-249 (1980).
13. F. Rossi Fanelli, O. Riggio, C. Cangiano, A. Cascino, D. De
    Conciliis, M. Merli, M. Stortoni, and G. Giunchi (Coordinator
    L. Capocaccia), Branched-Chain amino acids vs lactulose in
    the treatment of hepatic coma. A controlled study. Dig. Dis.

Sci 27: 929 (1982).

14. H. O. Conn and M. M. Lieberthal, The hepatic coma syndromes and
    lactulose, Williams & Wilkins, Baltimore (1979).

15. R. D. Adams, J. M. Foley, The neurological disorder associated
    with liver disease, Res. Publ. Assoc. Res. Nerv. Ment. Dis.
    32: 198 (1953).

16. L. E. Early, Conclusive remarks and presentation of diagnostic
    criteria of the hepato-renal syndrome, in: "Hepato-renal
    Syndrome", E. Bartoli, L. Chiandussi eds., Piccin Medical
    Books, Padova, pp. 494-499 (1980).

17. M. G. Buse and M. Reim, Leucine, a possible regulator of protein
    turnover in muscles, J. Clin. Invest. 56: 1250 (1975).

18. H. Freund, H. C. Hoover, S. Atamian, and J. E. Fischer, Infusion
    of the branched chain amino acids in postoperative patients,
    Ann. Surg. 190: 18 (1979).

19. P. B. Soeters and J. E. Fischer, Insulin, glucagon, amino acid
    imbalance and hepatic encephalopathy, Lancet 2: 880 (1976).

20. C. Cangiano, V. Calcaterra, A. Cascino, and L. Capocaccia, Bound
    and free tryptophan plasma levels in hepatic encephalopathy,
    Rend. Gastroenterol.8: 186 (1976).

21. C. Cangiano, F. Rossi Fanelli, A. Cascino, and L. Capocaccia,
    Tryptophan and hepatic encephalopathy, Gastroenterology 77:
    203 (1979).

22. J. Ono, D. G. Hutson, R. S. Dombro, J. U. Levi, A. Livingstone,
    and R. Zeppa, Tryptophan and hepatic coma, Gastroenterology
    74: 196 (1978).

23. F. Salerno, S. D. Dioguardi, and R. Abbiati, Tryptophan and
    hepatic coma, Gastroenterology 75: 769 (1978).

24. F. Rossi Fanelli, H. Freund, R. Krause, A. R. Smithy, J. H.
    James, S. Castorina-Ziparo, and J. E. Fischer, Alterations
    of plasma amino acids, amines and metabolites in hepatic
    coma, Gastroenterology 83: 664 (1982).

25. A. R. Smith, F. Rossi Fanelli, V. Ziparo, J. H. James, B. S.
    Berenice, A. Perelle, and J. E. Fischer, Induction of coma
    in normal dogs by the infusion of aromatic amino acids and
    its prevention by the addition of branched chain amino acids,
    Ann. Surg. 187: 343 (1978).

26. F. Rossi Fanelli, J. Escourrou, A. R. Smith, and J. E. Fischer,
    in: "Noncatecholic Phenylethylamines" part 2, A. D. Mosnaim
    and M. Wolf eds., Marcel Dekker, Inc., New York, p. 231
    (1980).

27. A. H. Lockwood, J. M. McDonald, R. E. Reiman, A. S. Gelbard,
    S. J. Laughlin, T. E. Duffy, and F. Plum, The dynamics of
    ammonia metabolism in man, J. Clin. Invest. 63: 449 (1979).

28. J. H. James, V. Ziparo, B. Jeppsson, and J. E. Fischer, Hyper-
    ammonemia, plasma AA imbalance and blood brain amino acid
    transport: an unified theory of portal systemic encephalo-
    pathy, Lancet 2: 772 (1979).

PROPHYLAXIS OF HEPATIC ENCEPHALOPATHY AFTER PORTA-CAVAL

ANASTOMOSIS USING BRANCHED CHAIN AMINO ACID MIXTURES

A. Puglionisi, F. Ceriati, I. R. Marino, C. Cavicchioni,
G. De Luca, A. Roncone and E. Di Cera

Department of Surgical Pathology, Università Cattolica
del Sacro Cuore, Rome, Italy

INTRODUCTION

Bleeding esophageal varices in cirrhotic patients is a cause
of death in 40-50% of cases at its first occurring, and in 80% at
its second occurring. This complication can effectively be prevented
by porta-caval anastomosis. However, this kind of surgery is frequently responsible for the appearance of symptoms of hepatic encephalopathy (HE).

The syndrome is essentially treated with the administration of
lactulose, antibiotics, hypertonic glucose solutions, and BCAA-
enriched solutions.

This study is aimed at verifying the effectiveness of BCAA
solutions in the prevention and treatment of HE consequent to portal-
systemic shunt.

MATERIALS AND METHODS

We have studied 20 patients admitted to our Department for
elective porta-caval shunt. They were divided into 2 random groups
of 10 each (Table 1).

All the patients suffered from esophageal varices, with previous
hemorrhages. Ascites was present in 8 cases.

Three blood samples were taken, the first before the operation,
the second three days later, and the third seven days later.

Before surgery the patients were on a low-protein diet (0.8 g/kg

345

Table 1.

	Patient	Age	Sex	P.O.HE	CHILD CLASS
	1) C.B.	56	M	NO	A
	2) C.S.	62	M	NO	A
	3) F.P.	49	F	NO	B
	4) L.B.G.	71	M	NO	B
Group A	5) N.F.	66	M	NO	B
(Treated)	6) R.G.	60	M	NO	A
	7) M.F.	54	F	NO	B
	8) F.G.	46	M	NO	B
	9) P.M.	51	F	NO	A
	10) P.L.	62	F	NO	B
	11) C.A.	48	F	NO	A
	12) D.P.L.	65	M	GRADE 3*	A
	13) E.J.	52	M	NO	B
	14) I.A.	57	F	NO	A
Group B	15) L.F.	53	M	NO	B
(Untreated)	16) N.A.	15	M	NO	A
	17) P.A.	47	M	NO	A
	18) V.A.	70	M	NO	B
	19) R.M.	58	M	GRADE 2	B
	20) D.M.A.	48	F	NO	B

*Dead three days after surgery.

Among more recent techniques, we will mention spleno-renal selective portal shunting,[3] porta-caval anastomosis with arterialization of the portal vein,[4] coronary-caval anastomosis by interposed graft,[5] and direct operations on esophageal varices.[6]

Though these methods partly respond to the assumptions of the pathogenetic etiology, they seem unable to change substantially the post-surgery course, which can be affected by a late portal-systemic flow excess. As to the "metabolic" definition of the disease, the importance of ammonia having been reconsidered, credit is now given to the hypothesis of an unbalance in neurotransmitters due to a change of the BCAA/AAA ratio.

In performing the porta-caval anastomosis we prefer the side-to-side shunt, as, in our opinion, besides being effective in reducing the risks of serious recurrent bleeding, it also allows to perform a "gauged" anastomosis (7-10 mm $\emptyset$).

b.w.); all treatment of lactulose or antibiotics was suspended in all of them three days before the first sample was taken.

The samples were assayed for aminoacids, ammonia, acid-base balance.

Routine blood tests were performed daily. The presence of HE was assessed by the Number Connection Test, EEG, test of evoked auditory and visual potential, and automatic audiometry. Neurologists were not informed which treatment was given.

Treatment A (Group A): a solution containing only BCAA and 16% dextrose was given i.v. through a centrally inserted catheter during the three days following surgery; an aminoacid enriched solution was administered in the next four days (Table 2).

Treatment B (Group B): electrolyte and 6% glucose solutions were given throughout the seven-day study.

RESULTS

Table 3 shows a comparison between aminoacid values in the treated (A) and untreated (B) groups.

In Figure 1 are indicated the mean molar ratios BCAA/AAA in the two groups, before surgery, 72 hours and seven days after surgery.

Our evaluations for the diagnosis of post-surgery HE allowed to detect the syndrome in 2 cases of Group B namely, one case of second grade coma two days after the operation, and one case of third grade coma three days after the operation.

The syndrome was not found in any of the patients of Group A.

DISCUSSION

The notion that portal-systemic shunting can be a direct cause of HE, due to a decreased portal flow to the liver, has long since been critically reexamined.[1,2]

A fundamental role for the occurring of the syndrome seems to be played by the degree of the hepatic failure, possibly made more serious by the flow change due to the shunt.

This is why, on the one hand, more selective surgical techniques should be sought, able to ensure an effective decrease of the portal blood pressure, without substantial modifications of the blood flow to the liver; and, on the other hand, it is necessary to give a "metabolic" definition of the syndrome, related to the hepatic insufficiency.

Table 2.   Composition of the two synthetic ammonia-free mixed
           amino acid solutions used in the treated group.

	BS 692 Gm/500 ml	BS 666 Gm/500 ml
Essentials		
L - isoleucine	6,428	4,500
L - leucine	7,857	5,500
L - lysine		3,800
L - methionine		0,500
L - phenylalanine		0,500
L - threonine		2,250
L - tryptophan		0,380
L - valine	6,000	4,200
Nonessentials		
L - alanine		3,750
L - arginine		3,000
L - histidine		1,200
L - proline		4,000
L - serine		2,500
L - glycine		4,500

For HE prevention and treatment, the BCAA solutions we employed proved useful.

Our study's results bring about the following remarks:

1) Before the operation, the aminoacid pattern is in accordance with the patients chronic liver disease. Later, BCAA undergoes a definite increase. A substantial change of the BCAA/AAA ratio can be seen around 72 hours after surgery. In tests made seven days after the operation, values are back to pre-operation levels.

2) The duration of treatment seemed sufficient to prevent an immediate HE onset. Controls on the same patients several months after the study showed a normal course, comparable to the average of cirrhotic patients.

3) HE percentage in untreated patients can be compared to the average of a large number of cases. This observation, and the fact that no HE occurred in the treated group, suggest that the BCAA solutions we used were an effective therapy.

4) Finally we may conclude that the administration of BCAA mixtures as described in this paper in post-operation TPN is useful. In fact, our data from this research suggest that the intake of BCAA is advisable for nutrition sakes and to prevent post-operation HE.

Table 3.   Comparison between group A (treated) and group B
           (untreated):average AA plasma levels (μm/1)

		PRE		72h POST		7 DAYS POST
VAL	B	140,528	(B)	121,677	B	99,997
	A	141,295	(A)	254,05	A	107,66
ILEU	B	89,582	(B)	93,996	B	66,487
	A	80,545	(A)	243,151	A	66,862
LEU	B	99,394	(B)	116,312	B	87,629
	A	102,299	(A)	316,85	A	72,412
TYR	B	96,563	(B)	116,204	B	84,966
	A	114,465	(A)	88,77	A	108,153
PHE	B	137,415	(B)	167,181	B	124,034
	A	156,924	(A)	112,086	A	123,218

5) In our opinion, AA solution treatments should have a duration
of 7 days. The first 72 h are mainly directed at preventing the
risk of HE, while in the next period problems related to nutrition
intake acquire a major importance.

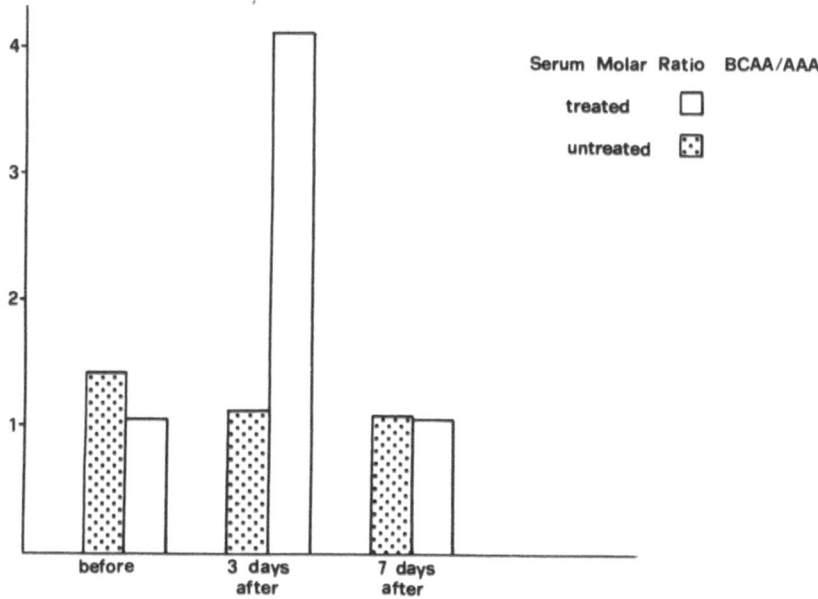

Fig. 1.   Behaviour of BCAA/AAA in the treated and untreated patients
          before and after surgery.

Acknowledgements

We are grateful to Sisters Franca Baiguera, Annunciata Beni
and Savina Zanchi, for their expert technical help.

REFERENCES

1. J. E. Fischer and R. J. Baldessarini, Pathogenesis and therapy
    of hepatic coma, in: "Progress in Liver Disease", H. Popper,
    F. Schaffner, eds., Grune and Stratton, New York, pp. 363-
    397 (1976).
2. H. Freund, J. Dienstag, J. Lehrich, N. Yoshimura, R. R. Brad-
    ford, H. Rosen, S. Atamian, E. Slemmer, J. Holroyde, and J.
    E. Fischer, Infusion of branched chain enriched amino acid
    solution in patients with hepatic encephalopathy, Ann. Surg.
    196: 209 (1982).
3. W. D. Warren, R. Zeppa, and J. J. Fomon, Selective trans splenic
    decompression of gastroesophageal varices by distal spleno-
    renal shunt, Ann. Surg., 166: 437 (1967).
4. R. J. Adamson, K. Butt, S. Iyer, J. De Rose, C. R. Dennis, M.
    Kinkhabwala, D. Gordon, and E. Martin, Porta-caval shunt with
    arterialization of the portal vein by means of a low flow
    arterio-venous fistula, Surg. Ginecol. Obstet., 146: 869
    (1978).
5. K. Inokuchi, M. Kobayashi, A. Kusaba, Y. Ogawa, M. Saku, and
    T. Shiizaki, New Selective decompression of esophageal va-
    rices by a left-gastric venous-caval shunt, Arch. Surg. 100:
    157 (1970).
6. M. Sugiura and S. Gutagava, A New technique for treating eso-
    phageal varices, J. Thor. Cardiovasc. Surg. 66: 677 (1973).

EFFECTIVE TREATMENT OF LATENT PORTO-SYSTEMIC ENCEPHALOPATHY WITH

ORAL BRANCHED CHAIN AMINO ACIDS *

E. H. Egberts,° H. Schomerus,° W. Hamster,°° P. Jürgens°°°

°Dept. I Med. Univ. Klinik, Tübingen; °°Neurologische
Poliklinik, Tübingen; °°°Allgemeines Krankenhaus, St.
Georg, Hamburg, West Germany

INTRODUCTION

About 60% of patients with portal hypertension without clinical
signs of porto-systemic encephalopathy (PSE) and with normal EEG
show substantial cerebral functional impairments[1,2,3,4,5]

The nature and extent of these impairments are such as to put
the aptitude to drive a car into doubt.[5] This degree of PSE which
ranges between grade 0 and grade 1 of the conventional classification, has been named latent PSE.[1]

It appears reasonable to treat a patient with latent PSE who
might put himself and others into danger when driving. Such a treatment would be long term in a patient who has little subjective
symptoms. It therefore should be free of objective and subjective
side effects. The conventional treatment of PSE with protein restriction, antibiotics and/or lactulose does not fulfil these criteria.
Based on the concept of Fischer and Baldessarini[6] treatment of
hepatic coma with branched chain amino acids (BCAA) enriched infusions has been introduced.

In a previous paper we could show that infusion of BCAA leads
to an improvement of cerebral function in latent PSE.[7] As infusions
are not practicable in outpatient treatment, we investigated the
effect of oral BCAA treatment in latent PSE.

---

*Paper selected for publication.

MATERIALS AND METHODS

Patients: 22 ambulatory cirrhotics, without clinical signs of PSE, but with impairment of driving fitness according to psychometric results were included in a randomized double blind cross-over trial. The study was approved by the local ethic committee.

Study design: all patients were admitted for at least 3 weeks to one hospital ward. Medications were kept constant for at least 10 days prior to and during the study. A defined diet providing 1 g of protein and 35 cal/kg/day was given. The actual food intake was measured daily. After 3 days of this diet, treatment was started with 0.25 g/kg/day of Verum or Placebo (Table 1) divided into 4 doses. The treatment lasted for 7 days followed by 7 days of the complementary medication (Figure 1). Psychometric tests, EEG recordings and ammonia profiles were done before and on the last days of each treatment period. EGG and psychometric tests were repeated 4 weeks after the end of the trial. Serum amino acids were determined in the fasting state as indicated in Figure 1. Urine was collected throughout the study for nitrogen determination to establish a semiquantitative nitrogen balance.

Compliance control: all medications was taken in the presence of a nurse. In addition the study compounds contained vitamin B_6 which was later on determined in the urine.[8]

Amino acid concentrations were determined by a multichrome M auto-analyser (Beckman instruments). Free and total tryptophan was measured.[9] Ammonia was determined enzymatically (Dupont).

Nitrogen was determined in 24-hour - urine according to Kjeldahl. Dominant and mean dominant EEG frequency were measured by visual assessment.[10] An extensive psychometric program was employed testing for intellectual function (3 tests) mnestic function (1 test), attention under different degrees of stress (3 tests), psychomotor functions (tests evaluating the Fleischmann factors of motor skill[11]) and reaction time. The tests were always given in the morning following the above sequence by the same investigator (W.H.). Three experts assessed driving fitness by a blind rating procedure.[5]

Paired t-tests were employed to evaluate overall changes during treatment periods and 4 weeks thereafter. To separate treatment effects and period effects (e.g. training effects in psychometric tests) and interactions between these and to estimate the extent of these influences, a special statistical model taking into account the cross over design[12] was applied. All reported significance levels refer to two tailed p values.

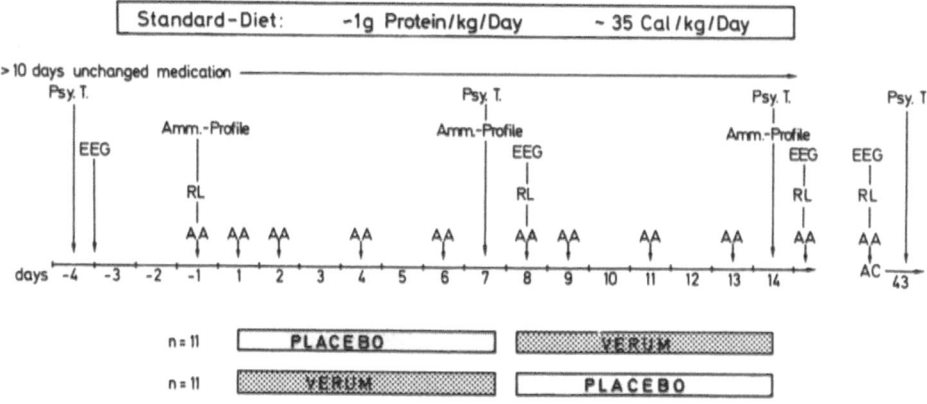

Fig. 1.   Study design. Psy.T. = psychometric tests, RL = routine
         laboratory, Amm. = ammoniak, AA = amino acid determination
         in serum, AC = ambulant control.

RESULTS

    When breaking the code the groups were comparable in clinical
and laboratory parameters as outlined in Table 2.

    The actual food intake was comparable in both groups throughout
the study. Estimated nitrogen balance improved from the pretreatment
to the treatment periods. Taking both groups together, the nitrogen
balance was significantly better during treatment with BCAA compared
with casein. Vitamin B_6 excretion in the urine increased significantly during medication in all patients indicating a good compliance.

    Mean ammonia concentration as derived from 6 ammonia determi-
nations on the day before treatment, day 7 and day 14 decreased under
treatment with BCAA. A mean decrease of 20.8 µmol/l (p = 0.087) could
be estimated as a treatment effect. The mean treatment effect on Val
level +37   µmol/l (p < 0.0005), on Leu concentration +11   µmol/l
(p < 0.005), on total Try -12 µmol/l (p < 0.0005), on free Try -5
µmol/l (p < 0.0005), on Tyr -6 µmol/l (p< 0.0005), on Phe -20 µmol/l
(p < 0.001). It is noteworthy that these values were obtained in the
fasting state about 10 hours after the last medication. When determining amino acid profiles during the day under oral BCAA the changes
observed are in the same direction, but much more pronounced as could
be shown in a pilot study.[7] All laboratory parameters related to
liver function remained unchanged throughout the study. For psychometric variables the following treatment effects could be estimated

Table 1. Composition of verum and placebo

Verum		Placebo	
L-Leucin	1.290 g		
L-Isoleucin	0.855 g	Casein	3.000 g
L-Valin	0.855 g		
Vitamin B_6	0.003 g	Vitamin B_6	0.003 g

Table 2. Clinical data

	Group 1 n = 11	Group 2 n = 11
Sex	7 ; 4	9 ; 2
Age in years (range)	51 + 6 (40–59)	52 + 10 (37–65)
Weight in kg	70 + 12	66 + 12
Etiology		
Alcohol	9	10
Hepatitis	2	1
Diagnosis		
Clinical	2	2
Biopsy	9	9
Esophageal varices	8	8
Ascites	7	8
Therapy		
Diuretics	7	8
Lactulose	7	7
Laboratory values		
Albumin (%)	46 + 8	46 + 9
γ-globulin (%)	32 + 8	31 + 7
Prothrombin index (%)	61 + 16	57 + 13
Indocyanin green half life in min.	18 + 5	20 + 7
Driving fitness		
with restriction	7	5
unfit	4	6

considering the cross over design: line tracing –11 sec (p < 0.0005),
tapping +20 hits (p = 0.007), steadiness error duration –4sec
(p = 0.033), auditory reaction time –3/100 sec (p = 0.012), digit

table -66 sec (p = 0,031), Digit symbols +3 points (p = 0,055),number connection test -16 sec (p = 0,044). Training effects seem probable in the Number Revision Test, +13 points (p = 0,066) and in the Number Connection Test -14 sec (p = 0,066), the latter showing a treatment effect as well. Mnestic function and the Multiple Choice Vocabulary Test remained unchanged.

DISCUSSION

Since the proposal of the hypothesis of Fischer and Baldessa-rini[6] a number of reports have been published on the effect of BCAA infusions in hepatic coma. Considering the fact that many patients in grade III to IV coma have very poor and deteriorating liver function and that this is the main factor determining the outcome, they may not represent the ideal group to test a new treatment, which is aimed at symptoms and not at the underlying disease.

The situation is different in patients with low grade or latent PSE which appears to be the most common form of PSE. As in these patients liver function is relatively stable and usually no life-threatening complications are present, they appear to be more apt to demonstrate the effect of a new therapeutic principle. The apparent necessity of long term treatment in these patients largely excludes the employment of protein restriction and neomycin as these may have unfavourable side-effects when applied over longer duration. Lactulose therapy appears to be a reasonable alternative, but in our experience the subjective side effects such as taste and abdominal discomfort lead to poor compliance in the long run.

Up to now no objective or subjective side effects have been reported with BCAA treatment and they are not to be expected on theoretical grounds.

Our results have shown that with infusion and with oral application of BCAA a measurable improvement of cerebral function can be obtained in lower grade PSE patients. In addition a positive nitrogen balance can be achieved which we - as others - consider highly important in chronic liver disease. Furthermore increased nitrogen intake by BCAA substitution was accompanied by a decrease in ammonia levels, possibly due to an anabolic effect of BCAA.

Our results correspond to the first observation of Freund,[13] and to the results of a controlled trial by Horst et al.,[14] and to a study by Langnans et al.[15] Contrary to these findings, Eriksson et al.[16] reported no improvement of PSE in a cross over trial including 5 patients and 2 outpatients. But in view of the small number of patients the probability of a type II error in this trial appears to be fairly high. Two tests of their psychometric program (Digit Symbol and Number Connection) which proved to be highly sensitive in our investigations seem to show a favourable tendency in their study too. As in our studies the Benton Test was not altered.

Tests similar to their Bourdon-Wirsma test proved not to be very
sensitive and show a training effect in our experience.

The correspondence between the improvement of the deranged
amino acid pattern with the improvement of psychometric tests in
our study and in others corresponds well to the Fischer hypothesis.
Nevertheless, we rather hesitate to enter into the discussion of
the pro's and con's of this pathophysiologic concept. But even
considering treatment with BCAA as empirical, it appears to be promising especially in the long term treatment of latent PSE. Therefore a long term study is actually in preparation.

REFERENCES

1. H. Schomerus and W. Hamster, Latent portasystemic encephalo-
    pathy, Digestion 14: 5 (1976).
2. S. Rehnström, G. Simert, J. A. Hansson, G. Johnson, and J. Vang,
    Chronic hepatic encephalopathy. A psychometrical study,
    Scand. J. Gastroent. 12: 305 (1977).
3. L. Rikkers, P. Jenko, D. Rudman, and D. Freides, Subclinical
    hepatic encephalopathy: detection, prevalence and relation-
    ship to nitrogen metabolism, Gastroenterology 75: 462 (1978).
4. P. Elsass, Y. Lund, and L. Ranek, Encephalopathy in patients
    with cirrhosis of the liver. A neuropsychological study,
    Scand. J. Gastroent. 13: 241 (1978).
5. H. Schomerus, W. Hamster, H. Blunck, U. Reinhard, K. Mayer, and
    W. Dölle, Latent portasystemic encephalopathy, Dig. Dis. Sci.
    26: 622 (1981).
6. J. E. Fischer and R. J. Baldessarini, False neurotransmitters
    and hepatic failure, Lancet II: 75 (1971).
7. E. H. Egberts, W. Hamster, and P. Jürgens, Effect of branched
    chain amino acids on latent portasystemic encephalopathy,
    in: "Metabolism and Clinical Implications of Branched Chain
    Amino and Ketoacids," Walser, Williamson, eds., Elsevier
    North-Holland, New York, pp. 453-463 (1981).
8. S. Udenfried, "Fluorescence Assay in Biology and Medicine,"Aca-
    demic Press, New York and London, pp. 252-263 (1962).
9. W. D. Denckla and H. K. Dewey, The determination of tryptophan
    in plasma, liver and urine, J. Lab. & Clin. Med. 69: 160
    (1967).
10. J. Laidlaw and A. E. Read; The EEG in hepatic encephalopathy,
    Clin. Sci. 24: 109 (1963).
11. E. A. Fleishman, A factor analysis of psychomotor abilities,
    J. Exp. Psychol. 46: 95 (1962).
12. B. Schneider, Some problems of repeated measurements, Rome:
    European Symposium on Medical Statistics, (1980).
13. H. Freund, N. Yoshimura, and J. E. Fischer, Chronic hepatic
    encephalopathy. Long-term therapy with a branched chain amino
    acid-enriched elemental diet, JAMA 242: 347 (1979).
14. D. Horst, N. Grace, and H. O. Conn, A double-blind randomized

comparison of dietary protein and an oral branched chain amino acid (BCAA) supplement in cirrhotic patients with chronic portal-systemic encephalopathy (PSE), Chicago: AASLD (1981).

15. W. Langhans, E. Holm, U. Staedt, and M. Hartmann, Diätische Anwendung verzweigtkettiger Aminosäuren bei Patienten mit Leberzirrhose, Z. Gastroenterol. 14: 495 (1981).

16. S. Erikkson and J. Wahren, Failure of oral branched-chain amino acid administration to improve chronic hepatic encephalopathy, in: "Metabolism and Clinical Implications of Branched Chain Amino and Ketoacids," M. Walser, J. R. Williamson eds. Elsevier North-Holland, New York, pp. 481-485 (1981).

EFFECT OF VEGAN AND MEAT PROTEIN DIETS IN MILD CHRONIC PORTAL-SYSTEMIC ENCEPHALOPATHY (*)

B. Jeppsson, A. Kjällman, U. Åslund, A. Alwmark, P. Gullstrand, and B. Joelsson

Departments of Surgery and Psychiatry, University of Lund, S-221 85 Lund, Sweden

INTRODUCTION

Patients with liver impairment tend to develop protein intolerance, and excess protein intake may in these patients precipitate encephalopathy. The etiology of hepatic encephalopathy is closely linked to the altered protein metabolism in liver disease.[1] There is some evidence to suggest that tolerance to protein diets in liver disease may vary depending on the nature of the diet. Fenton et al.[2] demonstrated that patients with portal-systemic encephalopathy (PSE) tolerate a milk diet better than a similar amount of protein given as meat. More recently Greenberger et al.[3] reported results suggesting that patients with encephalopathy tolerate vegetable protein better than meat protein. There may be several reasons for this difference such as different generation of ammonia and different amino acid profiles in various types of protein.

The following study was undertaken to investigate alterations in nitrogen metabolism and neuropsychologic status in patients with stable liver cirrhosis and a history of PSE under two different nutritional regimens.

Material and methods

Eight patients with liver cirrhosis and a history of PSE participated in the study (Table 1). No acute precipitating factors were found in the immediate prestudy period. During the study the

_____

(*)Paper selected for publication.

patients did not receive any other medical therapy. The design of
the study is outlined in Table 2. All bound tests were drawn after
an overnight fast. The psychometric tests were performed in the
mornings under equivalent conditions by the psychologist, who was
not informed which diet the patient was receiving. The urinary
excretion of urea and creatinine was followed daily throughout the
study. The order of the diets was randomized by the dietitian. Some
representative diets of each type are described in Tables 3 and 4.
Patients received the same amount of calories and protein during
the two weeks of study. The mean daily protein intake was 59.1 g
(58.0-60.0 g). The caloric intake varied individually with age, sex
and physical activities. The mean caloric intake was 1920 (1670-
2210).

     The psychometric tests utilized in the study are in general use
at the Department of Surgery, University of Lund, in diagnosing
organic brain damage. The tests were carried out individually by
each patient within one hour. Different versions of the tests were
used on each test occasion in order to avoid a training effect. The
tests were designed to evaluate both sensory functions and motor
functions. Lowered performance on these tests can reflect a slowing
of general response and inattentiveness, typical of diffuse brain
injuries. The following tests were used:

a. Digit symtol test, a subtest of WAIS, is a visual motor test.[4]
   The patient is given a list of symbols associated with digits
   from 1 to 9, and should fill the blanks with symbols that correspond to each number.

b. Dot-test. A modified version of the Bourdon-Wirsma vigilance test
   was used to test perceptual speed.[5]

c. Trail making test A and B.[6] These tests measure cognitive motor
   abilities. It consists of connecting numbers and letters arranged
   in a circle requiring the patient to deal with two dimensions.

d. Simple reaction time test. The patient is instructed to respond
   to a visual signal by pressing a switch with their finger tips
   as fast as possible. 96 stimuli were given over five minutes.
   Calculation was made for each one-minute period in order to
   analyze changes in performance over time.

e. Manual dexterity. The test consists of lifting cylindrical knobs
   from one board, placing them in holes in another identical board.
   The number of knobs correctly placed were recorded.

     Standard statistical methods have been employed (Snedecor and
Cochran),[7] using the paired t-test when applicable.

Table 1. Clinical and laboratory data for the patients.

Age yrs	Sex	Etiology of Cirrhosis	Bilirubin[a]	ALP[b]	Prothrombin[c]	ASAT[d]
34	M	Cryptogenic	21	10	65	3.4
70	M	Alcoholic	18	4.8	110	0.5
37	F	Alcoholic	50	4.7	45	1.9
47	M	Alcoholic	13	5.3	85	0.6
62	M	Alcoholic	72	3.9	70	0.9
42	F	Alcoholic	16	3.3	75	0.6
62	M	Alcoholic	15	4.4	70	0.8
34	M	Alcoholic	13	3.1	85	0.4

[a] Normal value 3–20 μmol/l.

[b] ALP (alkaline phosphatase), normal value 0.8–4.6μkat/l.

[c] Prothrombin index, normal value 80–120.

[d] ASAT (aspartate aminotransferase), normal value< 0.67 μkat/l.

Table 2. Design of the study.

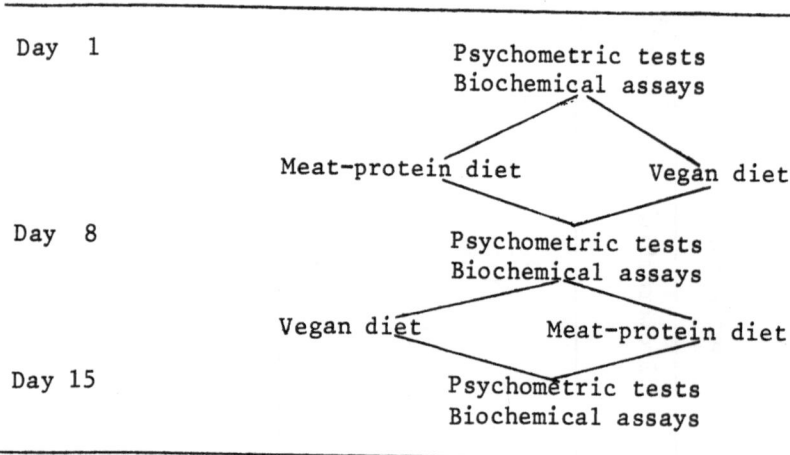

Day 1   Psychometric tests
                                      Biochemical assays

              Meat-protein diet   Vegan diet

Day 8   Psychometric tests
                                      Biochemical assays

         Vegan diet   Meat-protein diet

Day 15   Psychometric tests
                                      Biochemical assays

Results

The two protein diets were well tolerated by all patients. Liver function tests remained unchanged during the study. Venous plasma ammonia rose from 50+6 μmol/l before the study to 60+8 after meat protein diet and 61+2 after vegan diet with no statistically significant difference between the groups. Plasma urea and creatinine were unchanged. The mean daily urinary excretion of urea decreased significantly (p < 01) from 260+44 mmoles during the week with meat protein diet to 198+29 during the vegan diet week. There was a similar significant (p < 0.5) decrease in urinary excretion of creatinine from 14.8+1.7 to 13.1+1.4. The plasma amino acid pattern was altered in a fashion similar to what has been described previously in patients with liver cirrhosis or portal-systemic shunting, with decreased levels of branched-chain amino acids and increases of aromatic amino acids (Table 5).[8] The plasma concentrations of valine, leucine, tryptophan and phenylalanine decreased slightly during the study. The only significant alteration, however, was a decrease of plasma tyrosine after vegan diet. The results from the psychometric testing before the trial and after the two diets are presented in Table 6. The results obtained with either diet as compared to the pre-study values revealed significant improvements in the case of four of the psychometric tests (trail making A and B, Bourdon-Wirsma and digit symbol). For one test there was a significant difference between the two diets. If two patients, who were not considered encephalopathic at the start of the study, are excluded, five patients had improved psychometric test after vegan diet and only one after meat protein diet.

Table 3.   Composition of typical meat-protein diet.

	Amount (g or ml)	Calories	Protein (g)
1. Breakfast			
Oatmeal	25	96	3.3
Apple sauce	30	36	0.1
Low fat milk	150	57	5.1
Bread	50	143	4.0
Margarine	10	75	-
Cheese	15	60	4.3
Orange marmalade	20	49	-
Orange juice	100	45	0.7
2. Lunch			
Roast beef	60	82	13.1
Gravy	12	35	0.5
Green beans	50	14	0.9
Pickles	30	35	0.5
Potato	120	114	2.0
Orange soup	106	87	0.8
Biscuits	10	50	0.6
Fruit punch	200	126	-
3. Dinner			
Chicken	40	70	7.2
Rice	7	25	0.5
Peas, corn, pepper	35	25	1.2
Lettuce, tomato	30	7	0.4
Sauce	53	45	1.7
Bread	37	117	2.9
Margarine	10	74	-
Fruit punch	200	126	-
Fruit	100	45	0.2
4. Snacks			
Bread	67	222	5.5
Margarine	10	74	-
Sausage	15	56	2.4
Marmalade	20	49	-
TOTAL		2039	57.9

Table 4. Composition of typical vegan diet.

	Amount (g or ml)	Calories	Protein (g)
1. Breakfast			
Bread	85	232	6
Margarine	10	75	–
Veg. paste	70	169	4.9
Cucumber	50	8	0.5
Orange juice	100	45	0.7
2. Lunch			
Potato	200	174	3.0
Lentils	40	133	9.8
Millet	40	129	3.9
Mushroom	50	12	0.9
Veg. broth	5	5	1.0
Cabbage	50	12	0.6
Green pepper	30	10	0.4
Veg. oil	10	88	–
Peas, carrots	70	39	2.0
Fruit	100	61	0.7
3. Dinner			
Kale	100	52	6.0
Potato	150	143	2.2
Onion	50	19	0.8
Veg. broth	5	5	1.0
Bread	60	160	3.8
Margarine	10	75	–
Veg. paste	50	121	3.0
Orange juice	150	68	1.1
4. Snacks			
Graham rusks	36	156	3.9
Orange	100	50	1.0
TOTAL		2041	57.7

Table 5. Venous plasma amino acid concentrations. Data are
given as mean ± SEM.

	Normal values	Patients		
		Before study	During meat-protein diet	During vegan diet
Valine (µmol/l)	213	165+18	139+21	144+13
Isoleucine	58	42+4	44+5	39+4
Leucine	115	86+10	77+12	78+9
Methionine	20	38+4	38+3	37+3
Tryptophan	41	65+6	58+5	60+4
Tyrosine	56	124+14	124+17	109+10[a]
Phenylalanine	54	77+10	72+5	73+3

[a] $p < .05$, as compared to values before study and during meat-protein diet.

Discussion

The present study was designed to evaluate the effect of vegan
diet on cerebral function in patients with liver cirrhosis and
chronic encephalopathy. There was an improvement in the patients'
response to psychometric tests after vegan diet as compared to meat
protein diet. These findings are in accord with a previous report
by Greenberger.[3] There are several possible explanations to account
for the beneficial effects of vegan diet. The vegan diet in the
study by Greenberger lowered plasma methionine and thereby possibly
resulting in decreased production of mercaptans, which may be toxic
to the brain.[1] Plasma methionine levels were, however, unchanged
during the two diets of this study. Vegan diet may contain smaller
amounts of the aromatic amino acids tryptophan, phenylalanine and
tyrosine implicated in the causation of PSE.[9] There was a decrease
of plasma tyrosine after vegan diet in this study, while tryptophan
and phenylalanine were unchanged. It is also possible that the
increased fiber content of the vegan diet resulted in decreased
production and absorption of ammonia or other putative materials
from the gut, that are important in the pathogenesis of PSE. A change
in bowel transit time during the vegan diet may increase fecal loss
of urea and partly explain the reduced urinary excretion. Plasma
ammonia levels remained unchanged during the study weeks, and in
this study there was no evidence for decreased production of ammonia
by vegan diet, as has been proposed previously.[3,10]

Table 6. Psychometric test results. Data are given as mean
          $\pm$ SEM.

	Before study	During meat-protein diet	During vegan diet
Trail making A (sec)	60+9	51+7[a]	50+7[a]
Trail making B (sec)	89+15	79+11[a]	76+12[a]
Bourdon-Wirsma (sec)	199+22	184+22[a]	172+16[a] [b]
Digit symbol (No. correct)	42+6	47+7[a]	48+7[a]
Manual dexterity (No. correct)	64+6	68+6	66+7
Reaction time (msec)	26.6+2.7	27.7+3.4	26.7+3.1

[a] $p < .01$, as compared to the corresponding measurement
    before the study.
[b] $p < 0.5$, as compared to the corresponding measurement
    during meat-protein diet.

The study does not provide a clear-cut explanation for the
observed beneficial effect of vegan diet in PSE. One explanation
may be that the vegan diet contains lower amounts of amino acids
and other putative materials which may be important in the pathogenesis of PSE. Furthermore this diet may be superior in tolerating
and conserving nitrogen. The results are preliminary and further
controlled trials should be undertaken with vegan diet, maybe with
addition of lactulose or neomycin.

REFERENCES

1. L. Zieve, Hepatic encephalopathy: summary of present knowledge
    with an elaboration on recent developments, in:"Progress in
    Liver Diseases,"H. Popper, ed., vol. VI. Grune and Stratton,
    New York, p. 327 (1979).
2. J. C. B. Fenton,E. J. Knight, and P. L. Humpherson, Milk and
    cheese diet in portalsystemic encephalopathy, Lancet i: 164
    (1966).
3. N. J. Greenberger, J. Carley, S. Shenker, I. Bettinger, C.
    Stamnes, and P. Beyer, Effect of vegetable and animal protein

diets in chronic hepatic encephalopathy, Am. J. Dig. Dis. 22: 845 (1977).

4. A. Mirsky and C. Kornetsky, On the dissimilar effects of drugs on the digit symbol substitution and continuous performance tests, Psychopharmacologia 5: 161 (1964).

5. J. Weckroth, Studies in brain pathology and human performance. On the relationship between severity of brain injury and the level and structure of intellectual performance, Psych. & Soc. Res. 12: 1 (1965).

6. R. M. Reitan, Validity of the trail making test as an indicator of organic brain damage, Percept. Mot. Skills 8: 271 (1958).

7. G. W. Snedecor and W. G. Cochran, "Statistical Methods", 6th edn. Iowa State University Press, Ames (1967).

8. H. M. Rosen, N. Yoshimura, H. M. Hodgman, and J. E. Fischer, Plasma amino acid patterns in hepatic encephalopathy of differing etiology, Gastroenterology 72: 483 (1977).

9. J. H. James, B. Jeppsson, V. Ziparo, and J. E. Fischer, Hyperammonemia, plasma amino acid imbalance, and blood-brain amino acid transport: an unified theory of portal-systemic encephalopathy, Lancet ii: 772 (1979).

10. D. Rudman, J. T. Galambos, R. B. Smith, A. A. Salam, and W. D. Warren, Comparison of the effect of various amino acids upon the blood ammonia concentration of patients with liver disease, Am. J. Clin. Nutr. 26: 916 (1973).

$[^{14}C]$-L-VALINE BINDING TO POST MORTEM FRONTAL CORTEX HOMOGENATES

IN HEPATIC ENCEPHALOPATHY *

P. Riederer, Elisabeth Kienzl,
K. Jellinger and G. Kleinberger

Ludwig Boltzmann Institute of Clin. Neurobiology
Lainz-Hospital, Vienna, and Department of Medicine I
University School of Medicine, Vienna, Austria

SEROTONIN RECEPTORS IN HEPATIC COMA

In hepatic encephalopathy (HE) the plasma aromatic amino acid (AAA) concentrations are increased, while branched chain amino acid (BCAA) levels are reduced. Increased availability of AAA in particular of tryptophan (TRP) at brain uptake sites will influence brain synthesis and turnover of neurotransmitters like serotonin (5-hydroxytryptamine; 5-HT). In HE increased TRP, 5-HT and 5-hydroxyindole acetic acid (5-HIAA) concentrations and enhanced 5-HT turnover have been demonstrated in human post mortem brain studies with kynurenine synthesis being more pronounced in plasma than in the brain.[1] Treatment with BCAA and in particular L-valine (VAL) frequently lead to awakening of patients from hepatic coma[2,3] and this effect has been suggested to correlate with normalization of 5-HT disturbances in the brain.[1] Corresponding changes in 5-HT receptor activity occur in HE and may be influenced by the administration of VAL. Using radioreceptor ligand binding techniques with ^{3}H-5-HT and ^{3}H-spiroperidol (R 50-656 as unlabeled ligand to define unspecific binding) it has been shown in human post mortem frontal cortex that 5-HT-1 receptors (labeled by ^{3}H-5-HT) lose binding density with a slight increase in affinity (total specific binding; B_{max}: - 58%, K_{D}=-35%) while treatment with VAL normalizes both 5-HT-1 receptor density (B_{max}: -4%) and affinity (K_{D} = 0%) ex vivo.[4] These results have been confirmed by in vitro studies using either control tissue or tissue (frontal cortex) from patients dying from severe hepatic failure.

---

* Paper selected for publication.

Brain tissue obtained from hepatic coma patients with endogenous
ammonia levels being in the range of 4,3 to 5,2 nmol/g tissue is
much more sensitive to in vitro incubation of VAL.[5] 5-HT-1 receptor
density increased from a reduced level of -68% up to +180% at the
low concentration of 0.1 mM VAL while higher concentrations of VAL
did not show this effect (Table 1). Studies performed with control
tissue revealed a significant reduction of 5-HT-1 receptor density
after incubation with 10 or 30 mM ammonia, while additional administration of 1 to 60 mM VAL antagonized this effect (Table 1)

    In contrast to these findings 5-HT-2 receptor activity measured
in human post mortem frontal cortex was unchanged indicating a
different response of both receptor sites to functional disturbances
by neurotoxic substances originating from degenerated liver and
passing a disturbed blood brain barrier (BBB).[6]

$[^{14}C]$-L-VALINE BINDING SITE

    VAL increases subnormal 5-HT-1 receptor densities in HE ex vivo[1]
and in vitro.[5] Furthermore, VAL leads to a significant reduction of
serum ammonia (NH_4^+),[2,3,1,7] CSF NH_4^+ [7] and human brain NH_4^+ concentration.[8] In addition VAL is able to antagonize the 5-HT-1 receptor
density diminishing effects of NH_4^+. Modulation of 5-HT receptors by
VAL suggests direct action of VAL on 5-HT-1 receptor units. For
further characterizing this interrelationship $[^{14}C]$-VAL binding has
been studied in HE using post mortem frontal cortex. Therefore we
have set up an assay and have characterized the biochemical and
pharmacological properties. These data are given elsewhere.[6,9]
Patients with liver failure (liver cirrhosis without coma; hepatic
coma) exhibit a significant increase in $[^{14}C]$-VAL binding density
with no change in affinity, while our preliminary data give evidence
for a reduction of binding number in hepatic coma treated with VAL
(Table 2).

    Although the nature of this binding type remains to be further
studied, modulation of 5-HT-1 receptor function by VAL might be a
regulatory principle of basic pathophysiological importance in HE.
This is also indicated by its preferential localization in synaptic
membranes and its different distribution in human brain areas with
predominance of frontal cortex, hippocampus and amygdaloid nucleus.[9]
It is concluded that the beneficial effects of VAL in HE are in
part due to this specific effect on postsynaptic receptor membranes.
In this respect the action of VAL can be distinguished from LEU,
which induces protein synthesis to a much higher degree than VAL[10]
but has only 1/5 to 1/10 of binding sites compared to VAL.[6] Thus
amino acid mixtures with high concentration of VAL[3] might improve
the mental stage of patients with hepatic coma to a higher degree
than infusion with high supply of LEU.

Table 1. Influence of ammonium ions and L-valine on serotonin receptor binding in human post mortem frontal cortex[a]

Patients	NH_4^+ mM	L-valine mM	High affinity spec. binding % B_{max} (fmol/mg protein)	K_D (nM)	Total spec. binding % B_{max} (fmol/mg protein)	K_D (nM)
Controls	-	-	100	100	100	100
	10	-	45	54	64	40
	10	15	95	136	98	87
	30	-	59	74	75	67
	30	1	340	329	112	174
	30	15	340	371	135	202
	30	60	235	430	99	70
Coma hepaticum	E	-	68[b]	51[b]	58[b]	30[b]
	E	0.1	180	303	125	365
	E	15	70	263	70	357
	E	30	0	0	34	253

[a] means of 60 single determinations
[b] compared to controls. This is the 100% value for hepatic coma.

E = endogenous NH_4^+ (4.3 to 5.2 nmol/g tissue)
Kienzl et al.[3]

Table 2. ^{14}C-L-valine binding to human post mortem frontal cortex

	Coma stage	B_{max} (pmol/mg protein)	B_{max} (% control)	K_D (µM)
Controls	(8)	—	229 ± 12	100	7.6 ± 0.75
Liver cirrhosis without coma	(2) I/I	534/518	233/226	12.0/ 6.4
Hepacic coma	(5) IV	396 ± 49.8[a]	173	9.4 ± 5.9
Hepatic coma (Wernicke S.)	(1) IV	452	197	7.5
Hepatic coma + VAL	(2) IV–I	220/47	96/21	4.9/7.8

Means ± SEM; number of brains in parenthesis;

[a] $P < 0.001$ compared to controls.

REFERENCES

1. P. Riederer, P. Kruzik, E. Kienzl, G. Kleinberger, K. Jellinger, and W. Wesemann, Central aminergic function and its disturbance by hepatic disease: current status of L-valine pharmacotherapy in metabolic coma, in "Transmitter Biochemistry of Human Brain Tissue", Riederer P., E. Usdin eds.; Macmillan Publ. Ltd., London-Basingstoke, 143-182 (1981).

2. G. Kleinberger, R. Dudczak, P. Ferenci, H. Pamperl, P. Riederer, and K. Widhalm, Parenteral Ernährung bei schwerer Leberinsuffizienz, Z. Gastroenterol. Suppl. 16: 99 (1980).

3. G. Kleinberger, P. Riederer, P. Ferenci, and H. Binder, Complete parenteral nutrition and intravenous administration of L-valine in hepatic coma, in "Aminosäuren- und Ammoniakstoffwechsel bei Leberinsuffizienz". E. Holm ed.; Witzstrock, Baden-Baden, Köln, New York, pp. 220-225 (1982).

4. N. Arold, Ph. D. Thesis, Philipps-Universität, Marburg, GFR, (1982).

5. E. Kienzl, P. Riederer, K. Jellinger,and G. Kleinberger, Antagonisierung der Ammoniakwirkung auf Serotoninrezeptoren durch L-valin, Leber.Magen.Darm.12, Nr. 5: 179 (1982).

6. P. Riederer, E. Kienzl, K. Jellinger, H. Noller, and G. Kleinberger, General properties of ^{14}C-L-valine-binding to human brain tissue, Journal of Neural Transm. Suppl.in press (1982).

7. M. Rössle, R. Herz, G. Lehmann, M. Luft, and W. Gerok, Therapie der hepatischen Enzephalopathie, Infusionstherapie 9: 256 (1982).

8. M. Weiser, P. Riederer,and G. Kleinberger, Human cerebral free amino acids in hepatic coma, J. Neural. Transm. Suppl. 14: 95 (1978).

9. E. Kienzl, P. Riederer, K. Jellinger, and G. Kleinberger, $\left[^{14}C\right]$-L-valine binding to membranes of the frontal cortex in hepatic encephalopathy, J. Neural. Transm. 55: in press (1982).

10. A. L. Goldberg and M. E. Tischler, Regulatory effects of leucine on carbohydrate and protein metabolism, in "Metabolism and Clinical Implications of Branched Chain Amino and Ketoacids". M. Walser, J. R. Williamson, eds., Elsevier, North Holland, New York, pp. 205-216 (1981).

11. J. Wahren, J. Denis, P. Desurmont, S. Eriksson, J. M. Escoffier, A. P. Gauthier, L. Hagenfeldt, H. Michel, P. Opolon, J.C. Paris,and M. Veyrac, Is i.v. administration of BCAA effective in the treatment of hepatic encephalopathy? A multicenter study. Abstract FC 47, ESPEN Congress, Maastrich, 1981.

REGIONAL ANALYSIS OF NOREPINEPHRINE, DOPAMINE AND AMINO ACIDS IN THE

BRAIN 18 HOURS AFTER HEPATECTOMY AND INFUSION OF BRANCHED-CHAIN

AMINO ACIDS

M. Herlin, J.H. James, C.A. Nachbauer and J.E. Fischer

Department of Surgery, University of Cincinnati Medical
Center, Cincinnati, Ohio 45267, USA

INTRODUCTION

Fulminant hepatic failure is accompanied by an increase of the
concentrations of most amino acids in plasma and brain except the
branched-chain amino acids.[1-4] Norepinephrine (NE) levels in the
brain are low in rats with hepatic devascularization[5] or hepatectomy[6]
and in dogs with portacaval shunt and encephalopathy.[7] Dopamine (DA),
the precursor of NE, has been observed to be near normal in rats
with hepatectomy[6] and decreased in dogs with portacaval anastomosis[7]
or in humans with hepatic coma.[8]

Fischer and Baldessarini[9] have proposed that inhibition of catecholamine synthesis in the brain in hepatic failure may occur due
to high concentrations of phenylalanine which may inhibit the synthesis of dopa from tyrosine by competing with tyrosine for the enzyme
tyrosinase. High levels of phenylalanine and tyrosine may also result
in increased synthesis of neuroactive amines which may displace NE
from vesicles. Parenteral administration of a solution rich in the
BCAA to dogs with hepatic encephalopathy improved encephalopathy and
normalized amino acid concentrations both in plasma and in CSF[11] as
well as decreasing CSF concentrations of octopamine and phenylethanolamine. Since the group of large neutral amino acids share a
common transport system at the blood-brain barrier, the BCAA compete
with other neutral amino acids for blood-brain transport[12] and may
therefore reduce the accumulation of aromatic amino acids in the
CNS. In the present studies the effect of BCAA on the depletion of
catecholamines in various regions of brain after hepatectomy was
examined.

---

*Paper selected for publication.

MATERIALS AND METHODS

Male Sprague-Dawley rats were used and all surgical procedures were carried out under ether anesthesia. Hepatectomy was performed in three stages similar to the technique described by Holmin et al.[13] In the first stage (I), the inferior vena cava was divided between two ligatures above the renal veins. In the second stage (II), four weeks later, an end-to-side portacaval shunt was performed without ligation of the pancreaticoduodenal vein. In the third stage (III), one week later, all the liver parenchyma was removed after ligation of the hepatic artery, the biliary duct and the inferior vena cava. Group A (n = 12) and Group B (n = 12) underwent total hepatectomy while Group C (n = 8) underwent stage I and II as above but at stage III a sham operation was performed. Group D (n = 8) underwent stage I as above but the animals were sham operated at stage II and III. The animals were infused with a solution containing 10% glucose and electrolytes. Groups A, C and D received the solution above. Group B received the solution above with 0.24 mol/l BCAA added (0.08 mol/l of each valine, leucine and isoleucine). The solutions were infused at a rate of 0.9 $\pm$ 0.01 ml/h and 100 g body weight. The rate were warmed by proximity to a heating lamp and rectal temperature was maintained at 35-37°C.

Following 18 hours of infusion all rats were sacrificed by decapitation and blood from the cervical wound was collected into heparizinized cups. The brain was removed and dissected into the following regions: cortex (2 hemispheres), hypothalamus, striatum, hippocampus, mesencephalon, diencephalon, pons-medulla, and cerebellum.

Plasma cerebral cortex free amino acids were determined by using a Beckman 121-MB amino acid analyzer.

NE and DA were assayed by liquid chromatography with electrochemical detection from each region.

Data were subjected to analysis of variance and Newman-Keul's test.

RESULTS

Seven of twelve rats of each hepatectomized group survived 18 hours of infusion. In Group A five of seven rats were in coma (no response to tail pinch) at sacrifice, and in the BCAA-treated group two of seven rats were in coma.

Following hepatectomy and glucose infusion (Group A) compared to Group C, plasma concentrations of isoleucine and valine were lower whereas leucine, tryptophan and glutamate were unchanged. The plasma levels of all other amino acids were significantly higher in

Group A than in Group C. In brain of rats in Group A concentrations of aspartate and glutamate were lower than in Group C while the BCAA and tryptophan were unchanged. The remaining amino acids in brain were significantly higher in Group A than in Group C.

Compared to Group A, infusion of BCAA (Group B) resulted in lower plasma concentrations of phenylalanine, tyrosine, tryptophan, histidine, methionine, threonine, and lysine, whereas BCAA, alanine, glutamine, and aspartate were higher. Concentrations of BCAA and glutamate were higher in brain of Group B whereas phenylalanine, tyrosine, tryptophan, histidine, methionine, threonine, and lysine in Group B were lower as compared with Group A.

No significant differences either in DA or NE levels were observed between the control groups C and D in any region.

Following hepatectomy and glucose infusion (Group A) DA levels were significantly lower in striatum and higher in pons-medulla than in either group C or D. Concentrations of NE were lower in all brain regions of Group A than of either Group C or D except in striatum in which they remained unchanged. Infusions of BCAA (Group B) resulted in higher levels of DA in striatum and in higher levels of NE in hypothalamus, cortex and mesencephalon compared to Group A.

DISCUSSION

In the present studies we infused hepatectomized rats with the BCAA, thus preventing the massive increase in brain levels of histidine, methionine, phenylalanine, tryptophan, and tyrosine which normally follows hepatectomy. This effect of BCAA appeared to be a result of reduced accumulation of these neutral amino acids in the circulation and competition for blood-brain transport via the neutral amino acid transport system. The study shows that with respect to competition for neutral amino acid transport the blood-brain barrier seems to be functional 18 hours after hepatectomy.

BCAA infusion after hepatectomy was associated with significantly higher brain levels of NE in hypothalamus, cortex and mesencephalon and higher DA levels in striatum as compared with hepatectomized rats receiving glucose. In the remaining regions NE levels were still low after infusion of BCAA. If it is assumed that levels of phenylalanine and tyrosine in cortex are close to the levels of those amino acids in other brain regions as has been reported for rats with portacaval shunt by Bucci et al.,[14] then it is unlikely that high levels of tyrosine or phenylalanine (or their metabolites) in brain are the only cause of low brain NE levels after hepatectomy.

Thus, the present results suggest that the reduction in brain NE after hepatectomy seems to be unrelated to high concentrations of phenylalanine and tyrosine in most regions. Depletion of NE could

Table 1. Amino acids in plasma of hepatectomized or control rats 18 hours after surgery.

Treatment:	Hepatectomy		PCA	Sham
	Glucose	Glucose+BCAA	Glucose	Glucose
Group (n):	A(7)	B(7)	C(8)	D(8)
Alanine	856+53	5016+321 **	382+38 **	369+22 **
Aspartate	87+12	222+26 **	16+1 **	10+2 **
Glutamate	77+6	94+6	60+7	53+6
Glutamine	3306+208	8865+390**	854+40**	541+23**
Histidine	394+28	205+16**	76+4**	55+2**
Isoleucine	20+1	1252+253**	37+3**	44+2**
Leucine	63+3	1281+197**	68+3	83+4
Lysine	1672+80	898+64**	324+21**	346+19**
Methionine	158+17	34+9**	51+2**	49+3**
Phenylalanine	420+30	110+20**	83+5**	76+2**
Threonine	325+23	69+9**	135+7**	141+10**
Tryptophan	43+4	16+2**	47+3	44+3
Tyrosine	403+16	177+14**	96+5**	64+4**
Valine	75+5	1939+250**	102+6*	111+11*

Values are $\bar{x}$ $\pm$ SEM. *P <0.05 and **P < 0.001 compared to Group A.

Table 2. Amino acids in brain of hepatectomized or control rats 18 hours after surgery.

Treatment:	Hepatectomy		PCA	Sham
	Glucose	Glucose+BCAA	Glucose	Glucose
Group (n):	A(7)	B(7)	C(8)	D(8)
Alanine	2340+553	2546+414	530+15***	578+10***
Aspartate	1952+74	2047+140	3100+195**	3336+146***
Glutamate	8041+453	9753+398**	11525+312***	11663+290 ***
Glutamine	25300+1200	26300+1200	9200+400***	4300+200***
Histidine	745+27	101+12***	142+8***	73+3***
Isoleucine	23+5	342+50***	20+1	18+1
Leucine	85+13	407+43***	57+2	51+2
Lysine	491+21	318+22***	175+10***	142+13***
Methionine	226+10	16+4***	83+3***	56+4***
Phenylalanine	631+20	48+12***	146+8***	71+2***
Threonine	749+32	137+10***	471+21***	428+16***
Tryptophan	50+4	---a	52+3	30+1***
Tyrosine	686+50	87+17***	183+10***	76+6***
Valine	82+12	454+37***	61+2	61+2

Values are $\bar{x}$ $\pm$ SEM. *P < 0.05, **P < 0.01 and ***P < 0.001 compared to Group A. a = non-detectable.

Table 3. Norepinephrine (NE) and dopamine (DA) in various regions of the brain in rats with hepatectomy or in controls 18 hours after surgery.

Treatment:	Hepatectomy		PCA	Sham
Group (n):	Glucose A(7)	Glucose+BCAA B(7)	Glucose C(8)	Glucose D(8)

Brain region (ng/g)

Region		A(7)	B(7)	C(8)	D(8)
Hypothalamus	DA	430+35	525+25	451+23	444+31
	NE	838+28	998+59 *	1655+60***	1531+54 ***
Cortex	DA	64+13	96+23	54+17	53+12
	NE	139+25	214+34 *	254+15 **	260+11 **
Striatum	DA	8333+316	10416+696 *	11127+496 **	10391+310 *
	NE	101+16	145+19	123+11	116+8
Hippocampus	DA	118+26	239+85	176+75	66+18
	NE	148+26	181+38	368+34 ***	313+12 ***
Mesencephalon	DA	258+31	291+23	216+9	230+7
	NE	287+27	351+29 *	493+16 ***	464+10 ***
Diencephalon	DA	1647+228	1592+192	1118+309	1544+101
	NE	364+27	419+37	610+26 ***	616+18 ***
Pons-medulla	DA	113+16	122+10	60+2 **	70+6 **
	NE	374+25	399+29	555+13 ***	505+30 ***
Cerebellum	NE	142+20	148+21	208+10 *	211+19

Concentrations of NE and DA expressed as $\bar{x}$ + SEM. * $P < 0.05$, ** $P < 0.01$ and *** $P < 0.001$ compared to Group A.

results from enhanced release and breakdown of the transmitter or from a block of the hydroxylation of DA to yield NE. The higher concentrations of NE in 3 brain regions of hepatectomized rats receiving BCAA compared to glucose infused hepatectomized rats suggest that some effect of BCAA infusion tended to prevent depletion of NE in these regions.

REFERENCES

1. E. V. Flock, G. M. Tyce, and C. A. Owen, Utilization of U-^{14}C glucose in brain after total hepatectomy in the rat, J. Neurochem. 13: 1389 (1966).

2. A. M. Mans, S. J. Saunders, R. E. Kirsch, and J. F. Biebuyck,
    Correlation of plasma and brain amino acid and putative neuro-
    transmitter alterations during acute hepatic coma in the rat,
    J. Neurochem. 32: 285 (1979).
3. P. M. Herlin, Z. Gimmon, C. A. Nachbauer, J. H. James, and J. E.
    Fischer, Infusion of branched chain amino acids (BCAA) after
    hepatectomy in the rat reduces the accumulation of aromatic
    amino acids in plasma and brain, Surg. Forum 32: 191 (1981).
4. C. O. Record, B. Buxton, R. A. Chase, G. Curzon, I. M. Murray-
    Lyon, and R. Williams, Plasma and brain amino acids in
    fulminant hepatic failure and their relationship to hepatic
    encephalopathy, Eur. J. Clin. Invest. 6: 387 (1976).
5. J. M. Dodsworth, J. H. James, M. C. Cummings, and J. E. Fischer,
    Depletion of brain norepinephrine in acute hepatic coma,
    Surgery 75: 811 (1974).
6. G. M. Tyce and C. A. Owen, Dopamine and norepinephrine in the
    brains of hepatectomized rats, Life Sci. 22: 781 (1978).
7. B. A. Faraj, V. M. Camp, J. D. Ansley, J. Scott, F. M. Ali, and
    E. J. Malveaux, Evidence for central hypertyraminemia in
    hepatic encephalopathy, J. Clin. Invest. 67: 395 (1981).
8. K. Jellinger, P. Riederer, W. D. Rausch, and E. Kothbauer, Brain
    monoamines in hepatic encephalopathy and other types of me-
    tabolic coma, J. Neural. Transm. (Suppl.) 14: 103 (1978).
9. J. E. Fischer and R. J. Baldessarini, Pathogenesis and therapy
    of hepatic coma, in: "Progress in Liver Diseases", H. Popper,
    F. Schaffner, eds., Grune & Stratton, N.Y. pp. 363-397
    (1976).
10. M. Karobath and R. J. Baldessarini, Formation of catechol com-
    pounds from phenylalanine and tyrosine with isolated nerve
    endings, Nature 236: 206 (1972).
11. A. Smith, F. Rossi-Fanelli, V. Ziparo, J. H. James, B. A.
    Perelle, and J. E. Fischer, Alterations in plasma and CSF
    amino acids, amines and metabolites in hepatic coma, Ann.
    Surg. 187: 343 (1978).
12. W. H. Oldendorf, Brain uptake of radiolabelled amino acids,
    amines and hexoses after arterial injection, Am. J. Physiol.
    6: 1629 (1971).
13. T. Holmin, C. D. Agardh, G. Alinder, and P. Herlin, Some effects
    of total hepatectomy upon the metabolic state of the rat
    brain, in: "Amino Acids, Ammonia, and Energy Metabolism in
    Hepatic Failure and Neoplastic Diseases", E. Holm ed.,
    Verlag Gerhard Witzstrock, pp. 108-111 (1982).
14. L. Bucci, M. Cardelli, R. Chiavarelli, M. Massoti, and G. Morri,
    Behavioral, electroencephalographic, and biochemical changes
    in porta-cava shunted rats, Int. J. Neurosci. 10: 129 (1980).

COMMENT TO ORAL BCAA TRIALS

H. Schomerus

Dept. I Med. Univ. Klinik, Tübingen, West Germany

Three papers presented during the meeting concerned double blind placebo controlled trials evaluating the effect of oral branched chain amino acids (BCAA) on portal-systemic encephalopathy (PSE). Two of these carefully designed trials[1,2] arrived at the conclusion that BCAA do have a favorable influence on low grade and latent PSE. Contrary to this, Eriksson et al.[3] in an equally elaborate trial did not find any significant differences. To reconcile these divergent statements a few comments are necessary: the first comment is a numerical one. Both Egberts and Horst included more than 20 patients in their respective studies, whereas the study of Eriksson et al. concerned only 7 patients. Conclusions derived from small size studies such as this can be valuable if the study is carefully designed and if statistically significant differences are found. However, if statistically significant differences are not found, the conclusions to be drawn from the results are extremely limited. Certainly, the general conclusion that there is no difference can not be drawn. This is due to the fact that the probability of a type II error - i.e. the non-detection of a true difference - increases for decreasing number of patients included in the study. Thus, any conclusion derived from statistical significant differences in a study including 22 patients can not be contradicted on the basis of negative results in 7 patients. As pointed out by Freiman et al.[4] most clinical trials arriving at negative results are too small, and due to the high probability of a type II error are far from justifying the conclusion that there is no difference.

Another comment concerns the way to evaluate a study. The trial of Horst et al. was conducted with two independent groups, one receiving treatment, the other placebo. This justifies an evaluation with conventional t-statistics. Eriksson et al., and Egberts and

381

co-workers employed a cross-over design, in which each patient serves as his own control, going through a treatment and a placebo period in randomized sequences. Such a design has the disadvantage that the starting point for the treatment period is different, depending on whether the treatment preceeds or follows the placebo period and that overall changes due to training or hospitalization may mask small treatment effects. Thus, the sequence of treatment is of central importance and has to be considered when evaluating such a trial. It is therefore inadequate to group together all placebo and all treatment periods, irrespective of the sequence as has been done by Eriksson et al. There are statistical methods available which take into account the cross-over design and permit the separation between treatment effects and period effects and they should be employed whenever a cross-over design is chosen.

The last comment concerns the results of the study of Eriksson et al. Although there are only a few mean values and standard errors and no individual patient data, it is noteworthy that comparing the reported results of Eriksson et al. with those of Egberts et al., there are the following interesting parallels: in the Eriksson trial significant changes were found only in those variables (number connection test, digit symbols) which showed also significant treatment effects in the study of Egberts et al. The Benton visual retention test showed no change at all in both studies. Most pronounced treatment effects in the Egberts study were found in psychomotor variables, such as line tracing, which appeared to be most specific for PSE.[5] However, psychomotor variables were not tested at all in the trial of Eriksson et al. Thus, one might even speculate that the study of Eriksson et al. including three times the number of patients and adding psychomotor tests would probably arrive at the same results as did both other studies.

REFERENCES

1. D. Horst, N. Grace, H. O. Conn, E. Schiff, S. Schenker, A. Viteri, D. Law, and C. E. Atterbury, A double-blind randomized comparison of dietary protein and an oral branched chain amino acid (BCAA) solution in cirrhotic patients with chronic portal-systemic encephalopathy (PSE), AISF Symposium on Hepatic Encephalopathy, Rome, Nov. (1982).
2. E. H. Egberts, W. Hamster, H. Schomerus, and P. Jürgens, Effective treatment of latent porto-systemic encephalopathy (PSE) with oral branched chain amino acids (BCAA), AISF Symposium on Hepatic Encephalopathy, Rome, Nov. (1982).
3. S. Eriksson and J. Wahren, Failure of oral branched chain amino acids to improve chronic hepatic encephalopathy, in: "Metabolism and Clinical Implications of Branched-Chain Amino and Ketoacids", M. Walser, R. Williamson, eds., Elsevier North Holland, New York, pp. 381-385 (1981).
4. J. A. Freiman, T. C. Chalmers, H. Smith, and R. Kubbler, The

importance of beta, the type II error and sample size in the design and interpretation of the randomized controlled trial, New Engl. J. Med. 299: 690 (1978).

5. W. Hamster and H. Schomerus, Selection of appropriate psycho-metric tests for clinical use in latent porta-systemic encephalopathy (abstract), AISF Symposium on Porta-Systemic Encephalopathy, Rome, Nov. (1982).

CONTRIBUTORS

(Number in parentheses indicate the pages on
which the authors' contributions begin.)

G. Agolini (193)   Istituto di Patologia Medica, Università di
Trieste, Trieste, Italy

A. Alwmark (359)   Departments of Surgery and Psychiatry, University of Lund, Lund, Sweden

M. Anzà (183)   Istituto di Patologia Chirurgica IV, Università di Roma, Roma, Italy

U. Åslund (359)   Departments of Surgery and Psychiatry, University of Lund, Lund, Sweden

J. P. Aubin (301)   Clinique des Maladies de l'Appareil Digestif
and Laboratoire de Biochimie B, Hôpital
Saint Eloi, Montpellier, France

F. Balsano (239)   Istituto di Clinica Medica I, Università di
Roma, Roma, Italy

M. Baraldi (25)   Istituto di Farmacologia, Università di Modena, Modena, Italy

L. Battistin (115)   Clinica Neurologica, Università di Padova,
Padova, Italy

H. Bellet-Hermann   Laboratoire de Biochimie B, Faculté de Méde-
(127, 301)   cine, Montpellier, France

E. Beretta (95)   Clinica Chirurgica V, Università di Milano,
Milano, Italy

G. P. Bianchi (149,   Istituto di Patologia Medica I, Università
209)   di Bologna, Bologna, Italy

J. Bircher (275)   Department of Clinical Pharmacology, University of Berne, Berne, Switzerland

A. Borghetti (229)   Istituto di Semeiotica Medica, Università di
                            Parma, Parma, Italy

L. Borghi (229)   Istituto di Semeiotica Medica, Università di
                            Parma, Parma, Italy

P. Bories (127, 301)   Clinique des Maladies de l'Appareil Digestif,
                            Hôpital Saint-Eloi, Montpellier, France

V. Bua (209)   Istituto di Patologia Medica I, Università di
                            Bologna, Bologna, Italy

M. Bührer (275)   Department of Clinical Pharmacology, Univer-
                            sity of Berne, Berne, Switzerland

C. Cangiano (71, 87,   Clinica Medica III, Università di Roma, Roma,
183, 335)   Italy

L. Capocaccia (239,   II Cattedra di Gastroenterologia, Università
335)   di Roma, Roma, Italy

P. Cardelli-Cangiano   Istituto di Biochimica, Università di Roma,
(71)   Roma, Italy

G. Casalgrandi (221)   Istituto di Clinica Medica III, Università
                            di Modena, Modena, Italy

A. Cascino (87, 183,   Clinica Medica III, Università di Roma, Roma,
335)   Italy

M. Cassanelli (221)   Istituto di Clinica Medica III, Università
                            di Modena, Modena, Italy

S. Cassarani (209)   Istituto di Patologia Medica I, Università
                            di Bologna, Bologna, Italy

C. Cavicchioni (345)   Istituto di Patologia Speciale Chirurgica,
                            Università Cattolica del Sacro Cuore, Roma,
                            Italy

F. Ceriati (345)   Istituto di Patologia Speciale Chirurgica,
                            Università Cattolica del Sacro Cuore, Roma,
                            Italy

C. Collini (245)   Istituto di Clinica Medica III, Università
                            di Modena, Modena, Italy

C. Cortesini (41)   Clinica Chirurgica, Università di Firenze,
                            Firenze, Italy

J. E. G. de Boer (137)   Departments of Surgery and Biochemistry, St. Annadal Hospital, University of Limburg, Maastricht, The Netherlands

M. Dell'Oca (95)   Clinica Medica III, Università di Milano, Milano, Italy

S. Del Signore (87)   Clinica Medica III, Università di Roma, Roma, Italy

G. De Luca (345)   Istituto di Patologia Speciale Chirurgica, Università Cattolica del Sacro Cuore, Roma, Italy

L. Demelia (213)   Istituto di Medicina Interna, Cattedra di Patologia Speciale Medica II, Università di Cagliari, Cagliari, Italy

E. Di Cera (345)   Istituto di Patologia Speciale Chirurgica, Università Cattolica del Sacro Cuore, Roma, Italy

C. Dondi (149, 209)   Istituto di Patologia Medica I, Università di Bologna, Bologna, Italy

E. H. Egberts (351)   Dept. I Med. Univ. Klinik, Tübingen, West Germany

G. Elia (229)   Istituto di Semeiotica Medica, Università di Parma, Parma, Italy

L. S. Eriksson (287)   Departments of Medicine and Clinical Physiology, Huddinge University Hospital, Stockholm, Sweden

L. Faccini (193)   Istituto di Patologia Medica, Università di Trieste, Trieste, Italy

B. Feneyrou (127)   Clinique des Maladies de l'Appareil Digestif, Hôpital Saint-Eloi, Montpellier, France

P. Ferenci (121)   I. Universitätsklinik für Gastroenterologie und Hepatologie, Vienna, Austria

F. Fiaccadori (87, 229, 323)   Cattedra di Malattie Infettive, Università di Parma, Parma, Italy

A. Fiori (71)   Istituto di Biochimica, Università di Roma, Roma, Italy

J. E. Fischer (53, 61,   Department of Surgery, University of Cincin-
311, 375)   nati Medical Center, Cincinnati, Ohio, U.S.A.

M. Frezza (193)   Istituto di Patologia Medica, Università di
Trieste, Trieste, Italy

P. Gentilini (239)   Istituto di Clinica Medica II, Università
di Firenze, Firenze, Italy

F. Ghinelli (87, 229,   Divisione Malattie Infettive, Ospedale Re-
323)   gionale di Parma, Parma, Italy

P. Gibertini (221,   Istituto di Clinica Medica III, Università
323)   di Modena, Modena, Italy

J. Giordan (127)   Clinique Chirurgicale C, Hôpital Saint-Eloi,
Montpellier, France

G. Giunchi (239)   Istituto di Clinica Medica III, Università
di Roma, Roma, Italy

D. Giuntini (193)   Istituto di Patologia Medica, Università di
Trieste, Trieste, Italy

G. F. Guarnieri   Istituto di Patologia Medica, Università di
(193)   Trieste, Trieste, Italy

P. Gullstrand (359)   Departments of Surgery and Psychiatry, University of Lund, Lund, Sweden

W. Hamster (351)   Neurologische Poliklinik, Tübingen, West
Germany

P. M. Herlin (375)   Department of Surgery, University of Cincinnati Medical Center, Cincinnati, Ohio,
U.S.A.

E. Holm (161)   Department of Pathophysiology, I Med. Clinic
Mannheim, University of Heidelberg, West
Germany

P. Incerti (95)   Clinica Medica III, Università di Milano,
Milano, Italy

S. Jacob (161)   Department of Pathophysiology, I Med. Clinic
Mannheim, University of Heidelberg, West
Germany

J. H. James (61,   Department of Surgery, University of Cincin-
375)   nati Medical Center, Cincinnati, Ohio, U.S.A.

M. A. Janssen (137)   Departments of Surgery and Biochemistry, St. Annadal Hospital, University of Limburg, Maastricht, The Netherlands

K. Jellinger (369)   Ludwig Boltzmann Institute of Clin. Neurobiology, Lainz-Hospital, Vienna, Austria

B. Jeppsson (61, 359)   Department of Surgery, University of Cincinnati Medical Center, Cincinnati, Ohio, U.S.A.

B. Joelsson (359)   Departments of Surgery and Psychiatry, University of Lund, Lund, Sweden

E. A. Jones (121)   Liver Disease Section, Niaddk, NIH, Bethesda Md, U.S.A.

T. Jonung (61)   Department of Surgery, University of Cincinnati Medical Center, Cincinnati, Ohio, U.S.A.

P. Jürgens (351)   Allgemeines Krankenhaus St. Georg, Hamburg, West Germany

E. Kienzl (369)   Ludwig Boltzmann Institute of Clin. Neurobiology, Lainz-Hospital, Vienna, Austria

A. Kjällman (359)   Departments of Surgery and Psychiatry, University of Lund, Lund, Sweden

G. Kleinberger (369)   Department of Medicine I, University School of Medicine, Vienna, Austria

H. Leweling (161)   Department of Pathophysiology, I Med. Clinic Mannheim, University of Heidelberg, West Germany

G. Lombardi (41)   Istituto di Farmacologia, Università di Firenze, Firenze, Italy

A. Lucchesi (193)   Laboratorio Ospedale Pediatrico di Trieste, Trieste, Italy

R. Lupino (183)   Istituto di Patologia Chirurgica IV, Università di Roma, Roma, Italy

G. Marchal (127)   Clinique Chirurgicale C, Hôpital Saint-Eloi, Montpellier, France

G. Marchesini (149, 209)   Istituto di Patologia Medica I, Università di Bologna, Bologna, Italy

R. Marini   (193)   Istituto di Patologia Medica, Università
                             di Trieste, Trieste, Italy

I. R. Marino (345)   Istituto di Patologia Speciale Chirurgica,
                             Università Cattolica del Sacro Cuore, Roma,
                             Italy

A. Melli (209)   Istituto di Patologia Medica I, Università
                             di Bologna, Bologna, Italy

M. Merli (183, 335)   II Cattedra di Gastroenterologia, Università
                             di Roma, Roma, Italy

E. Messori (245)   Clinica Oculistica, Università di Modena,
                             Modena, Italy

M. T. Meuwese-Arends   Department of Medicine, Division of Gastro-
    (107)   enterology, St. Radboud Hospital, University
                             of Nijmegen, Nijmegen, The Netherlands

H. Michel (127, 301)   Clinique des Maladies de l'Appareil Digestif,
                             Hôpital Saint-Eloi, Montpellier, France

D. Mirouze (127, 301)   Clinique des Maladies de l'Appareil Digestif,
                             Hôpital Saint-Eloi, Montpellier, France

G. Moneti (41)   Centro di Spettrometria di Massa della Fa-
                             coltà di Medicina, Università di Firenze,
                             Firenze, Italy

A. Montanari (229)   Istituto di Semeiotica Medica, Università
                             di Parma, Parma, Italy

M. Y. Morgan (255)   Department of Medicine, Royal Free Hospital
                             School of Medicine, Hampstead, London, U.K.

F. Moroni (41)   Istituto di Farmacologia, Università di Fi-
                             renze, Firenze, Italy

M. Muscaritoli (87)   Clinica Medica III, Università di Roma, Roma,
                             Italy

C. A. Nachbauer (375)   Department of Surgery, University of Cincin-
                             nati Medical Center, Cincinnati, Ohio, U.S.A.

A. Novarini (229)   Istituto di Semeiotica Medica, Università
                             di Parma, Parma, Italy

R. J. Oostenbroek   Departments of Surgery and Biochemistry, St.
    (137)   Annadal Hospital, University of Limburg,
                             Maastricht, The Netherlands

L. Pagliaro (239)   Istituto di Patologia Medica, Università di
                          Palermo, Palermo, Italy

C.S. Pappas (121)   Liver Disease Section, Niaddk, NIH, Bethesda,
                          Md., U.S.A.

S. Parco (193)   Laboratorio Ospedale Pediatrico di Trieste,
                          Trieste, Italy

G. Pedretti (229,   Cattedra di Malattie Infettive, Università
   323)   di Parma, Parma, Italy

D. Pellegrini (41)   Istituto di Farmacologia , Università di Fi-
                          renze, Firenze, Italy

G. Pelosi (87, 229,   Divisione Malattie Infettive, Ospedale Re-
   323)   gionale di Parma, Parma, Italy

A. Penne   (245)   Clinica Oculistica, Università di Modena,
                          Modena, Italy

A. Pietrangelo (221)   Istituto di Clinica Medica III, Università
                          di Modena, Modena, Italy

G. Pinelli (245)   Istituto di Clinica Medica III, Università di
                          Modena, Modena, Italy

E. Pisi (239)   Istituto di Patologia Medica I, Università
                          di Bologna, Bologna, Italy

G. Pomier-Layrargues   Clinique des Maladies de l'Appareil Digestif,
   (127, 301)   Hôpital Saint-Eloi, Montpellier, France

G. Pozzato (193)   Istituto di Patologia Medica, Università di
                          Trieste, Trieste, Italy

A. Puglionisi (345)   Istituto di Patologia Speciale Chirurgica,
                          Università Cattolica del Sacro Cuore, Roma,
                          Italy

P. Ricci (245)   Istituto di Clinica Medica III, Università
                          di Modena, Modena, Italy

P. Riederer (369)   Department of Medicine I , University School
                          of Medicine, Vienna, Austria

O. Riggio (183, 335)   II Cattedra di Gastroenterologia, Università
                          di Roma, Roma, Italy

P. Rigotti (61, 115)   Istituto di Clinica Chirurgica III, Università
                         di Padova, Padova, Italy

E. Rocchi (221, 323)   Istituto di Clinica Medica III, Università
                         di Modena, Modena, Italy

A. Roncone (345)   Istituto di Patologia Speciale Chirurgica,
                         Università Cattolica del Sacro Cuore, Roma,
                         Italy

F. Rossi Fanelli   Clinica Medica III, Università di Roma, Roma,
   (87, 183, 335)   Italy

D. Sacchini (87, 229,   Divisione Malattie Infettive, Ospedale Regio-
   323)   nale di Parma, Parma, Italy

D. Salassa (115)   Istituto di Clinica Chirurgica III, Univer-
                         sità di Padova, Padova, Italy

F. Salerno (95)   Clinica Medica III, Università di Milano, Mi-
                         lano, Italy

H. Schomerus (351,   Dept. I Med. Univ. Klinik, Tübingen, West
   381)   Germany

R. Situlin (193)   Istituto di Patologia Medica, Università di
                         Trieste, Trieste, Italy

P. B. Soeters (137)   Departments of Surgery and Biochemistry, St.
                         Annadal Hospital, University of Limburg,
                         Maastricht, The Netherlands

A. Solinas (213)   Istituto di Medicina Interna, Cattedra di Pa-
                         tologia Speciale Medica II, Università di
                         Cagliari, Cagliari, Italy

U. Staedt (161)   Department of Pathophysiology, I Med. Clinic
                         Mannheim, University of Heidelberg, West
                         Germany

M. Stortoni (183,   Clinica Medica III, Università di Roma, Roma,
   335)   Italy

J. P. Striebel (161)   Department of Pathophysiology, I Med. Clinic
                         Mannheim, University of Heidelberg, West
                         Germany

R. Strom (71)   Istituto di Biochimica, Università di Roma,
                         Roma, Italy

A. Tangerman (107) — Department of Medicine, Division of Gastro-enterology, St. Radboud Hospital, University of Nijmegen, Nijmegen, The Netherlands

G. Toigo (193) — Istituto di Patologia Medica, Università di Trieste, Trieste, Italy

F. Uggeri (95) — Clinica Chirurgica V, Università di Milano, Milano, Italy

M. Uribe (267, 279) — Liver Unit, Instituto Nacional de la Nutricion Salvador Zubiran, México, D.F.

J. H. M. Van Tongeren (107) — Department of Medicine, Division of Gastro-enterology, St. Radboud Hospital, University of Nijmegen, Nijmegen, The Netherlands

P. Vassanelli (115) — Clinica Chirurgica III, Università di Padova, Padova, Italy

E. Ventura (25, 221, 239, 245, 323) — Istituto di Clinica Medica III, Università di Modena, Modena, Italy

J. Wahren (287) — Departments of Medicine and Clinical Physiology, Huddinge University Hospital, Stockholm, Sweden

G. Zanchin (115) — Clinica Neurologica, Università di Padova, Padova, Italy

M. L. Zeneroli (25, 245, 323) — Istituto di Clinica Medica III, Università di Modena, Modena, Italy

L. Zieve (5, 15, 239) — Hannepin County Medical Center, University of Minnesota, Minneapolis, Mn., U.S.A.

V. Ziparo (183) — Istituto di Patologia Chirurgica IV, Università di Roma, Roma, Italy

M. Zoli (149, 209) — Istituto di Patologia Medica I, Università di Bologna, Bologna, Italy

INDEX